The Nurse Apprentice, 1860–1977

The Nurse Apprentice, 1860–1977

Ann Bradshaw

Routledge
Taylor & Francis Group
LONDON AND NEW YORK

First published 2001 by Ashgate Publishing

Published 2017 by Routledge
2 Park Square, Milton Park, Abingdon, Oxfordshire OX14 4RN
711 Third Avenue, New York, NY 10017, USA

First issued in paperback 2017

Routledge is an imprint of the Taylor & Francis Group, an informa business

British Library Cataloguing-in-Publication Data
Bradshaw, Ann
The nurse apprentice, 1860–1977. — (The history of medicine in context)
1. Nurses — Training of — Great Britain —History — 19th century. 2. Nurses — Training of — Great Britain —History — 20th century. 3. Nursing students — Great Britain — History —19th century. 4. Nursing students — Great Britain —History — 20th century.
I. Title
610.7'3'0941'0904

US Library of Congress Cataloging-in-Publication Data
Bradshaw, Ann
The nurse apprentice, 1860–1977 / Ann Bradshaw.
p. ; cm. — (The history of medicine in context)
Includes bibliographical references and index.
1. Nursing—Great Britain—History. 2. Nursing—Study and teaching—Great Britain—History. I. Title. II. Series.
[DNLM: 1. History of Nursing—Great Britain. 2. History of Nursing—United States. 3. Education, Nursing—history—Great Britain. 4. Education, Nursing—history—United States. WY 11 FA1 B812n 2001]
RT11 .B73 2001
610.73'0941—dc21 00-042042

ISBN 13: 978-1-138-25747-4 (pbk)
ISBN 13: 978-0-7546-0172-2 (hbk)

Contents

Introduction

This book examines the apprenticeship model of nurse training from its inception at St Thomas's Hospital in 1860, until its ending in 1977, the date of the last syllabus published by the General Nursing Council (GNC) for England and Wales. Thereafter, following the Act of 1979, the GNC was replaced by the United Kingdom Central Council for Nurses, Midwives and Health Visitors; a new preparation for nursing practice was developed which was no longer based on the apprenticeship method of learning how to nurse.

Where this book differs from other contemporary nursing histories is in its central theme, the systematic analysis of the framework of principles and values which have underpinned the apprenticeship mode of training. Since the 1960s nursing histories have tended to minimise the significance of the vocational tradition for the development of the nursing profession and the motivations of individual nurses. This book questions that interpretation. In order to understand the impact of this tradition on the parlous state of early nineteenth-century nursing care, and to appreciate its subsequent development in the twentieth century, the beliefs, values and assumptions that have underpinned it need clear exposition. By moral, intellectual and practical learning of appropriate knowledge, skills and techniques, the student nurse was initiated into a practical tradition of service. The ward sister was its guardian. Through apprenticeship training the nurse was taught to see the patient as central to all her learning.

Chapter 1 examines the principles and practices of nursing in historical context by clarifying the origins of the apprenticeship training between 1860 and 1896. It considers the nature of apprenticeship and its principles, as envisaged by Nightingale in her writings, and shows how this developed over the century at St Thomas's Hospital. This chapter demonstrates how the apprenticeship training was intended to prepare nurses with biomedical knowledge, technical skill and a virtuous character.

In Chapter 2, I consider the views of nurse leaders from 1874 to 1982, and examine the content of contemporary training, by a systematic analysis of nursing textbooks. The aims and objectives of teachings were fourfold: to develop moral character; to teach technical knowledge and skill; to perpetuate the method of apprenticeship learning by the example of the ward sister; and to encourage the professional etiquette of right relationships. This apprenticeship system of nursing was the core structure for the development of the profession for a century.

The political and parliamentary context of nursing from 1888 to 1925 is set out in Chapter 3. This chapter examines debates in Parliament concerning the nature and purpose of the nurse's role, and the much disputed issue of professionalisation, which led to the Nurses' Registration Act in 1919. This Act, in turn, led to the setting up of the General Nursing Council, and its purpose of public protection. The prescribed national syllabus of training, developed by the GNC, was intended to fulfil this purpose. Chapter 3 examines the factions involved in the dispute, highlights the reasons for conflict and shows where consensus was reached.

Chapter 4 considers the further development of the apprenticeship training and contextual factors from 1923 to 1948. The first nationally prescribed syllabus was followed by several governmental and professional reports concerning the nature of nursing, nursing recruitment and the method of training nurses. These reports are critically reviewed with particular reference to the significance and implications of the apprenticeship method of training nurses for patient care.

In Chapter 5, I examine the British nursing tradition and the American influence from 1948 to 1960. The views from both inside and outside the profession on the proper role of the nurse, and how she should be prepared for this role, are considered in detail. The discussion brings to light evidence that North American nursing ideas began to influence British nursing leaders, and shows why several nursing leaders were concerned with this development. Debates centred on whether 'basic' bedside care, together with training in technical skills and techniques, should remain the province of the British registered nurse. The counter-argument was that apprenticeship training should be replaced by a college-based North American model of education which would prepare the nurse to take on a more specialist function, and leave bedside care to the less qualified.

Chapter 6 involves an analysis of the years from 1960 to 1972, and a detailed examination of the process which led up to the professional consensus breaking. The apprenticeship model of nursing, its values and presuppositions, began to be strongly challenged. Radical change was proposed by the influential Briggs Committee, although evidence from the period, known to Briggs, including their own commissioned data, raises important questions about the analysis of the report and its recommendations.

Chapter 7 looks behind the scenes of the 1960s, at hitherto unexamined evidence in the form of correspondence, articles and editorials in nursing journals. This body of evidence reveals a deep tension between those nurses who wanted to retain the values and methods of the apprenticeship training, and those nurses who argued that this traditional approach was outdated. That changes were being questioned at all levels, is further supported by studies of nurses' and patients' opinions, which provide additional insight into the motivations of nurses and the effectiveness of nursing during this period.

Finally, the period from 1972 to 1979, which marked the beginning of the end of the nurse apprentice, is considered in Chapter 8. Ideological changes at the General Nursing Council during the 1970s led to the ending of the national prescribed syllabus and record of instruction for state registration, and brought fundamental legislative change to nurse education in the following decades. This change in ethos is examined in order to cast light on the movement away from apprenticeship training towards college-based education, and to highlight the possible consequences for the future preparation for, and practice of, nursing.

For simplicity, and because throughout this period the vast majority of nurses in general nursing were women, the feminine gender will be used to refer to the nurse. This should not, however, be seen to exclude the minority of nurses who were male.

Chapter 1

The principles and practices of nursing in historical context: the Nightingale tradition of nursing, 1860–1896

From 1860 until 1977 nurses were inducted into an apprenticeship tradition of care. This tradition, which rested on a vocational ideal of service to humanity as the primary Christian virtue, originated with religious orders and was remodelled and rearticulated by Florence Nightingale to make it acceptable to her contemporary context. This chapter will examine Nightingale's principles of nursing, and seek to understand to what extent they formed the self-understanding of the nursing profession as it developed at St Thomas's Hospital. The analysis will take account of modern revisionist interpretations which have questioned the influence of Nightingale's training school, her own motives, and the effectiveness of nursing reforms.

Nightingale's influence on the development of modern nursing

In 1939 the eminent historian Lord Elton, in a BBC radio talk printed in *Nursing Times*, described Florence Nightingale as the creator of the profession of nursing, and even of the Army Medical Service.[1] To both the public and the profession the perception was clearly that Nightingale was responsible for the development and ethos of modern nursing. According to a recent historian of the Nightingale Training School, Roy Wake, Nightingale's work in 'inventing nursing' as a secular and organised profession needs careful scrutiny and modification.[2] In medieval Europe, religious orders were responsible for Christian charity, nursing the sick and giving alms to the poor. After the Reformation this became the obligation of secular Protestant philanthropy. In England, the religious revival of the nineteenth century led to the foundation of several nursing orders by High Church, as well as evangelical, Christian movements, that pre-dated Nightingale. Elizabeth Fry, for example, a Quaker, founded an Institute of Nursing in 1840.[3] Both Elizabeth Fry and Florence Nightingale were deeply influenced by their visits to a Lutheran religious foundation, Kaiserswerth, for the care of the sick.[4] What Nightingale may have found lacking amongst the religiously motivated, that is a scientific system,[5] she brought together with their vital moral tone. Nightingale made nursing a synthesis of both art and science.[6]

The question at issue is the extent to which this vision of Nightingale's influenced the development of nursing, particularly in her training school at St Thomas's Hospital. In appraising the evidence, Wake has taken account of the seminal work conducted by Monica Baly,[7] whom he describes as the first major revisionist.[8] Wake thinks there is some justification for Baly's argument that in its first ten years the Nightingale School achieved very little, but he believes that the early years of famous institutions have a tendency to show mistakes and fluctuations.[9] Yet, there is ample evidence, according to Wake, of Nightingale's continued, 'real but uneven', interest and concern in her training school.[10] This involved not only 'intrigue and plotting' but a close scrutiny of the registers and report books completed by ward sisters on the performances of probationers as well as the diaries kept by the probationer nurses themselves. Her unshakeable view that patients came first and last and were 'honoured guests' remained in the perceptions of nurses trained at her school for over a century.[11]

Often the real does not reflect the ideal; and it may be, as Baly argues, that training at the Nightingale School became too often inadequate and erratic, because ward sisters rarely had time to be good teachers.[12] This does not, however, diminish the ideal which future generations of nurses and their leaders would constantly strive to live up to. Nightingale's principles did not only affect the Nightingale School. Through the school's far-reaching influence, they would form the shared self-understanding and perception of the nursing profession in Britain for a century, as the evidence in the following chapters will reveal. Whatever Nightingale's actual influence really was, the principles that she articulated would become normative for the nursing profession.

The Nightingale ideal: fitting the nurse for her purpose

Nightingale had a strong Christian faith, although her technical theology was amateur and less than coherent.[13] As Quinn and Prest have written: 'Florence Nightingale's life was predicated upon her faith in God.'[14] There can be little doubt that Nightingale's work was shaped by her religious faith and her conviction that nursing must be more than an occupation. It had to be a calling: 'Like it or not, the clear analogy with religious Orders [sic] is inescapable; to take up nursing was the equivalent of a religious vow. Nursing was an art and required vision and idealism, making it among the most exalted vocations.' Nursing, which involved important scientific attributes, had to be based on this moral foundation.[15] It should be concerned with principle rather than personality: the principles of character formation, efficient management, hygiene and sanitation, which required organised obedience and discipline.[16]

Nightingale's approach to nursing began to take shape in 1851, when she worked at a Kaiserswerth. There she realised that the demanding work of nursing depended for its quality and standards on moral motives: love rather than money. This conviction would underpin her motivation to change the haphazard nursing system in England, where: 'We see the nurses drinking, we see the neglect at night owing to their falling asleep. Where women undertake so toilsome an office, for hire, and not for love, it cannot be otherwise.'[17] The spur to Nightingale's later work was the Crimean War. In 1854 *The Times* reported that there was an absence of reputable, trained, nurses to treat the wounded, sick and dying soldiers, unlike the French army who had nursing nuns. An editorial and correspondence followed. The question was posed: 'Why have we no Sisters of Charity?'[18]

By 1860 Nightingale had a clear picture of the kind of system she wanted to adopt.[19] Women who were nursing the sick at this time were of three types. The active religious orders produced women who, although of unblemished character, were deficient in technical proficiency and theoretical knowledge. Next, there were 'ladies', women with respectable characters but entirely incompetent, having a sentimental view of nursing and eschewing hard work. These were the 'brow-soothers' in the Crimea much disparaged by Nightingale. Lastly, there were the uneducated domestic servant nurses, the usual type of lay nurses in British hospitals, who could be morally weak and had low technical skill. There is some evidence that medical staff were already attempting to give some training to this group in a haphazard and unsystematic way.[20]

Nightingale set out her principles in two articles for a medical textbook, *A Dictionary of Medicine*, which was published in three editions from 1882 to 1902. The nature and purpose of nursing and its underpinning principles were clear: the effective, efficient and morally exemplary service of care to the patient. The needs of the patient, be they physical, emotional, social, or, indeed, spiritual, were central. The patient was expected to be the epicentre of all the nurse's thought:

> The nurse must have simplicity and a single eye to the patient's good. She must make no demand upon the patient for reciprocation, for acknowledgement or even perception of her services; since the best service a nurse can give *is* that the patient shall scarcely be aware of any – shall perceive her presence only by perceiving that he has *no* wants. The nurse must always be kind, but never emotional. The patient must find a real, not forced or 'put on,' centre of calmness in his nurse.[21]

Because the central purpose of nursing was clear to Nightingale, she assumed that the method of preparing nurses was to fit them for this purpose. The nurse needed to be a certain kind of person, the attributes of which were enshrined in the term 'character': 'A woman cannot be a good and intelligent nurse without being a good and intelligent woman.'[22] This was fundamental to her training, a scientific, practical preparation which was also a moral, educative process. As she stated:

> Nursing is, above all, a progressive calling. Year by year nurses have to learn new and improved methods, as medicine and surgery and hygiene improve. Year by year nurses are called upon to do more and better than they have done. It is felt to be impossible to have a public register of nurses that is not a delusion. Further, year by year, nursing needs to be more and more of a moral calling.[23]

The nurse needed to be sober, in spirit as well as drink, temperate in all things. She needed to be honest, not accepting bribes from patients or friends. She should be truthful in attention and observation, in memory and power of expression, in order to report and remember accurately what she observed. She should be trustworthy, carrying out directions intelligently and perfectly, unseen as well as seen. She needed to be chaste, in the sense of the Sermon on the Mount, because as Nightingale pointed out, 'Remember this great and dangerous peculiarity of nursing, and especially of hospital-nursing, namely, that it is the only case, queens not excepted, where a woman is really in charge of men.'[24]

She should be punctual and orderly, having everything ready and prepared before beginning a dressing on a patient: 'Punctual to a second, and orderly to a hair ... Quiet, yet quick; quick without hurry; gentle without slowness; discreet without self-importance, no gossip.' She should be cheerful, hopeful, not allowing herself or her patient to become discouraged by unfavourable symptoms or anticipation of an unfavourable result. She should be exquisitely clean, neat and ready.[25]

Nightingale repeated the same ideas in letters to probationers in her training school written from 1873 to 1900: 'It is what she *is* in *herself*, and what comes out of herself, out of what she *is* – that exercises a moral or religious influence over her patients. No set form of words is of any use.'[26] The character of the nurse was self-knowledge, a knowledge and confidence in the creator and the moral order, expressed in 'heroic' virtues: trustworthiness, punctuality, quietness and order, cleanliness, neatness, patience, cheerfulness and kindliness.[27]

As early as 1851 Nightingale defended the importance of intellectual knowledge: 'What then? Shall we have less theory? God forbid. We shall not work better for ignorance. Every increase of knowledge is a benefit, by shewing us more of the ways of God. But it was for the increase of "wisdom", even more than of knowledge, that David prayed – for wisdom is the practical application of knowledge.'[28] Hence, she believed it was vital to use the mind. In her letter to her probationers, dated May 1872, Nightingale wrote:

> For the obedience of intelligence, not the obedience of slavery, is what *we* want. The slave obeys with stupid obedience, with deceitful evasion of service, or with careless eye service. Now we cannot suppose God to be satisfied or pleased with stupidity and carelessness. The free woman in Christ obeys, or rather *seconds* all the rules, all the orders given her, with intelligence, with all her heart, and with all her strength, and with all her *mind*.[29]

Although Nightingale, herself, was sometimes obstinate in the face of scientific evidence, for example in her refusal to accept the germ theory of infection, she believed firmly that the moral purpose of nursing involved the intelligent application of knowledge.[30] An adequate medical knowledge in subjects such as chemistry, anatomy and physiology, was to be learned from a medical instructor, and examined both orally and in writing, in order that the nurse's powers of expression to train others would thereby be developed. Careful jottings of doctors' comments and notes of cases were to be recorded, so that the nurse learned to observe and understand her own cases and 'learn the reason of what is done', enabling her to teach others.[31]

A good nurses' library of professional books was important, to be used under the guidance of the medical instructor and class-mistress. The ward sister was responsible for supervising, teaching and ensuring that the probationer knew 'the reason why'.[32] Nightingale was scathing about sloppy and unintelligent practice: 'A young nurse, dressing an ulcerated leg, has been known to wipe it with the sheet, and alleged that she had seen it done elsewhere!'[33] It was for every ward sister to show every new probationer how to do her work, not only how it should be done, but also to guard against how it should not be done.

The moral purpose of nursing was inseparable from its practical outworking; dealing with the intimate bodily needs of patients was a spiritual matter, a true calling. Order, method and structure were vital to achieve good practical care. Tasks and procedures involved diligence and precision, the manner of performance was crucial. Nightingale described these tasks and procedures in minute detail. Seemingly unimportant and insignificant matters, such as how urinals should be washed out, how chamber utensils should always be kept covered when not in use and when carried, and that urinals should never be left under the bed but beside the patient and emptied immediately after use, were the vital details that differentiated good care from bad. Hygiene of the nurse's skin, including short nails, and careful washing and scrubbing of surgical instruments and dressing forceps were crucial to prevent infection.[34]

According to Nightingale, nurses needed to operate within a community of care. The key factor to mutual cooperation, for the sake of patients' welfare, was the exercise of authority and the following of rules. This involved respect for the matron and ward sisters. Nightingale took pains to explain exactly what she meant by this: 'She who rules best is she who loves best: and shows her love not by foolish indulgence to those of whom she is in charge, but by taking a real interest in them for their own sakes, and in their highest interests.'[35]

The matron was to have absolute authority for the whole nursing staff, but as a corollary, the ward sisters were to be the matron's lieutenants, and the linchpin for the training of the probationers. On this cardinal point Nightingale's opinions never wavered. As she wrote to a newly appointed sister at St Thomas's thirty years later, 'You have my very best wishes that you should succeed as one of the keystones under the Matron – as one of the great influences over Staff Nurses, Probationers, Wardmaids and patients both technically and morally.'[36] Indeed, she believed passionately in the correct management of nursing under a female head.[37]

Authority also involved respect for doctors. Although the nurse was expected to obey the physician's or surgeon's directions, this was an intelligent obedience using discretion. Responding to the physician's or surgeon's orders, the nurse had to realise that these orders were conditional: 'To obey *is* to understand orders, and to understand orders really is to obey.'[38] Loyalty to orders could not be without 'independent sense or energy of responsibility' which alone made for real trustworthiness. To be loyal to the doctor and his medical knowledge was to be loyal to the purpose of nursing: to 'keep the health-mechanism prescribed to her in gear'.[39] Loyalty was emphatically not a blind mechanical obedience, as Nightingale made clear:

> Yet no *man*, not even a doctor, ever gives any other definition of what a nurse should be than this – 'devoted and obedient.' This definition would do just as well for a porter. It might even do for a horse. It would not do for a policemen. Consider how many women there are who have nothing to devote – neither intelligence, nor eyes, nor ears, nor hands. They will sit up all night by the patient, it is true; but their attendance is worth nothing to him, nor their observations to the doctor ... But let no woman suppose that obedience to the doctor is not absolutely necessary. Only, neither doctor nor nurse lay sufficient stress upon *intelligent* obedience, upon the fact that obedience *alone* is a very poor thing.[40]

The key to authority, in having control over others, according to Nightingale, was to have control over oneself. Moreover, it was considered important that such control should be by 'the silent power of a consistent life'. Here there could be no pretence or dissimulation. In exercising authority nurses should not 'try to "seem" anything, but to *be* what we would *seem*'.[41] The root of this authority was in fulfilment of the Christian calling: 'And the highest "authority" which a woman especially can attain among her fellow women must come from her doing God's work here in the same spirit, and with the same thoroughness, that Christ did, though we follow him but "afar off".'[42]

Nightingale expressed many forward-thinking ideas, including a belief in the importance of health promotion and improved methods for recovery from sickness, so that hospitals, an 'intermediate stage of civilisation', would no longer be required.[43] She also suggested both a model of hospital organisation and a paradigm for health care that were prescient. She argued that hospital organisation needed a good lay administration with a chief executive officer, a civilian chairman, advised by businessmen, forming a board that would oversee the whole financial administration and supervision of the hospital. This board would take into account the opinion of medical officers, who would not have executive powers. Similarly, nurses would be responsible to the matron, who would herself be responsible to the board. The nursing tradition, affirmed by Nightingale, had within it seeds to bear the fruit of progress. The past, present and future were regarded as a continuum sustained by an unchanging moral tradition. Development and change were part of this progress.

According to one eminent reviewer of her *Notes on Nursing*, first published in 1860, Nightingale's views on hygiene were sensational innovations. It was radical to suggest that women should concern themselves with the laws governing their own bodies and the physical environment of their children including the importance of ventilation, cleanliness and proper drainage: 'It was accepted that the very poor lived in miserable squalor. To exhort and educate them was a seemly Christian duty.'[44]

Medical diagnosis and treatment were rudimentary in these days before medical and surgical advances, when contagious diseases often necessitated amputation and excision. The nurse's job was to fortify the patient's will and courage, and support his constitution during the period of slow recovery and tedious confinement. Gentle, sensitive and constantly watchful, the nurse's strength and skill was to be interposed between the patient and his enemy. The nurse needed to think for the patient, to save his energy and even his thought. She respected the integrity of the patient's personality.

No subterfuges should be practised in cheering the sick, or in making light of the dangers. Neither did Nightingale want to make light of illness itself, and she condemned the suspicious attitude to illness which advocated the sick learning self-control by choosing to dismiss painful thought which aggravated their disease: 'Believe me, almost *any* sick person, who behaves decently well, exercises more self-control every moment of his day than you will ever know till you are sick yourself.'[45]

This moral and religious purpose of nursing was so fundamental to Nightingale that she was impatient with contemporary ideology: 'jargons' of the 'rights of women'. She was dismissive of both extremes of argument: that women should do all that men do, including medical and other professions; and that women should do nothing that men do, because women's work differed from men's: 'Surely woman should bring the best she has, *whatever* that is, to the work of God's world, without attending to either of these two cries.'[46]

Nightingale's approach to nursing was far-reaching. In Chicago in 1893 her paper was read at a conference. Delegates were told that nursing was a vocation, a calling, not a money-getting profession, it was not about book-learning and lectures, but 'an apprenticeship, a workshop practice'.[47] Nursing was not articulated or written about, it was lived as a 'service of the good'. Being a nurse involved method, self-sacrifice, watchful activity, love of the work, devotion to duty, the courage and coolness of the soldier, the tenderness of the mother, the absence of the prig. She was a virtuous person:

> It is said that you give examinations and certificates to plumbers, engineers, etc. But it is impossible to compare nurses with plumbers, or carpenters, or engineers, or even with gardeners. The main, the tremendous difference is that nurses have to do with these living bodies and no less living minds; for the life is not vegetable life, nor mere animal life, but it is human life – with living, that is, conscious forces, not electric or gravitation forces, but human forces. If you examine at all, you must examine all day long, current examination, current supervision, as to what the nurse is doing with this double, this damaged life entrusted to her.[48]

The high value that Nightingale placed on character training was at the root of her opposition to any form of registration. She felt there was a danger of worshipping examinations and making the passing of these more important than anything else. Book-learning, without developing the moral heart, was outward show. Performance had to be 'unseen' as well as 'seen', dependent on the inner woman:

> Now, there is a danger in the air of our becoming Parasites in Nursing (and also Midwifery) of our becoming Nurses (and Midwives) by deputy – a danger now when there is so great an inclination to make School and College education, all sorts of Sciences and Arts, even Nursing and Midwifery, a book and examination business, a profession, in the low, not the high sense of the word. And the danger is that we shall be content to let the book and the theory and the words do for us ... It is not the

> certificate which makes the Nurse or the Midwife. It may *un-make* her. The danger is lest she let the certificate be *instead of* herself, *instead of* her own never ceasing going up higher as a Woman and a Nurse.[49]

But it would be quite untrue to assume that Nightingale undervalued theoretical proficiency. In her school she endeavoured to have the theoretical teaching as good and as thorough as possible, but she gave a higher priority to the training of character. Highly educated as a child, she retained a strong interest in statistics, and had tried, unsuccessfully, with Benjamin Jowett, Master of Balliol College, Oxford, to found a chair of statistics at the university. But she also argued that statistics were no use if they were not used for their purposes. As she wrote to Jowett, she was frustrated at the amount of statistics collected that merely gathered dust on administrators' shelves.[50] Nursing was ultimately practical work.

To be a nurse was to have a vocation. This was much wider than a specific religious calling from God, although it could be this, as it was for Nightingale. Vocation implied a way of serving humanity by following timeless values involved in the moral imperative to love one's neighbour as oneself. To follow the vocation, to become a nurse, involved responding to a moral demand of altruistic service. Genuine moral commitment involved nurses attending even to such matters as disposing of the patient's excreta, a task that usually fell to household servants: 'If a nurse declines to do these kind of things for her patient, "because it is not her business," I should say that nursing was not her calling.'[51] And this impetus was often preconceptual, unarticulated and non-specific.

It has been argued that Nightingale offers a case study in the development of vocation.[52] The religious call motivated her creative energy and was a certain kind of charismatic power, with all the inherent dangers and corrupting influences of self-importance that can accompany it. But because of its religious associations, the exercise of charismatic power in a vocational sense is *de facto* rooted in self-knowledge, humility and love.

The Nightingale Training School: putting the ideal into practice

Nurse training was intended to develop a threefold interest in the trainee: 'an intellectual interest in the case, a (much higher) hearty interest in the patient, a technical (practical) interest in the patient's care and cure. She must not look upon patients as made for nurses, but upon nurses as made for patients'.[53] A compassionate and genuine interest in and for the patient was to accompany the intellectual interest needed to learn about and understand the nature and progress of the patient's illness as it affected his life and relationships. The acquisition of practical skills and the subsequent mastery of techniques should follow. There was no compulsion, but religion was seen as the essential background to nurse training: 'Life is a shallow thing, and more especially *Hospital* life, without any depth of religion.'[54]

To achieve this, Nightingale believed that nurses should be technically trained in hospitals prepared for the purpose; and they should live in homes to fit them for moral life and discipline.[55] A trained matron or superintendent was to have undisputed authority over nurses and trainees. A planned course of theoretical and practical training was to be given, the latter in the hospital where the school was connected. And carefully selected probationers should live in a home attached to the hospital where a sister was to be responsible for their moral and spiritual character training.[56]

These principles became the basis for Nightingale's training school at St Thomas's Hospital, which began in 1860. The advertisement for the first matron in *The Times* read: 'Wanted, a Matron for a large provincial hospital. She must have had experience in the management of nurses, be of fair education, and possess firmness and gentleness on Christian principles to control a large establishment.'[57]

The new probationers were recruited by advertisements in the public papers in May 1860. Their course of instruction started in June and was almost exclusively practical, covering all that a nurse needed to know and to do at the bedside of the sick. A strict timetable of supervision and certification was imposed on probationers.[58] Applicants for training applied to Mrs Wardroper, who became the first matron of St Thomas's Hospital, and were considered for selection if they were aged from twenty-five to thirty-five. They needed a certificate of age as well as a testimonial of character. During their year of training probationers were to receive instruction from sisters and the Resident Medical Officer. At the end of their training year the probationers were expected to enter into service as hospital nurses.

The names of probationers were entered in a register, in which a record was kept of the conduct and qualifications of the nurse. At the end of every month this was submitted to the committee of the Nightingale Fund. At the end of a year those whom the committee found to have passed satisfactorily through the course of instruction and training would be entered on the register as certified nurses, and would then be recommended for employment. There were two classes of efficiency, at which nurses were certified, first and second class, and gratuities of £5 or £3 were given accordingly.

The term of the probationer's service was one complete year. They were expected to stay for the period but could withdraw on three months notice, in exceptional circumstances approved by the committee. They could be discharged by the matron at any time for misconduct, inefficiency or negligence in their duties. They would be eligible for permanent appointment at St Thomas's Hospital at the end of this year, upon proof of competency.

This system of classes of efficiency ceased after the first year, when, in November 1861, on the death of Arthur Clough, Henry Bonham Carter became Secretary of the Nightingale Fund. He saw no point in such classification. In 1875 Nightingale commented that it was invidious to make distinctions between nurses as first or second class.[59]

The regulations for probationers precisely specified how the progress of the probationer was to be ascertained. The duties of the probationer under the Nightingale Fund were listed under two headings.[60] Under the first, the nurse was required to be sober, honest, truthful, trustworthy, punctual, quiet and orderly, cleanly and neat. Under the second, the nurse was expected to be skilful in thirteen separate functions including dressings, the application of leeches, the administration of enemas, the management of trusses and of appliances in uterine complaints, friction to the body and extremities, the management of helpless patients, bandaging, bedmaking, attending at operations, sick cookery, ventilation of the ward, cleanliness of utensils, observations of the sick, and the management of convalescents.

During the year of training, lectures of a practical nature were given to the probationers by members of the medical staff. The chaplain gave a short lecture on a religious subject twice a week. At the end of the year Mrs Wardroper, and the resident medical officer, Mr Whitfield, who supervised the probationers, reported their approval of the 'general conduct and proficiency' of the probationers. The probationers who had completed the course, according to the report, 'have expressed their gratitude for the benefits they have derived, and the kind manner in which they have been treated'. The committee was satisfied at the matron and resident medical officer's work, and pronounced the scheme a success. Twelve new probationers were to be admitted to fill vacancies.

Uniform was provided for the probationers. Nightingale intended that probationers should be adequately (if not luxuriously) provided for, both financially and in terms of accommodation. As Seymer writes, in considering the setting up of the Nightingale School 'what strikes one above all else is that it was such an intensely *personal* enterprise'. They really were 'Florence Nightingale's nurses'.[61] It is also striking to note from the syllabus outlined above, the basic, menial service that was expected of these probationers: privileged women learning to cook, clean, and tend the bodies of others.

The syllabus of medical lectures was prescribed by Mr Croft in 1873, and published.[62] Twenty-two weekly lectures were given in February, March, May, June, July, October, November and December. These lectures included general subjects common to medical and surgical nursing, medical subjects and surgical subjects. Two years later, in January 1875, Mr Croft printed a reading list for all the medical and surgical subjects he taught. He also recommended Nightingale's *Notes on Nursing* and her introductory address. Mr Croft's own textbook prescribed twenty-four lectures, including all the above subjects, and also adding lectures on disinfection and artificial respiration.

Mrs Wardroper's 'Memorandum of Instructions', written at Easter 1879, offers an insight into the practical training of the probationer, and how Nightingale's principles were applied in practice. Every new probationer was shown, once or twice at least, by the ward sister or staff nurse how to do her work to the ward sister's satisfaction: 'to be shown not only what things are to be done, and how they are to be done; but guarded against how they are not to be done'. The sister, wrote Mrs Wardroper, needed to remember that the probationer 'cannot be made responsible for doing well what she did not know how to do'.[63]

The novice probationer was shown the cupboards where lint, tow, bandages and ointments were kept and the whereabouts of instruments and utensils. She was shown her ward work, how to dust, wash and clean the ward, equipment and furniture, including the lavatories, the urinals and gratings. The new probationer was to have the bedpan explained to her, how to empty it and how to disinfect it; and how to wash and cleanse helpless patients, especially men, without exposure, by washing them between blankets. She would see how to wash daily the axilla, flexures of thighs and so on, of patients between towels or blankets. The sister was to remember that the probationer, particularly the 'special' probationer: 'may never have handled or even seen such Patients before, and that a Probationer cannot be expected to know of herself one of the most important things she has to do' [sic].

The sister would show the probationer how to lift helpless patients, or turn them from side to side; how to clean, or make her patients clean, teeth, mouth and so on of every patient ill enough to be washed by a nurse; how to feed and how to administer medicine to helpless patients; how to prevent bedsores. And she was to be taught fully how they were caused. The probationer learned to report the first appearance of the first signs of bedsores to sister in order for her to report immediately to the physician or surgeon; how to make beds, change sheets and draw sheets, especially with patients in the bed; and how to undress accident or fever cases.

The probationer was taught how to do dressings, using two basins for washing wounds, and always dipping tow or cotton wool into one basin only; how to make and apply poultices at their proper temperature and also fomentation flannels; how to dress blisters; how to apply iodine and other paints and liniments. She learned how to give injections and enemata, nutritive and otherwise; how to pass catheters on women; how to take temperature, pulse and respiration; how to make and apply bandages, cover splints and how to use trusses on women; and how 'to use "friction" in the sense in which it is used by professional rubbers'.

Every probationer was to learn sick cookery and the use of cooking utensils as well as how to make beef tea and egg flip, when to use beer and wine, and the proportions, and how to make gruel and drinks for the sick. She was to be taught by the ward sister 'observation of the sick', explaining the reason why medicines were given and why they were altered, as well as the reasons for dressings and so on. The probationer was to be taught how to read 'cards' at the head of beds, and was to be questioned, if possible, on special cases after the round of the attending physician or surgeon. She was also to be taught to describe the different sorts of coated tongues and so on; the differences of sputum and so on; 'the *feeling* of pus or skin'.

She would need to learn the necessary precautions to prevent finger poisoning, and 'the carrying of contagion by want of cleanliness or want of fresh air'; and the art of ventilation, by night as well as by day. She was taught how to manage convalescent patients, particularly convalescence from typhoid, as well as cases such as chorea and hysteria; and how to prepare the dead for removal without exposure. By this method, wrote Mrs Wardroper, a probationer 'can thus best be taught how to wash between blankets, the living'.

Finally, according to Mrs Wardroper's memorandum, the sister was to instruct nurses how to instruct probationers. As it was impossible for the sister, with her sister's duties, to have time to show the probationers all she needed to know, the sister was to question the probationer: 'the Sister to question her, and see if she has been shown them, and *how* she does them – kindly remembering that it is of use to the Probationers to put it into words' [sic].

Sister was expected to take each new probationer on her rounds and ask her, for example, how she had washed the helpless case, how she had bandaged or made bandages. The sister needed to remember that the probationer's training constituted not only what the probationer did, but whether she had learned to do it correctly. A good nurse could be charged by the ward sister to teach the probationer, for example, to wash a helpless case; the sister was to question the probationer afterwards, 'kindly remembering that it is not for the Probationer to criticize the Nurse, nor for the Sister to reprove *ignorance* in the Probationer, but for the Sister to enquire what the Probationer has been taught'. Every probationer was to be encouraged not only to keep case papers, but to jot down at the time any special thing she had learned or done in the ward during the day.

Mrs Wardroper's memorandum embodied the practical and scientifically up-to-date approach to the training of nurses that characterised Nightingale's approach to nursing. Although Nightingale was to criticise Mrs Wardroper's judgement of character as often faulty, she was given a free hand in selecting candidates and, in essentials, she was the 'heart and soul for the Nightingale idea, and without her administrative gifts, her hard work and enthusiasm the whole precarious experiment might have foundered'.[64]

The training at the Nightingale School developed from 1873 to 1896. These years saw a steady increase in the scope of instruction given and in the number of certified nurses sent out to other schools. John Croft took over the medical instruction from Mr Whitfield, and his syllabus and reading list was worked out closely with Miss Crossland; according to Seymer, he 'discussed the training minutely with Florence Nightingale'.[65]

A Fund Council report for 1880 recorded how practical work formed the foundation of training. Skills were taught on the wards by ward sisters, who made detailed written records, weekly and monthly, of the nurse's daily practical work, such as washing helpless patients, cleansing utensils and ventilation of wards. The records showed what the nurse was taught, including attendance at lectures, as well as what she had done. At the end of each course was a written examination.[66]

The improved scheme of teaching was different for nurse-probationers and the 'lady' or 'special' probationers. The two grades of nurse were entirely original to the Nightingale School, but according to Seymer it was not, as some critics have asserted, snobbishness which influenced the creation of these grades. In 1860, ten years before the 1870 Education Act made education free and compulsory, there was a great difference between the education of the middle or lower-middle class and that of the upper-class woman. As Nightingale told her friend the statistician Dr William Farr, her principle was to get the best training possible for any woman of any class or religious sect, paid or unpaid, who had the requisite qualifications for the vocation of a nurse. She thought it unquestionable, however, that the better educated would rise to the post of superintendent, not because they were ladies, but because they were educated.[67]

The second reason for the two grades of nurse was financial. Nurse-probationers received their training free, earned a small salary, and were engaged by the Nightingale Fund for two or three years; ladies or specials paid £30 or even £50 for their year's board and training and received no salary. They were bound to serve only one year after completing their training. Nurse-probationers were called by their surname only, while the ladies were given the prefix 'Miss'. But they were a financial saving to the Nightingale Fund which could be used for other purposes. The small prestige given to the ladies, as Seymer has argued, had compensating responsibilities, for they were closely watched and criticised, and more was demanded of them.

Although all probationers attended consultants' lectures, the specials had more lectures and were gradually given more time for private study and professional reading. Both groups, from the outset, were required to keep casebooks or 'cases' and also diaries of what was done on the wards. These diaries were considered to be very important from the beginning, and are referred to by Mrs Wardroper in letters to Nightingale. The diary and casebooks were Nightingale's idea, and Mrs Wardroper commended it, sending copies for Nightingale to look at, and on which she commented thoroughly.[68]

The diaries were mentioned in the first register of nurses. Dr Whitfield commented, for example, that a probationer had reported all the chemical lectures very carefully: 'her diary is very good'; and again, of another probationer, that she was not sufficiently educated to feel herself capable of reporting the lectures or keeping a diary.[69] Indeed, in a memorandum to Nightingale in March 1863, Dr Whitfield observed that he did not approve of the combination of diary with casebooks as was sometimes occurring. They should be distinct: the diary from the start of training as a method of work and time organisation and enabling opinions to be drawn as to the capability of each probationer; the casebook required a 'higher order of mental cultivation, a more intimate knowledge of sickness, and above all a power of observation not given to all alike'.[70]

One such comment entered into a diary shows the ethos: 'As to the so-called menial work, I don't see how it can be separated from what is often far more trying in "nursing work." The one and the other are alike justified and made easy by the fact that all is done for the comfort and wellbeing of the sick.'[71]

Nightingale wanted the diaries to show how the training was given. She was critical of probationers who might think: 'We did what was right in our own eyes'. She did not want opinions at the end of diaries, showing the cheerfulness and amiable willingness of the trainee, but rather a record of the manner and amount of training she was receiving: 'We do not want her opinion, we want her facts'.[72]

Another diary, from 1890, records the duties of a special probationer. These ranged from washing patients, washing urine bottles and locker tops, making beds, attending the doctor and the sister, and included attendance at prayers morning and evening, in a day that began at 7.00 a.m. and ended at 8.30 p.m. with bed an hour later. It is interesting to note the ward work of the ward sister: the probationer records one of her duties as, 'Helped Sister to wash an unconscious patient'.[73]

Written examinations were set and corrected apparently by Mr Croft himself and other lecturers. Seymer cites evidence from 1879 that probationers came to examinations in relays. In Miss Crossland's view the nurse-probationers were more thoroughly taught than the lady probationers. The former had learned at schools where they had to compete with others, while the latter were taught by governesses and were without competition. A practical examination was introduced by Dr Sharkey, in which nine probationers sat in a semicircle and were questioned.

During Miss Crossland's twenty years at St Thomas's, clinical teaching was given by doctors to probationers on the wards. Seymer regrets that this custom was eventually allowed to lapse. From 1873 the improved scheme of teaching continued to be different for nurse-probationers and the lady or special probationers. Nurse-probationers attended more elementary lectures and were given more class teaching and 'drilling' by Miss Crossland, while the lady probationers had more advanced lectures fitting them to more responsible posts. On two afternoons a week they were relieved of ward duties to have a study period in which they were required to read textbooks, supplemented by revision classes from Miss Crossland.

Miss Crossland's purpose was to train probationers to be 'thorough, straightforward, brave, unselfish', not to seek for ease, to consider nothing too much trouble and to consider nothing beneath them. She enjoined them to exclude the word 'trouble' from the dictionary. And according to Seymer, Miss Crossland's influence on the students, by virtue of both her moral training as well as her teaching, was very much appreciated by her students, and made the training school what it was, and distinct from other hospital training schools.[74]

The probationer was strictly watched by her superiors and a report sheet was drawn up by Nightingale for the matron to fill in.[75] Details of the probationer's name, age, religion, marital state, the sisters under whom she had worked, the nature of duty, absences and illnesses were all recorded. Her moral character during training was assessed in three aspects: sobriety, honesty (especially as to taking petty bribes from patients) and truthfulness. There was either a positive assessment, or dismissal – no degrees of attainment were admissible. Her character was assessed monthly for punctuality, quietness, trustworthiness, personal hygiene and cleanliness and ward management. She was also assessed for her technical record under fourteen main headings, which also included subheadings: dressing, applying leeches, enemas, management of trusses and uterine devices, rubbing, helpless patients, bandaging, making beds, waiting on operations, sick cooking, keeping the ward fresh, cleanliness of utensils, management of convalescents, and observation of the sick.[76]

For Nightingale, the 'good' nurse was classless. After all, it was what was 'inside' that counted. The primary object was to produce a 'practical and scientific training' for women who desired to be hospital nurses.[77] This was, however, not the view of all nurses. Following discussion in the *British Medical Journal*[78] in 1879, about a new system of 'lady' nursing introduced by Margaret Burt, Matron of Guy's Hospital, a nurse, Margaret Lonsdale,[79] argued that this 'lady nurse' was a better class of person, both intellectually and morally superior to the kind of nurse that Guy's Hospital had employed previously. Indeed, she went so far as to accuse the medical establishment of preferring lower-status women because they were morally inferior and so would turn a blind eye to the moral turpitude of the medical men.

The medical men disagreed. The doctor needed to maintain control of the care of the patient, by virtue of his scientific and technical training and for the sake of the patient's best interest. They argued for a subsidiary, but nevertheless crucial role for the nurse within the team. But they also disputed Lonsdale's inference that 'lower class' women could not have the virtues necessary to become a nurse.[80]

Bonham Carter, Secretary to the Nightingale Fund, writing in the *British Medical Journal*, reiterated Nightingale's presuppositions about what counted as good nursing: order, obedience, behaviour and general conduct were essential for the proper working of the hospital system.[81] The matron was responsible for the efficiency of the nurses, but she was responsible to the medical officers that their orders for the treatment of the sick were carried out. This necessitated a partnership between the matron and the doctors. She needed to exercise her authority with judgement and discretion. If she failed she should be removed; conversely, she should be supported in her judgements by the medical staff. Lonsdale[82] replied to her critics, maintaining her central argument for the more intelligent system of nursing, but also agreeing that the doctor must remain 'absolutely supreme'.[83]

Two articles from the *Edinburgh Medical Journal*, from an anonymous doctor and nurse, supported this view.[84] The writers are claimed by Baly to have been the surgeon Joseph Bell, and the St Thomas's trained nurse, pupil and protégé of Nightingale, Angélique Pringle.[85] The good nurse was clever, dutiful, cheerful and kind, and needing to be preserved as 'a clear, steady glow of inward brightness', argued the nursing author. Plenty of clever, educated women offered themselves as nurses, as well as plenty of weak but kindly women. But not many had all the qualities needed to make a good nurse, and if the superintendent lacked judgement recruitment difficulties ensued. This, rather than doctors' opposition, was the problem. As Pringle concluded, the issue was 'not to talk of vocation, but to live one'.

Analysing and interpreting the evidence for the Nightingale tradition

The nineteenth-century system for training nurses, shaped by the Nightingale School, reflected a clear application of Nightingale's principles. These facts are not disputed, even by those who question Nightingale's own personal influence on her school, or indeed, the influence of the Nightingale nurses. Baly, for example, who began writing in the 1960s,[86] refers to the same historical material as Seymer.[87] Baly was critical of earlier biographers, such as Sir Edward Cook[88] and Woodham-Smith,[89] for eulogising the Nightingale

School probationers and exaggerating their virtues and the extent of the instruction they received. She thought that Seymer's analysis perpetuated the myth that the school was independent, which allowed it to hold fast to its educational ideals. Baly argued, on the other hand, that the school was predominantly a labour force for the hospital. According to Baly, the Nightingale nurses were not the mark of a revolution, they were a small number, and their significance was overstated; rather, writers of nursing history books were leaders of the profession and had an agenda to portray nursing as a homogeneous, educated profession. They sought to play up the break with a morally corrupt, Sairey Gamp past.

There may be some truth in Baly's view that the actual situation fell short of the ideal. As the Lady Superintendent of the Hospital for Sick Children at Great Ormond Street, Catherine Wood, wrote circa 1887, the influence of the Nightingale Training School was not yet widely established, and bad nursing continued.[90] Wood was a founder member of the British Nurses' Association,[91] which at the time of her writing was in bitter dispute with Nightingale and her supporters over the issue of nurse registration. This is likely to have affected her analysis of the contemporary state of nursing. Nevertheless, Wood held the same ideals as Nightingale. As Wood stated, her principle was to set nursing standards at the highest level of Christian service: 'Not with eye-service as men-pleasers, but as the servants of Christ, doing the will of God from the heart".'[92] Wood's argument was that these principles needed to be promulgated systematically, and in the following century this did occur.

Baly has perhaps, as Wake suggests, overstated the short-term weaknesses and minimised the long-term achievements of Nightingale's system.[93] The reason for this may lie in Baly's twentieth-century perspective which espoused different values to those of the Nightingale tradition. Hence, for Baly, few Nightingale nurses became notable leaders of the profession because, apart from Agnes Jones, none made their mark on nursing; moreover, as she points out, many probationers did not finish their training. But the reason many did not finish is because if they were considered to be morally or intellectually below par, they were dismissed. As Hector has shown, this was the predominant reason for leaving.[94] Many others died from diseases they caught in service.

The good nurse was a humble nurse, whose record of achievement may well have lain buried with her. As Baly has accepted, women went into nursing from spiritual and religious motives; status was not a significant goal for them.[95] What counted was the good of the community served. Self-effacement, and not self-enhancement, was the quality required. The history of nursing has to be set in this historical context of the vocation, its moral basis and practical outworking.

But modern historians of nursing have tended to minimise the relevance of this vocational ethic,[96] perhaps because they are unsympathetic to, and impatient of, what are perceived to be outdated values. This is certainly the view of Judith Moore, who has examined the nineteenth-century struggle of professional nursing, and the conflicts between doctors, nurses and administrators, at King's College Hospital, Guy's Hospital and St John's House.[97] As she argues: 'assumptions about class and religion have tended to blinker contemporary historians – perhaps feminist historians, whose investigative premises tend to be egalitarian and secular, more than others'.[98]

From these egalitarian and secular premises, modern nursing historians have interpreted the emphasis on morality as heteronomy, externally imposed constraints, rather than as the genuine cultivation of virtue. The biomedical focus of training has been argued to show an expectation that the brighter nurses would become ancillary doctors and take over the measuring and treatments previously done by doctors. Others would be left as the 'practical' labour force, and doctors would be able to give away some of their more tedious chores.[99] But in the light of the evidence another interpretation may reasonably be supposed: a curriculum containing anatomy and physiology was considered a prerequisite for nursing because a knowledge of biomedical science improved the nursing care of sick people, and preserved health.

From a twentieth-century perspective which emphasises autonomy, the issue of authority has also become problematic. At the heart of the Nightingale system was a fundamental trust in the importance of proper order and authority, neither autonomy nor the heteronomy of blind, mechanistic obedience. For Baly, the model of obedience engendered by this system did not encourage nurses to rebel and provided the greatest obstacle to change. Nightingale nurses were reared in an atmosphere of obedience and conformity, and according to Baly, the second and third generations clung tenaciously to the principles that had raised them, first to respectability then to admiration: 'Obedience is inimical to innovation.'[100]

A more sympathetic interpretation recognises that Nightingale sought to transcend the polarity of both autonomy and heteronomy. Obedience to authority was vested in justice, and considered necessary for the proper organisation of patient care, rather than because hierarchy, with its associated status and privilege, demanded it. Conformity to unchanging principles did not, as Baly thinks, inhibit change and prevent progress, and Nightingale's own work shows this vividly: she was a truly progressive radical whose practical ideas breached the deeply entrenched class system of the Victorian period. Nursing probationers came from all classes, the servant class as well as the privileged class, which is why they needed to be taught to read, and why they were provided with necessary physical requirements such as food and clothing. As Baly has acknowledged: 'Contrary to what is supposed Miss Nightingale gave nursing one portal of entry. Her school was open to "any woman from any class and from any Church" – the lady had to be educated with her cook – and she insisted that the training was the same'.[101]

This radicalism meant that not only did genteel high-born nurses work alongside the lower classes, but women used to luxurious living involved themselves, by choice, in work that was not only menial and onerous, but also extremely dangerous. A doctor, Octavius Sturges, responding to Lonsdale's article discussed earlier, showed very vividly the absolute dedication nursing required during this period. Far from being romantic or sentimental, nurses had an enthusiasm and ardour 'which they intimately connect with the highest religious duty'. This involved them in an endless routine of caring for extremely ill people:

> ... of the ingratitude of many patients, the actual violence of some; of the careful tending of those who have reached the very bottom of social degradation, and whose wounds and diseases are the direct result of their depravity. All this the hospital nurse endures week after week, with small money remuneration, limited prospect of promotion, scanty share in any credit which may accrue, and prompted only by a motive which, however it may find expression, is of the highest and noblest kind. The dignity of such service seems to me quite unequalled.[102]

From the beginnings of her own training in Kaiserswerth, Nightingale was anxious to replace the drunken women who were called 'nurses' in England, and who were entrusted with the care of the sick as a means of earning money. This purpose was sacrosanct so that even when she was in disagreement with individuals, as she was, for example with Mrs Wardroper,[103] her personal views took second place to the fulfilment of her vision. Hence her obituary of Mrs Wardroper was fulsome. 'No Mrs Gamp could live in her neighbourhood; Mrs Gamp is extinct for ever.' Mrs Wardroper had been responsible for opening a new calling for women of all classes. 'The state of what was, by ignorance called nursing when she began hospital work, the miserable state, moral and technical of the nurses, would scarcely now be credited'. A good judge of character, strong and generous: 'She was free from self-consciousness; nothing artificial about her. "She did nothing because she was being looked at, and abstained from nothing because she was looked at".'[104] All she did was done silently and only God knew it; her life was in her work.

Adulation was given to Nightingale in her lifetime. One such article, written in 1861 in *St James's Magazine* by Mrs S.C. Carter Hall, described Nightingale's achievements in the Crimea as attributable to the work of God, leavening the whole family of man. She adduced statistics from officially published evidence to support her analysis of Nightingale's remarkable achievements. And she described the new work at St Thomas's, which she had personally visited, and the need for donations to it. In conclusion, she quoted from Nightingale that the work was God's: 'His will be done on earth, as it is in heaven!'[105]

Anne Summers, in an essay on nursing charities from c. 1830 to c. 1860, has argued that the history of nursing from this period cannot be divorced from Victorian Christianity.[106] Nursing history itself formed a sub-plot to Victorian Christianity. And she believed that these real origins of the reform of nineteenth-century nursing, in the work of the religious sisterhoods preceding and alongside Nightingale, have tended to be obscured. Medical history took the expansion of hospitals for granted, and it was therefore assumed that such expansion led to the development of hospital nurse training schemes. But this assumption obscured the real origins. Because the end of the story was so at variance from its beginning, the beginning of the story has been misunderstood, and some 'convenient, rational, organizing principle' has been cast around for: 'We have "read back" narrative themes from a familiar social landscape: experimentation, secularization, modernization, professionalization'. But, according to Summers: 'None of these concepts is adequate to describe a movement which was fed by the desire to spread the Christian faith and preach a gospel of reconciliation.'[107] A similar position seems to have occurred with regard to the the contribution of Christianity to health care reforms after the Reformation, which has been marginalised. Instead reforms are attributed to economic and social determinism.[108]

According to Summers, this impetus in no way meant that nursing care was so focused on the patient's soul that practical physical care suffered. Even among the nursing sisterhoods, about which Summers wrote, at the time of Nightingale, religious and clinical imperatives did not appear to have come into conflict. The St John's Sisters, who had worked at King's College Hospital, and were obliged to leave in 1868 because of sectarian controversy, were not accused of physically neglecting their patients. Instead, the patient's physical care improved under their care. After the installation of the St John's sisters at Charing Cross Hospital in 1866, the food bills went up, as patients were given a higher quality of food (to the chagrin of the Financial Committee who believed they were being fed above their station). When such hospitals contracted out their services to the sisterhoods, they noticed a higher standard of cleanliness, invalid cookery, surgical skill and knowledge and night watching.

The moral and vocational impetus was central to the development of the Nightingale Training School over the next century. Susan Coventry, who trained as a nurse at St Thomas's in the early 1950s, remembers her interview with the matron who did not use the word 'vocation'. This was a relief because: 'I had no conscious vocation for nursing at all.'[109] But this nurse also described her regular involvement in religious services, both at work and off duty. This was the unconscious pattern of nurses' lives, a shared value system which provided security, respect and authority, and upheld standards.

The Nightingale School training was to have an immense impact. Cicely Saunders, the founder of the modern hospice movement, trained as a nurse at the Nightingale School in the 1940s. She commented in 1998 that her 'nurse training taught me attention to detail and courtesy to patients which has proved invaluable in my palliative care work'.[110] No less significant were the opinions expressed to Roy Wake by many Nightingale nurses which reflected a training of which most were very proud. Some, however, thought the rigorous training was too restrictive.[111]

Although the Nightingale probationers were supernumerary in the early years, the practical nature of training was to become fundamental.[112] The Nightingale Training School, as even Baly has admitted, inculcated a system of training based on a working apprenticeship, which became the orthodoxy for nurse training.[113] Under the direction of the matron, it formed the beginning of a system and career structure for nurses, who were accountable to nurses.

As modern nursing historians agree, Nightingale reconstituted nursing primarily as a moral activity.[114] What has been underestimated, however, is the long-term impact and significance of this development. Gradual conformity to this Nightingale system of training meant that it was to provide the apprenticeship model for training for the next hundred years. The quality of nursing care was directly dependent on the moral qualities of the nurse. She was self-motivated into being attentive to every need of her patients; an often hard and burdensome self-imposed standard, but one which led directly to better patient care.

The Nightingale tradition became ingrained into nursing's self-consciousness and practical reality. As the authors of a practical nursing textbook in the 1960s would write:

> Over the past century the image of the nurse has changed from that of Mrs Sairy Gamp [sic] to that of the well-trained ward-sister, but this is only because thousands of nurses have worked to maintain high standards of professional behaviour. Every new nurse inherits the public goodwill which has been built up for her over the years by her predecessors, and she in her turn will add something to the total picture of what nurses are like and how they behave.[115]

Conclusion

This chapter has described Nightingale's vision of nursing as a synthesis of art and science, which came to define the self-understanding of the profession for a century. As Wake has argued, although the training at the Nightingale School may not have been scrupulously carried out as laid down in theory, nurses were undoubtedly initiated into humility, service and the rigid insistence in carrying out the most lowly of tasks: a way of being and of working.[116] This was because assiduous devotion to the welfare of the patient was the absolute priority and sole purpose. To this end, nurses submitted themselves to the authority of rigid and objective standards; they were inducted into a moral and practical tradition and the virtues of very demanding altruistic care; they learned to be informed and practically competent; they acquired specific knowledge, skills and techniques through hospital training. Not just 'head' knowledge, it also involved the hands and the heart. No mere theory, this was a way of caring. Nursing was a unified practice, part of a community of care, with a clear purpose of contributing to the moral narrative of humanity. The Nightingale tradition was to spread throughout the world.[117]

Notes

1 Lord Elton, 'Florence Nightingale', *Nursing Times*, 1939, pp. 1442–1443, December 2.

2 R. Wake, *The Nightingale Training School 1860–1996*, London, Haggerston Press, 1998.

3 Ibid., pp. 33–34.

4 A. Bradshaw, *Lighting the Lamp*, London, Scutari Press, 1994.

5 F. Nightingale, letter to Julia Ann Elizabeth Roundell, 4 August, 1896, in Vicinus, M. and B. Nergaard (eds) , *Ever Yours, Florence Nightingale*, London, Virago Press, 1989, pp. 433–435.

6 K. Heasman, *Evangelicals in Action*, London, Geoffrey Bles, 1962, p. 235.

7 M.E. Baly, Florence Nightingale and the Nursing Legacy, London, Croom Helm, 1986.

8 R. Wake, *The Nightingale Training School 1860–1996*, London, Haggerston Press, 1998, p. 24.

9 Ibid., p. 65.

10 Ibid., p. 43.

11 Ibid., p. 85.

12 M.E. Baly, *Florence Nightingale and the Nursing Legacy*, London, Croom Helm, 1986.

13 F. Nightingale, *Suggestions for Thought to the Searchers after Truth among the Artizans of England*, in 3 vols, London, Eyre & Spottiswode, privately printed, 1860; A. Bradshaw, *Lighting the Lamp*, London, Scutari Press, 1994, pp. 125–139.

14 E.V. Quinn, J.M. Prest, *Dear Miss Nightingale*, Oxford, Clarendon Press, 1987, p. xxii.

15 R. Wake, *The Nightingale Training School 1860–1996*, London, Haggerston Press, 1998, p. 42.

16 Ibid., pp. 32,36.

17 F. Nightingale, *The Institution of Kaiserswerth on the Rhine, for the Practical Training of Deaconesses, under the Direction of the Rev. Pastor Fliedner, Embracing the Support and*

Care of a Hospital, Infant and Industrial Schools, and a Female Penitentiary, London, London Ragged Colonial Training School, 1851, p. 15.

[18] 'Arrival of the Wounded in the Bosphorus', *The Times*, 1854, p. 8, October 9; 'From our Own Correspondent', *The Times*, 1854, p. 7, editorial, *The Times*, 1854, p. 6, October 12; 'From our Own Correspondent', *The Times*, 1854, p. 8, October 13; 'Hospital Assistants in the East', letter, *The Times*, 1854, p. 7, October 14.

[19] 'The Function of the Training School is not only to Teach the Mind but to form the Character', *Nursing Times*, 1954, pp. 871–872, August 14.

[20] R. Dingwall, A.M. Rafferty, C. Webster, *An Introduction to the Social History of Nursing*, Routledge, London, 1988, p. 23.

[21] F. Nightingale, 'Nurses, Training of; Nursing the Sick' in Quain, R. (ed.), *A Dictionary of Medicine*, 1st edn, pp. 1038–1049 (part 2); 2nd edn, pp. 231–244. 'Nursing the Sick' in Murray, M. (ed.), *Quain's Dictionary of Medicine*, 3rd edn, 1097–1103, London, Longmans, Green, & Co., 1882, 1894, 1902. 1st edn, p. 1049.

[22] Ibid., 1st edn, p. 1039.

[23] Ibid., 3rd edn, pp. 1101–1102.

[24] Ibid., 1st edn, p. 1048.

[25] Ibid., 1st edn, p. 1049.

[26] F. Nightingale, *Letters and Addresses to the Probationer Nurses in the 'Nightingale Fund' School at St Thomas's Hospital and Nurses who were Formerly Trained There*, original letters and prints for private circulation held by University College, London, May 23, 1873.

[27] F. Nightingale, *Letters and Addresses to the Probationer Nurses in the 'Nightingale Fund' School at St Thomas's Hospital and Nurses who were Formerly Trained There*, original letters and prints for private circulation held by University College, London, July 23, 1874.

[28] F. Nightingale, *The Institution of Kaiserswerth on the Rhine, for the Practical Training of Deaconesses, under the Direction of the Rev. Pastor Fliedner, Embracing the Support and Care of a Hospital, Infant and Industrial Schools, and a Female Penitentiary*, London, London Ragged Colonial Training School, 1851, p. 6.

[29] F. Nightingale, *Florence Nightingale to her Nurses*, Nash, R. (ed.), London, Macmillan & Co., 1914, p. 11.

[30] R. Wake, *The Nightingale Training School 1860–1996*, London, Haggerston Press, 1998, p. 42.

[31] F. Nightingale, 'Nurses, Training of: Nursing the Sick' in Quain, R. (ed.), *A Dictionary of Medicine*, 1st edn, pp. 1038–1049 (part 2), p. 1040.

[32] Ibid., p. 1042.

[33] Ibid., p. 1046.

[34] Ibid., p. 1046.

[35] F. Nightingale, *Letters and Addresses to the Probationer Nurses in the 'Nightingale Fund' School at St Thomas's Hospital and Nurses who were Formerly Trained There*, original letters and prints for private circulation held by University College, London, July 23, 1874.

[36] L.R. Seymer, *Florence Nightingale's Nurses*, London, Pitman Medical, 1960, p. 33.

[37] Ibid., pp. 32–33.

[38] F. Nightingale, 'Nurses, Training of; Nursing the Sick' in Quain, R. (ed.), *A Dictionary of Medicine*, 1st edn, pp. 1038–1049 (part 2), p. 1039.

[39] Ibid., p. 1043.

[40] F. Nightingale, *Notes on Nursing*, 1861, Skretkowicz, V. (ed.), London, Scutari Press, 1992, pp. 172–173.

[41] F. Nightingale, *Florence Nightingale to her Nurses*, Nash, R. (ed.), London, Macmillan & Co., 1914 pp. 12–13.

[42] Ibid., p. 21.

[43] Ibid., p. 37.

[44] P.D. James, 'A Breath of Fresh Air', *Times Literary Supplement*, 1975, p. 517, May 9.

[45] F. Nightingale, *Notes on Nursing*, 1st edn, London, Harrison, 1860, p. 35.
[46] Ibid., p. 76.
[47] F. Nightingale, 'Sick Nursing and Health Nursing', in Hampton, I.A. (ed.), *Nursing of the Sick*, 1893, pp. 24–37, New York, McGraw-Hill Book Co., 1949 p. 35.
[48] Ibid., pp. 33–34.
[49] F. Nightingale, *Letters and Addresses to the Probationer Nurses in the 'Nightingale Fund' School at St Thomas's Hospital and Nurses who were Formerly Trained There*, original letters and prints for private circulation held by University College, London, May 16, 1888.
[50] E.V. Quinn, J.M. Prest, *Dear Miss Nightingale*, Oxford, Clarendon Press, 1987, pp. 314–315.
[51] E.V. Quinn, J.M. Prest, *Dear Miss Nightingale*, Oxford, Clarendon Press, 1987, p. 13.
[52] D.M. Emmet, *Function, Purpose and Powers*, London, Macmillan & Co., 1958, pp. 269–284.
[53] F. Nightingale, 'Sick Nursing and Health Nursing', in Hampton, I.A. (ed.), *Nursing of the Sick*, 1893 pp. 24–37, New York, McGraw-Hill Book Company, 1949 p. 34.
[54] F. Nightingale, *Letters and Addresses to the Probationer Nurses in the 'Nightingale Fund' School at St Thomas's Hospital and Nurses who were Formerly Trained There*, original letters and prints for private circulation held by University College, London, May 23, 1873.
[55] R. Wake, *The Nightingale Training School 1860–1996*, London, Haggerston Press, 1998. p. 66.
[56] L.R. Seymer, M. Houghton, M.L. Wenger, 'Nursing', *Encyclopaedia Britiannica*, vol.16, pp. 791–795, Chicago, William Benton, 1971.
[57] *The Times*, 1860, p. 2, May 26.
[58] J. Jebb, 'Report of the Committee of the Council for the Year Ending 24th June, 1861', in Seymer, L.R., *Florence Nightingale's Nurses*, Appendix 1, London, Pitman Medical, 1960, pp. 151–154. 'Timetable for the Probationers under the "Nightingale Fund" (1862)' in Seymer, L.R., *Florence Nightingale's Nurses*, Appendix 3, London, Pitman Medical, 1960, p. 157.
[59] L.R. Seymer, *Florence Nightingale's Nurses*, London, Pitman Medical, 1960, pp. 17,156.
[60] J. Jebb, 'Report of the Committee of the Council for the Year Ending 24th June, 1861', in Seymer, L.R., *Florence Nightingale's Nurses*, Appendix 1, London, Pitman Medical, 1960, pp. 151–154.
[61] L.R. Seymer, *Florence Nightingale's Nurses*, London, Pitman Medical, 1960, p. 23.
[62] 'Syllabus of Mr. Croft's Lectures for 1873', Appendix 3; J. Croft, 'Reading List', January, 1875, Appendix 4, in Seymer, L.R., *Florence Nightingale's Nurses*, 1960, pp. 158–161; J. Croft, *Notes of Lectures at St Thomas's Hospital*, London, St Thomas's Hospital, Blades East & Blades, 1873.
[63] Mrs. Wardroper, 'Memorandum of Instructions by Matron to Ward Sisters on duties to Probationers', in Seymer, L.R., *Florence Nightingale's Nurses*, Appendix 6, London, Pitman Medical, 1960, pp. 163–165.
[64] L.R. Seymer, *Florence Nightingale's Nurses*, London, Pitman Medical, 1960, p. 26.
[65] Ibid., p. 67.
[66] R. Wake, *The Nightingale Training School 1860–1996*, London, Haggerston Press, 1998 pp. 78–79.
[67] L.R. Seymer, *Florence Nightingale's Nurses*, London, Pitman Medical, 1960, p. 38.
[68] R. Wake, *The Nightingale Training School 1860–1996*, London, Haggerston Press, 1998, pp. 75–76.
[69] L.R. Seymer, *Florence Nightingale's Nurses*, London, Pitman Medical, 1960, p. 39.
[70] Ibid., p. 40.
[71] Ibid., p. 74.
[72] Ibid., pp. 74–75.

[73] Appendix 2 in Baly, M.E., *Florence Nightingale and the Nursing Legacy*, London, Croom Helm, 1986, p. 232.

[74] Ibid., p. 79.

[75] Appendix 1, Baly, M.E., *Florence Nightingale and the Nursing Legacy*, London, Croom Helm, 1986, pp. 230–231.

[76] Ibid., p. 231; E.T. Cook, *The Life of Florence Nightingale*, volume 2, London, Macmillan & Co., 1913, p. 460.

[77] L.R. Seymer, *Florence Nightingale's Nurses*, London, Pitman Medical, 1960, pp. 41–42.

[78] 'The Nursing Question at Guy's Hospital', editorial, *British Medical Journal*, 1879, p. 871, November 29; 'The Nursing Staff at Guy's Hospital', editorial, *British Medical Journal*, 1879 p. 898, December 6; 'The Nursing Question at Guy's Hospital', editorial, *British Medical Journal*, 1879, p. 918, December 6; 'Nursing at Guy's Hospital', editorial, *British Medical Journal*, 1879, pp. 1027–1028, December 27.

[79] M. Lonsdale, 'The Present Crisis at Guy's Hospital' *Nineteenth Century*, 7, 38, 1880, pp. 677–684, April.

[80] J. Braxton Hicks, 'On Nursing Systems', correspondence, *British Medical Journal*, 1880, pp. 11–12, January 3; W.W. Gull, 'On the Nursing Crisis at Guy's Hospital I', *Nineteenth Century*, 7, 39, 1880, pp. 884–891, May; S.O. Habershon, 'On the Nursing Crisis at Guy's Hospital II', *Nineteenth Century*, 7, 39, 1880, pp. 892–901, May; A.G. Henriques, 'On the Nursing Crisis at Guy's Hospital III', *Nineteenth Century*, 7, 39, 1880, pp. 902–904, May; S. Messenger Bradley, 'Miss Lonsdale on the Present Crisis at Guy's Hospital', correspondence, *British Medical Journal*, 1880, pp. 605–606, April 17; C.H. Marriott, 'Guy's Hospital', correspondence, *British Medical Journal*, 1879, p. 1045, December 27; C.H. Marriott, 'Nursing Systems', correspondence, *British Medical Journal*, 1880, p. 73, January 10; W. Moxon, 'Miss Lonsdale on Guy's Hospital' *Contemporary Review*, 37, 1880, pp. 872–892; J.E. Neale, 'On Nursing Systems', correspondence, *British Medical Journal*, 1880, p. 90, January 17; F.T. Paul, 'Nursing Institutions', correspondence, *British Medical Journal*, 1880, pp. 125–126, January 24; E. Penny, 'The Nursing at Guy's Hospital', correspondence, *British Medical Journal*, correspondence, 1880, p. 230, February 7; S. Sharkey, 'Doctors and Nurses II', *Nineteenth Century*, 7, 40, 1880, pp. 1097–1104, June; O. Sturges, 'Doctors and Nurses I', *Nineteenth Century*, 7, 40, 1880, pp. 1089–1096, June; 'Nursing Difficulties', editorial, *British Medical Journal*, 1880, pp. 289–290, February 21; 'Nursing at Guy's Hospital', *British Medical Journal*, editorial, 1880, p. 374, March 6; 'The Nursing at Guy's Hospital', editorial, *British Medical Journal*, 1880, pp. 525–526, April 3; 'The Nursing at Guy's Hospital', editorial, *British Medical Journal*, 1880, p. 563, April 10; 'Miss Lonsdale and the Nursing at Guy's Hospital', editorial, *British Medical Journal*, 1880, pp. 706–707, May 8.

[81] H. Bonham Carter, 'Nursing Organisation in Hospitals', correspondence, *The British Medical Journal*, 1880, p. 225, February 7.

[82] M. Lonsdale, 'Doctors and Nurses III', *Nineteenth Century*, 7, 40, 1880, pp. 1105–1108, June.

[83] Ibid., p. 1105.

[84] 'Nurses and Doctors: Systems of Nursing, by a Nurse', *Edinburgh Medical Journal*, xxv, xi, 1880, pp. 1048–1050, May; 'Nurses and Doctors: Edinburgh Infirmary Nursing, by One of the Staff', *Edinburgh Medical Journal*, 25, 7, 1880, pp. 1051–1052, May.

[85] M.E. Baly, *Florence Nightingale and the Nursing Legacy*, London, Croom Helm, 1986, p. 196.

[86] M.E. Baly, 'The Reform of Nursing Education', *Nursing Times*, 1965: pp. 867–868, June 25; pp. 955–956, July 9; pp. 977–978, July 16.

[87] M.E. Baly, *Florence Nightingale and the Nursing Legacy*, Appendix 1, London, Croom Helm, 1986, pp. 3–4.

[88] E.T. Cook, *The Life of Florence Nightingale*, volumes 1 and 2, London, Macmillan & Co., 1913.

[89] C. Woodham-Smith, *Florence Nightingale*, Harmondsworth, Penguin, 1955.

[90] C.J. Wood, *A Handbook of Nursing for the Home and the Hospital*, preface, 8th edn, London, Cassell & Co., c. 1887, pp. iii–vi.

[91] A.M. Rafferty, *The Politics of Nursing Knowledge*, London, Routledge, 1996, pp. 47,48,76.

[92] C.J. Wood, *A Handbook of Nursing for the Home and the Hospital*, preface, 8th edn, London, Cassell & Co., c. 1887, pp. iii–vi.

[93] R. Wake, *The Nightingale Training School 1860–1996*, London, Haggerston Press, 1998, p. 65.

[94] W. Hector, *The Life of Mrs Bedford Fenwick and the Rise of Professional Nursing*, London, Royal College of Nursing, 1973, p. 20.

[95] M.E. Baly, *Florence Nightingale and the Nursing Legacy*, London, Croom Helm, 1986, p. 195.

[96] B. Abel-Smith, *A History of the Nursing Profession*, London, Heinemann, 1960; Baly, M.E., *Florence Nightingale and the Nursing Legacy*, London, Croom Helm, 1986; C. Davies (ed.), *Rewriting Nursing History*, London, Croom Helm, 1980; C.J. Maggs, *The Origins of General Nursing*, London, Croom Helm, 1983; A.M. Rafferty, *The Politics of Nursing Knowledge*, London, Routledge, 1996; F.B. Smith, *Florence Nightingale: Reputation and Power*, London, Croom Helm, 1982.

[97] J. Moore, *A Zeal for Responsibility*, Athens, University of Georgia Press, 1988.

[98] Ibid., p. xi.

[99] M.E. Baly, *Florence Nightingale and the Nursing Legacy*, London, Croom Helm, 1986, p. 160.

[100] Ibid., p. 222.

[101] Ibid., p. 223.

[102] O. Sturges, 'Doctors and Nurses I', *Nineteenth Century*, 7, 40, 1880, p. 1091, June.

[103] R. Wake, *The Nightingale Training School 1860–1996*, London, Haggerston Press, 1998, p. 69.

[104] F. Nightingale, 'The Reform of Sick Nursing and the Late Mrs Wardroper', *British Medical Journal*, 1892, p. 1448, December 31.

[105] S.C. Carter Hall, 'Something of What Florence Nightingale has Done and is Doing', *St James's Magazine*, vol. 1, 1861, pp. 29–40, April–July.

[106] A. Summers, 'The Costs and Benefits of Caring: Nursing Charities, c. 1830–c. 1860', in Barry, J. and C. Jones (eds), *Medicine and Charity before the Welfare State*, pp. 133–148, Routledge, London, 1991.

[107] Ibid., p. 145.

[108] O.P. Grell, 'The Protestant Imperative of Christian Care and Neighbourly Love', in Grell, O.P. and A. Cunningham (eds), *Health Care and Poor Relief in Protestant Europe 1500–1700*, pp. 43–65, London, Routledge, 1997.

[109] S. Coventry, *Images of a Nightingale*, Rustington, W. Sussex, Beauclerk Publishing, 1990, p. 10.

[110] C. Saunders, 'What Made the Nightingales so Special?', *Nursing Times*, 94, 20, 1998, p. 14, May 20.

[111] R. Wake, *The Nightingale Training School 1860–1996*, London, Haggerston Press, 1998, pp. 196–199, 149–150.

[112] L.R. Seymer, *Florence Nightingale's Nurses*, London, Pitman Medical, 1960, p. 40.

[113] M.E. Baly, *Florence Nightingale and the Nursing Legacy*, London, Croom Helm, p. 223.

[114] A.M. Rafferty, *The Politics of Nursing Knowledge*, London, Routledge, 1996, pp. 26–35.

[115] J. Darwin, J. Markham, B. Whyte, *Bedside Nursing*, London, William Heinemann Medical Books, 3 edns 1964–1971, p. 1.

[116] R. Wake, *The Nightingale Training School 1860–1996*, London, Haggerston Press, 1998, p. 115.

[117] B.M. Dossey, *Florence Nightingale: Mystic, Visionary, Healer*, Springhouse, Pennsylvania, Springhouse Corporation, 1999, p. 392.

Chapter 2

Voices from the Nightingale nursing tradition: views of nurse leaders, 1874–1982

Nightingale's vision caught on. To discover the full extent of this ethos, a comprehensive and systematic examination of hitherto unresearched reference textbooks, which provided the content of nurse training for a century, will be undertaken in this chapter. From the late nineteenth century through to the twentieth century, generations of nursing writers, who were also often practising ward sisters and matrons, as well as tutors, wrote textbooks as resources for the teaching content of nurse training. Textbooks followed the syllabuses of individual training schools and later, after it was published, the national syllabus.

Training the nurse: induction into the purpose and practices of nursing care

According to Seymer, Nightingale articulated the unchanging principles underlying all good nursing: the correct balance of theory and practice, an insistence on the thorough mastery of nursing techniques, and firmly supported 'above all with her high ethical ideals'.[1] Nursing textbook writers sought to apply these principles to their teaching for over a century. The aims and objectives of their teachings were fourfold: to develop moral character, to teach technical knowledge and skill, to perpetuate the method of apprenticeship learning by the example and tuition of the ward sister, and to encourage the professional etiquette of right relationships. The apprenticeship meant that nurses were initiated into a tradition and an organic community, of which ward sisters were the guardians, and which involved crucially the formation of character as its essence. That this was indispensable in nursing has been understood by a modern educationalist:

> The educator of nurses is more than just one who transmits nursing knowledge to new recruits; he/she is the guardian of a tradition about the meaning of nursing into which new nurses are inducted ... 'Education worthy of the name is essentially education of

> character', and the character of the nurse is as important as the knowledge that she possesses.[2]

Most textbooks began with an introductory chapter on the moral basis of nursing, and the importance of developing the nurse's virtuous character. Writers used the same language and approach as Nightingale. One of the earliest, included in the reading list for probationer nurses at St Thomas's Hospital by Mr John Croft in 1875,[3] was published by Florence Lees in 1874.[4] She was a superintendent who oversaw the care of the wounded in the Franco-Prussian War. Her textbook, *Handbook for Hospital Sisters*, had a preface by Sir Henry Acland, and was dedicated to Florence Nightingale. Her experience in France and Germany was influenced by the religious nursing work of Roman Catholic sisters and Protestant deaconesses, and she viewed the care of the sick in civilian life as occurring in a Christian environment.

Lees's introduction expanded on the purpose of nursing as the paramount duty of civilisation, concerned as it was with issues of life and death, and in which nurses were privileged to be involved. She listed the qualities nurses needed to learn in training school: cleanliness, neatness, obedience, sobriety, truthfulness, honesty, punctuality, trustworthiness, quickness and orderliness. The nurse was also to be patient, cheerful and kindly.[5]

A similar approach was taken by *Hints for Hospital Nurses* published in 1877 by two Nightingale nurses, Rachel Williams, of St Mary's Hospital, London and previously of Edinburgh Royal Infirmary, and Alice Fisher, of the Fever Hospital, Newcastle upon Tyne.[6] They began by entreating women not to enter nursing for love of notoriety, false sentiment, or even as just a means of earning a living. There was nothing so 'revolting' as this. Nursing had to be an 'inborn love' of the work which was sadly only given to a few.[7]

Nurses came from two classes: 'Respectable persons of the rank from which upper servants are usually taken, and a smaller number of more highly educated women, such as, for example, the daughters of professional, or naval and military men.'[8] In spite of very hard work and small pay much happiness was to be found in nursing. Nurses needed good health, healthy habits, 'nerve and constitutional cheerfulness'. They also needed 'to combine unselfishness, and a strong resolution not to be conquered by difficulties'.[9] Mutual forbearance was required, as were self-denial 'and frequent possibilities for the exercise of Christian charity';[10] and the nurse was told to rejoice in the Lord always, and work always in the knowledge of the presence of the 'Great Master'.[11]

The Lady Superintendent of the Hospital for Sick Children, Great Ormond Street, Catherine Wood, held a similar position.[12] The duties of the nurse and the signs and symptoms of disease provided her focus for the textbook, but she stated her intention as primarily 'to place the standard of nursing on the very highest level, as being the Christian work of Christian women'.[13] Although

Wood was not without criticism of systems of training, 'each teacher does what is right in her own eyes',[14] and keen for a more systematic approach, she acknowledged that service to the patient was the single purpose of both doctors and nurses. The nurse was not born but made, and needed six qualities: presence of mind, gentleness of heart and thereby of touch, accuracy, memory, observation and forethought. Like Nightingale, Wood stressed that the nurse must think only of the patient's comfort, not of herself, and that she should be conscientious and diligent, unseen as well as seen. Painstaking attention to detail was for the sight of God, rather than for the praise and reward of doctors, and could not be feigned:[15] 'Gentleness of the heart will teach gentleness to the hand and to the manners. I can give no better rule than to put yourself in your patient's place.'[16]

That care relied on a moral ethic was constantly reiterated, even if systems of training were contested. Eva Lückes, Matron of the London Hospital, argued that the personal qualities of the nurse were the absolute basis for nursing. Above all else the 'character' of the nurse made the 'real' nurse. She exhorted nurses to 'walk worthy of the vocation wherewith you are called' and held that indispensable qualities of this vocation were self-discipline, personal responsibility for learning, truthfulness, obedience, punctuality, loyalty and the kindliness of genuine compassion.[17] Unlike Wood, Lückes was to argue forcefully against moves to systematise training, because of her firm belief that the virtuous character was fundamental. Indeed, she suggested that complaints against nurses were rarely about failures in practical duties, rather that 'It is noteworthy that the grievance is almost always due to the lack of those personal qualities which are absolutely indispensable to real nursing':

> Mechanical nurses can be produced by machinery. But what kind of a substitute is a human machine for a tender-hearted woman, who from practical training and experiences is skilled in the services and attention which sick people require, and whose devotion to her work is inspired by a genuine love of, and satisfaction in helping, those who are in need of what she has to give.[18]

Similarly, the Matron of the Chelsea Hospital, Miss Mollett, argued that the mechanistic suppression of the person was harmful to both the individual and the community. Individuals had freely to choose to enter into the community as part of a living body, rather than be forced as 'mechanical adjuncts'. Training was to encourage self-discipline, in order that laziness and selfish ambition would be seen in their true light, and replaced naturally by unselfishness, devotion and self-abnegation.[19]

Alice Dannatt, Lecturer on Domestic Hygiene and Honorary Superintendent of District Nursing and formerly Lady Superintendent of the Royal Infirmary,

Manchester and Matron Superintendent of the Preston and County of Lancaster Royal Infirmary and Fever Hospital, published her book in 1893, which drew on an article published in 1888.[20] The efficient nurse must have knowledge, excellent qualities, and be morally, physically and mentally as perfect a person as was possible: unselfishness was the most essential quality for 'the making of a really good nurse ... An efficient nurse must, from the beginning of her training to the end of her working life, have an earnest purpose to be a kind, good, thorough nurse'.[21]

E.J.R. Landale, in 1893, also taught that nurses needed certain qualities: quietness, presence of mind, gentleness, accuracy, punctuality, memory, observation, forethought, promptness, unselfconsciousness, obedience, kindness and courtesy. Service before self was the only motivation suitable for the nurse. To escape the monotony of a narrow home life, to earn a living, or to raise social status were unacceptable reasons: 'Let, then, your first object in entering the profession of Nursing be that you may use the gifts God has given you, for His glory, in the service of the sick.'[22]

Similarly, at the turn of the twentieth century, Mary Annesley Voysey began her practical book with the nurse's qualities and motivations:[23] 'obedient, truthful, conscientious, careful, kind, and faithful, remembering Who has given us our highest motive: – "Inasmuch as ye have done it unto one of the least of these my brethren, ye have done it unto Me," and work without looking for results.'[24] The Matron of the Royal Hospital for Diseases of the Chest, Mary May, stated that duty held a real and serious meaning because it was the essence of service and thus of the nurse's calling, the basis of her honour and trust.[25] M.N. Oxford, a sister at Guy's Hospital, stressed the importance of virtuous qualities in her textbook of nursing lectures.[26] The nurse should be temperate, sober, careful, clean and busy, and in behaviour 'virtuous, loving, diligent'.[27] This was also the view of E. Margaret Fox, Matron of The Prince of Wales's Hospital, Tottenham.[28] Character was more important than cleverness: attributes such as reverence, gentleness, discretion and uprightness needed to be cultivated for the well-being of patients.

The approach to nursing did not change as the century progressed. This is evident in the textbooks of Margaret Riddell, Assistant Matron of the Royal Hospital for Sick Children, Edinburgh and later Matron of St Mary's Hospital, Hampton, first published in 1914.[29] It also evident in the writing of A. Millicent Ashdown, Lecturer to Nurses in Bandaging and Practical Work at King's College Hospital, London, Examiner in Nurse's Practical Work to St Mary's Hospital, Charing Cross Hospital, Paddington Hospital, East Suffolk and Ipswich Hospital, and Whipps Cross Hospital; and a former examiner to the General Nursing Council.[30]

Ashdown published *A Complete System of Nursing* in 1917. It was reprinted fifteen times before being revised in 1939 and 1943. She introduced her text by suggesting that the nurse's main qualification was a 'real love' for attending to the sick and helpless, a strong constitution and an equable temperament: 'Nurses should always remember the sacredness of their profession, and hold it in such respect that they will never bring discredit to their uniform.' Discipline and obedience, loyalty, generosity, tenderness, gentleness and cheerfulness were the basis of her work: 'They must look upon their patients as individuals to be cared for personally, not merely as "cases" to be treated medically.'[31]

Home Nursing, written in 1918 by Mildred Heather-Bigg, Matron of Charing Cross Hospital, and arranged according to the revised syllabus of the St John Ambulance Association, reiterated the same nursing values.[32] So did M. Vivian, the former Matron of Victoria Hospital, Deal and Princess Christian's Hospital, Weymouth, in 1920.[33] The nurse should strive against losing her sense of vocation. Nursing was not merely work that carried with it certain duties and consequent obligations, 'something more' was needed if the patient were to be considered first. The hardships that nursing involved, overwork and low pay, the lessons of self-denial, formed the nurse's character and method of thought. This made the 'rule of life' which gave nurses the highest possible ideals and standards of work.[34]

In 1929 E. Maude Smith, former Matron and Superintendent of Nurses, Withington Hospital, Manchester, certificated by St Bartholomew's Hospital and examiner for the General Nursing Council, reminded the nurse that she could not be a good nurse without being a good woman; all striving would be in vain unless 'we make practical use of our religion and show our belief in it in our lives'.[35] A year later, the Matron of Charing Cross Hospital, Mary Cochrane, wrote that despite the changes in nursing brought on by the First World War:[36] 'Many restrictions and apparent hardships are abolished, but the profession still calls for high principles and courage; in fact, all the essentials which went to make the first nurse.'

As the modern era approached and biomedical nursing knowledge progressed, the ethical basis remained. Esther Fisher, Matron of New End Hospital, Hampstead, introduced her book in 1937 by describing nursing as 'a sacred calling', its purpose to alleviate the sufferings of humanity, which should not, therefore, be taken up lightly. For this reason the qualities of the nurse were very important.[37] Evelyn Pearce, a former Senior Nursing Tutor at the Middlesex Hospital, a member of the General Nursing Council, and an examiner in Nursing, Fever Nursing and Epidemiology for the Diploma in Nursing, London University, restated this vision.

Her classic *A General Textbook of Nursing* was published in eighteen editions from 1937 to 1971, and dominated the training of generations of nurses.[38] With minor alterations over the thirty-four years, Pearce consciously saw nursing as evolving technically while maintaining the Nightingale tradition: 'The present generation of nurses has grown up entirely in the technological age of this century. The modern nurse, like the modern doctor is the product of an evolutionary process, but one where, nevertheless, her compassionate approach to patients remains unchanged'.[39] She, too, made explicit the importance of virtue for the nurse. In a later publication on the nurse–patient relationship[40] she taught, '*Character* is what we make of ourselves through the acquisition of moral virtues – the "cardinal virtues" of prudence, justice, temperance and fortitude'.[41]

Margaret Houghton's *Aids to Practical Nursing* reached ten editions between 1938 and 1965,[42] before it was revised by Margaret Clarke in 1971 and renamed *Practical Nursing*.[43] The first chapter started with a history of nursing and the Christian vocational tradition and delineated the qualities of character and mind that the nurse needed to develop or acquire during training. Such qualities included kindliness, sympathy, and a cheerful and pleasant manner to the patient to relieve anxiety and encourage confidence.

Such views were expressed in 1950 by two sister tutors from Guy's Hospital, Hilda Gration and Dorothy Holland, both also General Nursing Council examiners.[44] This textbook commenced with an introduction establishing the historical tradition of nursing as resting in the devotion of the nurse. While they agreed that patterns of nursing had changed, they argued that the nurse must not lose her idealism or need for self-discipline. Training started and should continue at the bedside. Patterns changed but virtues did not. These were imbibed through the example of others in the daily practices of care. In six editions of the book from 1944 until 1959 with wording barely changed, the virtues required of the nurse remained consistent. The good nurse was the kind nurse who took pleasure in spending time with her patient, and developed a relationship with him or her.

Lilian Darnell, Secretary of the Nursing Recruitment Service, King Edward's Hospital Fund, also commended the Nightingale nursing tradition. She introduced her book, *Nursing*, with a prologue on the Christian history of nursing, and suggested that Nightingale's list of the qualities required of a good nurse could not be improved upon.[45] What was implicit to Nightingale, Darnell suggested, was 'that the first necessity is a real interest in people and a desire to put that interest to practical use in their service. From that root will spring the kindness, consideration, tact, discretion and loyalty which can be read between the lines in this and other examples of her writings'.[46]

Winifred Hector, the Principal Tutor of St Bartholomew's Hospital, taught, in her *Modern Nursing* published between 1960 and 1982,[47] that the nurse needed not only mental and physical health but also reserves of spiritual strength as the foundation for her work. On this would be built knowledge, skill and experience. The nurse needed a good average intelligence and an adequate education to help her cope with the complicated techniques she must learn and the examinations 'in the scientific bases of her calling'. But most importantly, the nurse needed spiritual strength because she was exposed to 'the weaknesses, shames and humiliations of her patients', physical strain, and a responsibility for the safety and even the lives of others: 'she must be capable of carrying this burden with faithful assurance' and not be moved from her purpose, the loyal and meticulous performance of her duties, by hope of gain or the temptations of gossip.[48] The overwhelming testimony of nursing textbooks shows the foundational importance of character and virtue: from this sprang the very way of nursing practice.

Scientific knowledge and practical skill were no less important than attitude. Nursing textbooks all detailed the diseases, illnesses and infections which the nurse would meet in her patients, and which she needed to be prepared to care for in her nursing of them. Books were written according to the state of medical and scientific knowledge current at the time of writing, and were subject to its limitations. Textbooks went through many editions as science advanced and the skills and medical knowledge that the nurse needed changed. For example, J.K. Watson, House Surgeon at Essex and Colchester Hospital, wrote his *Handbook for Nurses* in 1899, which was revised through twelve editions until 1940.[49] In the preface to his first edition he admitted to abstaining from 'the vexed question as to how much medical knowledge we should impart to our nurses'.[50] Watson also wrote more detailed textbooks for senior nurses and midwives.[51]

Teaching of diseases and conditions was carried out by doctors, and many textbooks were written by them for nurses. The Nightingale School syllabus, from its earliest days, for example, recorded Mr Croft's textbook as well as a manual by a surgeon at the Royal Devon and Exeter Hospital, Edward Domville.[52] Medical and surgical lectures given to nurses in training at Addenbrooke's by Laurence Humphry, were published in 1889.[53] The content included anatomy and physiology, diseases and their nursing, baths, enemata, poultices, bandaging and dietetics. The author acknowledged Sir Dyce Bryceworth's notes of lectures to probationers at St Thomas's Hospital, and Mr Croft's hints on nursing surgical cases.[54] Wilfred Hadley, physician and pathologist at the London Hospital, lectured to nurses there, and wrote textbooks from these lectures which acknowledged Laurence Humphry, Honnor Morten[55] and M.N. Oxford.[56] Percy Lewis, Honorary Medical Officer to the Victoria Hospital, Folkestone, wrote a textbook which embodied the course of instruction he gave in a series of lectures at the Salop and Southampton Infirmaries.[57] In the twentieth century textbooks for nurses continued to be written, and regularly updated, by physicians and surgeons.[58]

Dannatt's practical book guided the reader through the application process to become a nurse and suggested reading material, including books on anatomy and physiology, and in particular Nightingale's *Notes on Nursing* and Williams and Fisher's textbook, both sources for her own book.[59] According to

Catherine Wood, much of the nurse's work was wearisome and tedious: the daily poulticing, the perpetual dressings, and the care of cases that were not just interesting and serious, but involved long-term chronic illnesses, a result of poverty, dirt, intemperance and so on.[60] She went on to detail the signs and symptoms of disease and how diseases like rheumatic fever, burns and amputations should be treated. With regard to contagious diseases, Wood admitted to 'humility' because the whole question of infection was vague, so many theories were then being floated. She suggested that bad air, bad drainage, impure water and contaminated milk played a role in the origins of infection.[61] Cholera, for example, originated in hot countries and was conveyed to more temperate climes in 'some mysterious manner'. Inhalation of bad smells and sewer gases, Wood thought, led to diptheria. Like Nightingale, her remedies were those of ventilation: the breathing of pure air to prevent and treat disease.

Wood, like Nightingale, was a woman of her time. Almost a century later, Evelyn Pearce provides an example of the constant updating that was necessary. A reviewer of her final textbook described her meticulous investigation of all the means whereby students could be exposed to the most up-to-date information.[62] Pearce acknowledged many authorities for the knowledge content including, in 1963, Doreen Norton, whose own research was to have a great influence on the care of the elderly.[63] Norton had found the commonly used cleansing material, tow, to be harmful and Pearce removed and substituted all references to it as a result.

Prevalent nursing treatments, described by Voysey in 1905, included the use of linseed, mustard, charcoal and starch poultices, leeches and setons (threads of silk passed through a fold of skin to make a wound that was intended to treat a local inflammation).[64] Over the next thirty years, A. Millicent Ashdown described prevalent diseases and their nursing care, including diabetes, tuberculosis, smallpox, typhoid fever, eczema and a variety of medical and surgical conditions.[65] In the prefaces to her 1940 and 1943 editions she described how the new edition was entirely revised to bring it up to date. New methods in the treatment of fractures, in the administering of oxygen, anaesthetics, blood transfusion and intravenous infusion all necessitated changes to the text. So, too, did new methods of radium treatment, as well as the new State Registration examination which now included bacteriology.

Like all the authors, Ashdown's purpose was to give the nurse an elementary knowledge of different diseases, symptoms, possible complications and medical treatment, for intelligent nursing to be carried out. This knowledge was necessary for both written and practical examinations. As with other textbook writers, the role of specialist doctors in advising the author was acknowledged.

Practical procedures were carefully detailed in each textbook. Precise descriptions and formats were laid down concerning, for example, the manner in which the patient should be washed, in what sequence his limbs should be moved, how he should be covered to prevent indignity, how bedpans should be given to avoid friction, how each task of care should be approached, in its correct ordering and in its carefulness. Attention to detail was considered to be paramount for the patient's comfort. Careful observation of the patient's condition and needs was crucial. They were part of the diligence of care and the personal qualities required of the nurse reflected this.

The main focus of Williams and Fisher's book was the anatomy and physiology of the human body, but practical hints for the nursing care of patients were crucial. For example, patients should be washed with the greatest gentleness possible, and as 'you would wish to be washed yourself'.[66] Knowledge could never take the place of those characteristics essential to real nursing. The organised, 'really methodical' nurse was expected to be so successful and effective in her management of care that even within the routines of hospital life 'every patient will feel that the arrangements have been specially adapted to his individual wants, and yet the general ward work will be steadily advancing and "done up to time" '.[67]

Textbooks were designed to be practical, and to be read by trainees. The skills and qualities needed by the new probationer nurse involved cleanliness, willingness to learn, conscientious carefulness, devotion and 'the putting away of selfishness', as Dannatt wrote. The nurse 'must cultivate an observant eye, a quiet manner, a gentle voice, a dextrous hand, a quiet foot (not a perfectly silent one; nothing is more trying to a nervous patient), unfailing patience, and very little thought about self'. These qualities were for the sake of the patient: a gentle voice was comforting and soothing, dextrous hands could make patients' beds, wash, dress and move them 'with the smallest possible amount of risk and pain'.[68]

The nurse needed sympathy for patients but should not 'spoil' them; she needed to carry out the doctor's directions; she needed to learn to notice, 'without seeming to notice, the flush of feverishness, the beads of weakness, the expression on the face of pain, the shiver, that danger-signal that must at once be mentioned to Nurse or Sister'. She needed skill to manage the helpless patient, skill for minor surgical dressings and much more besides. Training brought knowledge and, with it, confidence. Training helped the nurse learn 'to be calm in emergency and prompt in action; and how great a part *comfort*, simple comfort, plays in the well-doing of her patients'. Above all, the nurse learned the mysteries of life and death, and saw the power and love of God at work in the work of creation.[69]

Alongside these qualities the efficient nurse needed knowledge and understanding, skill and precision in all nursing procedures such as washing patients, in order to preserve dignity and comfort. She needed to know how to prevent bedsores, perform enemata, prepare for operations, apply dressings, administer medicines and injections, make bandages and splints, and so forth. She was to be concise and explicit in verbal and written communications, and also quietly confident, willing to turn her hand to any work that she saw needed doing: 'work, that some people term "menial," is not menial when done by her with that "tincture" which George Herbert says, makes even "drudgery divine." She *knows*, though she may not be always thinking about it, that "All true work is sacred" and that "Laborare est orare" .'[70]

There was no romantic sentimentality; all writers showed realism in considering the great difficulties nurses had to endure. Patients could be trying and difficult at times, wrote Landale. To help her cope, the nurse needed to think of St Paul's definition of 'charity'. Forethought was essential to precision in care: 'A good plan is to go over it in your mind, and then go to your Staff Nurse and ask her if you are right. Half the battle in Ward work is to know what you are going to do, what time you can do it in – and then do it'. Cleanliness, including rigorous handwashing after each procedure, tidiness and smartness, deference and politeness, willing and prompt loyalty and obedience, not 'eye-service' but cheerfully rendered, were all necessary for the smooth and successful running of the hospital and hence the standards of patient care.[71]

Some books were written jointly by a doctor and a nurse. Isla Stewart, Matron of St. Bartholomew's Hospital, and Herbert Cuff, Medical Superintendent of the North-Eastern Fever Hospital, Tottenham, together wrote *Practical Nursing*, which covered all aspects of ward work and practical nursing skills, techniques and biomedical knowledge.[72] The authors reiterated the common nursing ethos into which the nurse was trained. Accuracy, for example, was not limited to words but included the conscientious performance of duties. Training could strengthen these qualities, not produce them: 'Examinations, at the best, can only demonstrate that the candidate has learnt enough to enable her adequately to exercise her profession; they can never prove that this or that woman is a good nurse.' The essence of nursing was the patient, who must always be the nurse's first care. The nurse should be ever alert to anticipate his or her wants and needs. She could not go wrong if she 'always remembers the humanity of her patients, and makes their comfort and wellbeing her first thought ... Her manner towards her patients should be characterised by dignity and gentleness.'[73]

Textbooks give an insight into the conditions of patients from the period of writing, and hence what was expected of nurses, without distinction. For example, Stewart and Cuff taught the nurse to change the washing water several times, implying that the patient might be very dirty. The face was washed first, the body being taken in small sections afterwards, each area being carefully dried and covered with blankets. Hair washing needed to take into account the likelihood that the patient's hair might be extremely dirty and infested.[74]

From the same period, M.N. Oxford's text contained the substance of teaching given to probationer nurses at Guy's Hospital by lecturers in nursing, surgery and medicine. As the text stated, the better the education, the better the nursing care, and this involved the nurse's knowledge of the principles of her work, knowing the why and wherefore of the things she was expected to do for her patients, and something about the diseases they were suffering from, and of the drugs and other means that were used in hope of their alleviation.[75]

M.A. Gullan, Sister Tutor of St Thomas's Hospital, a member of the General Nursing Council, and a former examiner for both State Registration and the London University Diploma in Nursing, summarised the instruction given to nurses at the Nightingale School in a textbook published in 1920 which went through seven editions until 1961.[76] As the preface to her first edition stated, the lectures, which included medical and surgical nursing, anatomy and physiology, gynaecology and elementary science, together with subjects such as dietetics, enemata, observation of vital signs, administration of drugs, and infectious and contagious diseases, were expected to be augmented by experience, and supplemented with visual aids.[77] She, too, emphasised the importance of personal qualities, such as efficiency, loyalty, reticence, watchfulness, consideration, courtesy and adaptability.[78]

E. Maud Smith described how bedsores should be prevented, by avoiding friction, rubbing the skin with spirit and glycerine, keeping the sheet straight and clean, changing the patient's position frequently, removing pressure, and keeping the skin clean: 'Always bear in mind that patients are sometimes *made* incontinent by insufficient care and attention on the part of the nurse by not attending immediately to the patient's calls for the bedpan, etc., or by omitting to give the necessary utensils regularly to a patient who is unable to ask for them himself.'[79] Quoting Nightingale, Smith also stressed the importance of attention to detail: 'Look out for "these little things", and whatever is wrong put it right.'[80]

Pearce's textbooks were overwhelmingly concerned with the practical aspects of care. Bathing a patient meant that nurses could observe the patient and his condition, and record accurately what they could see, hear, feel and smell. This was no menial chore, but part of the real art of nursing. Nursing observation was crucial from the point of admission until discharge. The keenness and interest of the student should never lapse into routine. Attention to detail, scrupulous care, thoughtfulness, structure and supervision were ever vital for good nursing. The methodical attention given to each limb during the bedbath, the carefully organised procedure of the hairwash and mouth care were to be rigorously observed. Each task followed an ordered procedure. Nurses were to be scientifically informed but not mechanical.

The procedure for a bedbath, for example, was detailed. The patient was to be addressed, offered a bedpan or urinal, the windows closed, the curtains drawn, and bedclothes removed. Dignity was preserved at all times by the careful placing of towels. Touch was to be firm, steady and even, to avoid irritation. Each limb was to be washed and dried. Genital areas and pressure areas were to be carefully washed and dried. The patient would be encouraged to do as much as possible. Water was to be kept warm. Nails were attended to if necessary, mouth care and hair care was given. A drink and a hot water bottle might follow. All was done for the patient's comfort. Trolleys were laid up for all procedures, items needed were to be carefully placed. Hands were washed at regular intervals.[81]

Pearce described the reason for mouth care, including conditions that affected the mouth. Equipment was described and pictured, and the procedure detailed. The bed was protected, the mouth inspected 'and the treatment begun in some definite order'. Dentures were to be removed and brushed clean. The mouth was to be rinsed before being gently swabbed. The insides of the cheeks and the tongue needed special attention. All sordes and crusts should be gently removed. Each swab should be used once only.[82]

Pearce expanded her approach in 1953 in *Nurse and Patient* which was republished in 1963 and 1969.[83] Because the patient was not just a sick body but a human being, a person, the nurse needed to realise that the patient's needs were not merely bodily and mental, but spiritual as well. One of the greatest qualities for the nurse, therefore, was a genuine personal interest in the patient so that the performance of care would never be merely routine and menial: 'It is the *manner* in which every service is performed for a patient which is a thousand times more important, more valuable, than *what* is actually done for him.' Simple and unassuming tasks of care brought comfort: the careful tucking-in of the blanket, turning a pillow, adjusting clothes, ensuring papers and handkerchiefs were within easy reach, and the warm smile that expresses reassurance, was: 'a silent but eloquent language between two people brought together in a trouble shared. The patient's burden is lightened for he knows he is not completely alone'.[84]

'The Patient's Day', the title of the first chapter of Gration and Holland's textbook, was organised carefully for the best interest, safety and especially comfort of the patient.[85] On waking, the patient's curtains should be opened, face and hands sponged, mouthwash and dentures (if any) given. Routines were expected to accomplish this. Food and drink were to be presented attractively and the patient not kept waiting. Perhaps the patient would like to read his or her letters, or glance at a newspaper. The bedbath should be performed in such a manner as to keep the patient warm and comfortable. Clean nightclothes should be given, and the bed should have clean linen as necessary. Dentures and teeth should be cleaned, mouthwashes and bedpans given, with discretion, and eau-de-cologne offered. The dressings should be left until later in the morning when the patient would be more alert. Before any procedure certain requirements needed to be observed by the nurse; for example, before the patient was washed the temperature, pulse and respirations should be recorded, the window closed, and the bedpan given.

Every routine had a purpose and every step of the routine was for the patient's comfort. All equipment used was carefully laid out and cleaned before being put away afterwards. Nothing should be irksome for the patient. Far from being mechanical, wrote Gration and Holland, patients understood that routines made individual attention to detail possible. The human element counted most in the intimate care of the sick.

Bedside or 'basic' nursing care was seen as essential to patient care. In performing what might seem to be the more mundane elements of care, such as bathing and feeding, performing mouth care, disposing of excreta, the nurse was relating to the patient in the most intimate way. In carrying out this care she was also carefully observing the patient's condition, both physical and emotional. This was perhaps the most difficult aspect of care. It depended on the nurse's innate intelligence and the ability to reflect critically and creatively. But this form of care was not antithetical to the educated nurse. The opposite was in fact true. The nurse needed biomedical knowledge, the ability to think and understand, and to know the reason for the patient's treatment and the care she gave.

Procedures protected the patient because they were scrupulous. Each procedure was intended for the care, comfort and well-being of the patient. Careful informed observation of the condition of the patient, and prompt reporting of it to the ward sister, attention to the details of his or her comfort, and attentive supervision of nursing performance were part and parcel of the moral ethos. Although such rigorous procedures might later be deemed to be mechanistic and task-orientated, in fact they gave the nurse freedom and liberty. Secure in the performance of technical skills, so inculcated into her that they had become second nature, she did not have to think about the practical details of procedures, instead she could think about the individual needs of her patient. The nurse knew that if she carried out the procedure the way she had been taught, and as she constantly practised it, the patient was protected and his or her comfort ensured. She was freed then to think of the patient's individual nursing needs. As Wake has argued, with regard to the training in the Nightingale School, the transference of skills dominated training, so that, for example, perfection in sweeping and cleaning would lead to good care of patients and proper efficiency in theatre.[86] The science of nursing was also an art, the common goal, at many levels, of patient benefit.

The training of nurses was largely the responsibility of the ward sister, who led her nurses into the tradition of care. The sister was the trainer and must not only exhibit virtuous qualities in her own person, but, which was much harder, must try to cultivate these qualities in those placed under her: 'I know of no harder task, nor one requiring more Christian love and charity to fulfil it aright.'[87] Florence Lees taught that by precept and example from the sister the nurse was to learn Christian virtues, so that by her total obedience, truthfulness and trustworthiness, the patient's welfare would have absolute primacy. It was better for a nurse to be reprimanded, even by mistake, than that the patient should suffer through a mistake. Even so, Lees considered that love and charity should underpin all such discipline because the sister was not only responsible to her charges and the hospital authorities, but especially to God. And the person in ultimate charge, the superintendent, should not only be the mistress, but the mother, or rather, friend 'in the full sense of the word', as one who a nurse could go to in time of trouble or doubt, to find sympathy, advice and help.[88]

That virtues and skills were personally inculcated by lived example, not simply learned as theory, and that this process depended on the ward sister, was constantly reiterated by textbooks. Eva Lückes argued that the personal qualities of the sister were the absolute basis for nursing, and a good education was vital for their exercise: 'It is a mistake to suppose that there is no advantage in possessing a thorough education before entering upon Hospital work ... The cultivation of mind which is one of the best results of a good education, is certainly not of less value to a Hospital Sister than to women engaged in other work.'[89]

Catherine Wood argued that the ward sister should be the primary teacher, so that nurses learned correctly, and errors and inconsistencies were not promulgated.[90] Although training was variable in different institutions, according to Wood, the aim was to make nurses 'intelligent, conscientious attendants on the sick, handmaidens to the medical staff, a happy mean between the drudge that does all the dirty work, as in the olden time, and the quasi woman-doctor of modern times – the bane of the sisterhood and the plague of the doctors'.[91] Wood made clear that blind unthinking obedience was not intended. The nurse was taken round by the sister, to learn the nursing care of diseases, taught to listen to doctors' questions and answers received, and 'encouraged to ask the sister questions and to give the results of her observations; but above all things, she must be made to use her own mind, to think for herself, and not to get her knowledge ready made'.[92]

Each moment of the hospital day was ordered with specified procedures overseen by the ward sister. After breakfast patients were washed: 'Occasionally Sister has to remind her nurses of Miss Fisher's good advice: "Wash a patient as you would wish to be washed yourself." Whilst the washing progresses, Sister visits all her patients, observes their condition, and has a cheery good morning for each.'[93] Sister was expected to supervise all nursing practice, even in what might seem to be the minutest detail, and ensure, for example, that beds were made without wrinkles, because this might lead to bedsores. Prevention was crucial, noted Dannatt, because as all ward sisters knew, once bedsores arose they were very difficult to cure.

The central role of the ward sister in teaching and supervising nurses was fundamental to the apprenticeship. Lees's book, for example, was intended for nursing leaders, those in authority over nurses in training, especially the ward sisters, and its main purpose was to describe in detail the practical knowledge that ought to be taught by them, including bandaging, enemata and prevention of bedsores. Teaching was to be imparted in a moral context. As Angélique Pringle, one of Nightingale's students, and a Matron of St Thomas's Hospital wrote in *A Study in Nursing*, 'And above all these material attentions, inspiring and regulating them, is her [the sister's] moral attitude towards the patient. Our sister knows and she teaches her staff that she is there for the patients'.[94]

'The Probationer's Page', published in *Nursing Times* in 1912,[95] advised the reader: 'The kind of nurse she will make will depend not alone on what is taught her during the training period, but on the inner qualities of heart and life which she brought with her.' The writer asked:

> Can a nurse be trained to be kind if she is naturally thoughtless and inconsiderate? Under certain circumstances she can – not by any course of instruction, but under the power of example. Character is caught rather than taught. The character of the ward sisters and the matron will be more potent in the development of the spirit of kindness and the repression of what is sometimes termed 'mechanicalism,' than any other factor.[96]

The best way to teach nursing was by practical example, induction into a living way of caring. This was the reason why the apprenticeship method of training was considered essential, since it taught nurses how to behave ethically in every act they performed: giving medicines, making beds, giving baths and treatments, 'in conversations in both sickroom and corridor, into our unspoken attitude toward the institution and those in authority in it'.[97]

This was expanded on by Margaret Scales, former Ward Sister, Tutor and Night Sister at Guy's Hospital, and Tutor, Administrative Sister and Night Superintendent at Birmingham General Hospital and the Whittington Hospital, in her *Handbook for Ward Sisters*.[98] Writing in the 1950s, Scales emphasised that although there were plenty of reasons for taking up nursing, the vocational attitude was the most important.

Scales taught that the ward sister was the pivotal person on the ward, the trustee, handing on a living tradition. In charge of the ward, she was responsible for ensuring the friendly welcome to patients, and thoughtful attentions such as providing a newspaper, so that the patient would feel comfortable and secure. The ward sister needed to be sympathetic, genial and confident with a good memory, quick powers of observation, a lively imagination and good attention to detail. She needed to know and understand each individual nurse; she needed to teach and maintain a careful supervision of all that happened on the ward. She needed to be a diplomat, an administrator and a decision-maker: 'Lastly, if the Ward Sister is sufficiently fortunate to have an underlying, deeply religious conviction, her work becomes live and purposeful, her outlook on the ward and life in general is considerably broadened, and she herself is a serenely happy person.'[99]

The moral code was crucial to diligence in patient care. Scales argued: 'A student's moral code also needs attention, for why be content to teach the care of a patient's mouth if, day after day, the nurse does not willingly and punctiliously clean the mouth of her gastric patient and take trouble to examine the mouth of a patient who has a raised temperature?'[100]

There needed to be a balanced mix of staff to ensure nursing and training standard could be maintained and to preserve a sense of law and order. Standard methods should be taught to avoid confusion. The ward sister was responsible for teaching the nurse the principles underlying the procedures, and she needed to answer the student nurse's question, 'Why?' The ward sister wisely encouraged her nurses to put into practice the principles they learned during training. Questions should be encouraged and answered intelligently. Careless or slipshod work should not be treated leniently although understanding and help should be given.

The nurse's mastery of techniques was the ward sister's responsibility. She had to ensure that the nurse had the right approach to patients, a sensitive practical touch when carrying out treatments and dressings, including deft lifting and making comfortable of awkward patients. The nurse needed alert judgement, thoughtful imagination and even a good memory. All this was developed by continuous mental or practical experience. This art of nursing took time to acquire and involved much patience on the part of the ward sister to inculcate it into her nurses. Kindly, helpful attitudes had to be fostered from the start of the first year of training. The nurse needed to learn behaviour that was neither brusque nor a timid submission to authority: 'Good behaviour is really just a code of good manners and kindness, coupled with a quiet, professional way of conducting oneself.'

The ward sister also had to be a good nurse. For this she needed a knowledge and understanding of the individual, and a recognition of the physical, mental and spiritual needs of the patient. Knowledge, skill, purpose, kindness and a perfect administration were the pillars of good nursing. The ward sister must know how to nurse and do so whenever the occasion arose. Vigilance should never be relaxed or purpose clouded: 'nor must "learning by experience" be the excuse for indifferent treatment by inexperienced nurses'.

The hospital existed for the patient. No 'new schemes' should obscure this fact.

That good care signified good administration was assumed by all textbook writers: 'The personality of a hospital is largely dependent on the human contacts made through the goodwill and keen interest of the doctors and nurses who are the living spirit of the hospital.' The ward sister was fundamental to passing on the moral tradition and spirit of nursing:

> The principal concern of the ward sister [head nurse in 1969] is that all patient-care, down to the smallest detail, is being carried out with kindness and efficiency and with the greatest personal solicitude for the well-being of each individual; and, further, that every contact with members of the health team and other hospital personnel, inquiries and visits by relatives and friends, have been handled with the same understanding. [101]

The art and science of nursing was a living, practical tradition, naturally handed on and learned by the apprenticeship method. This centred on the ward sister, who was herself under the authority of the matron. The ward siter had final authority and control over her ward, and those who entered it, including perhaps eminent medical staff.

Right relationships, professional etiquette, transcended class barriers. This was a very remarkable phenomenon. Although the nineteenth century was a society divided by class, nurses were expected to live and work alongside each other irrespective of their social background or class. Writers such as Williams and Fisher were dismissive of suggestions of 'social embarrassment' made by those unfamiliar with hospital life:

> To this I can, from my experience, return a most emphatic negative. I have always seen the most perfect cordiality existing between the classes, and I think it is quite possible for both to derive great advantages from the close companionship into which, for a time, they must necessarily be thrown. [102]

Knowledge, sympathy and understanding of the classes was a two-way process by which both classes came to understand each other and learn from each other. With regard to 'menial duties', the writers were clear: some ladies felt a repugnance at having so many menial duties imposed on them, and thought others were more accustomed to perform these. They were apt to shirk them, or do them slowly. Pride was unacceptable, there was no place for 'vulgar self-assertion'. According to Landale, courtesy was basic: 'An important factor in the happiness of Hospital life is the behaviour of Nurses to each other. Be kind, be courteous; think of others before yourself.'[103]

According to Fox, hospital etiquette, courtesy in all relationships, whatever the class or professional status, was crucial for the well-being of the patient.[104] Respect for doctors, ward sisters and matrons was the ordinary rule of good manners. Reticence between nurses inhibited levity, gossip and criticism. Nurses could not be too careful what they said; even apparently unconscious patients could often hear what was said around them. The nurse required virtues of self-control and reserve; kindness but not familiarity; cheerfulness but not levity; obedience to rules and orders, upheld with pleasantness and without grumbling; loyalty to her hospital even if it was criticised by outsiders. The nurse should be tidy, punctual, intelligent and trustworthy. And Fox also argued:

> Theory is excellent; practice is good; systems, models, books, lectures, clinics – all the paraphernalia of hospital training schools have each their own appointed task in the shaping of the nurse; but unless surrounded on all sides by the sterner ethics of our profession, they are rather like rich furniture, left unprotected in the street ...[105]

Professional ethics were the moral principles by which the profession was governed and by which relationships were conducted. This conduct of right and wrong was neither separable nor different from the universal moral law embodied in the Ten Commandments; rather, it was a closer application of those laws to the peculiar circumstances of the lives of those occupied in the profession. Loyalty was the faithful allegiance to those in charge, for the sake of the patient: 'Many important things are left to the judgement and faithfulness of the nurse to carry out unseen, unknown to any except her own conscience.' Instructions should be carried out not only in spirit but to the letter in order to gain the confidence of both doctors and patients. Even though doctors were human and liable to err, to be loyal to them did not imply servility: 'True loyalty to order cannot be without the independent sense or energy of responsibility which alone secures real trustworthiness.' The moral character needed careful nurturing in an organic society existing for patient care.

Relationships between doctors and nurses required respect and loyalty for the sake of patients. Hence Catherine Wood argued, at the end of the nineteenth century, that nursing should not be independent of medical authority in a hospital, 'a danger into which I fear we are drifting', because the ultimate responsibility of the patient's treatment should rest with properly qualified medical staff: 'any woman, however experienced, taking upon herself these responsibilities is committing a grave error, and is entering a course destructive of the peaceful working of the hospital'.[106]

According to Miss Mollett, many nurses had difficulty in subordinating their own will to that of others. She agreed that, in the wrong hands, the exercise of power could become intolerable petty tyranny. Yet, the working of a large institution was impossible without proper discipline. Individual enthusiasm could never sustain the effort needed for the organisation to function. Success depended not on individual units but on the organic unity of the body working under a proper system:

> See how much more smoothly the work runs, how much more easily extra pressure is borne in a ward that is well organised, where each nurse knows what her exact work is and for what she is responsible, than in a ward in which there is no proper supervision, where much is left to the individual discretion, or indiscretion, of the nurses, and where, consequently, the unpleasant little details are either entirely left, or shifted from one to the other until they fall upon the junior probationer.[107]

Nurses were like soldiers, wrote Dannatt, fighting for life against death. Like them, they needed obedience, 'the keynote of hospital life'. This insistence on obedience might seem severe, she suggested, but it ensured that the responsibility, which in hospital life was often great, should be born by those whose duty, appointment, education and experience fitted them to bear it.[108]

The good of the patient was central to the way relationships were to be ordered. From her first edition in 1937, Evelyn Pearce specified how much depended on the nurse's attitude towards the patient. By kindness and thoughtful sympathy, Pearce taught, fears could be dispelled. Patience, gentleness, tact, confidence and cheerfulness could be displayed in the small acts of care: 'in accomplishing good team work and not in blind obedience. But loyalty to the orders and wishes of physicians, surgeons, matrons and sisters is necessary, and obedience to the rules which have been made to safeguard human life is imperative.'[109]

Later Pearce revised this introductory chapter and added her comments that nursing was a science, an art and a vocation: the doctor was the hospital director but the nurse (the ward sister) was the '*captain of the team*'.[110] She reminded nurses to see the patient as an individual, a person with a body, mind and soul. Referring to the Nightingale nursing tradition, Pearce implored nurses to keep their vocation alive in order to serve: 'in the spirit which asks *not* What do you want? but What can I do for you? How can I help you?' In the seventeenth edition of the book Pearce described the kind of care that should be given to patients as '*total patient care* realizing that human nature is constituted of body, mind and spirit'.[111]

This view prevailed over the decades of the twentieth century. Pearce, for example, wrote: 'It is essential that the nurse–doctor relationship should enable the nurse to discuss her patients in this way, and a thoughtful medical officer will appreciate it.' Each person was important as part of a team rather than as an isolated and competing individual: 'Each one accepts their responsibility in a common purpose – the welfare of mankind. The nurse acts as a sort of moral "prop", quick to notice any pull away from and direct it back again to the centre, the Patient.'[112]

Marjorie Houghton also used the idea of hospital etiquette for her teaching of nursing ethics.[113] The nurse was expected to show loyalty and obedience and even deference to those in authority. Medical staff as well as patients needed to be addressed correctly by their proper titles, as a matter of courtesy and good manners. The nurse should be loyal to her patients by giving ungrudging loyalty, respecting confidentiality and being trustworthy and reliable. She should be open to guidance and, if necessary, correction.

The term 'professional etiquette', frequently used by nursing writers, was a concept used to convey right manner and behaviour, a borderline away from 'professional ethics'.[114] Dorothy Emmet, the well-known philosopher, has suggested that etiquette is necessary to maintain 'affective neutrality', the emotional detachment needed to safeguard the professional relationship from being affected by personal preferences which may cloud judgements.

The professional relationship was related to the vocation, exemplified by Nightingale.[115] Nursing writers reflected this same secular vocation: the way of doing one's duty in a lawful way of life according to accepted norms, but doing it with a sense of religious responsibility. Wider than the specific religious calling, vocation meant the responsibility of the individual to live according to his or her role and function towards other people; to work for the sake of the good of society; and to accept the call to live an authentic life.

Leaders with power, informed and guided by their sense of vocation, should not use their power to dominate others into submissiveness, but rather should seek to be aedificatory: to use their power to build up subordinates. As Nightingale had envisaged, and as nurse teachers upheld, this was a different kind of relationship from the relation of a dominant charismatic character to submissive followers. In a similar way, rigorous routines and structures of the ward were intended to bring order and method to the patient's care, rather than to oppress or dominate.

Progress could only come with perseverance and self-control. The true professional spirit was manifested in friendliness to all without familiarity and a readiness to minister to all without regard to social distinctions, race or creed. These were the foundations for the qualities of observation, judgement, discrimination, foresight, swift action, accuracy, the ability to organise and manage, which a good training would develop. Above all, professional etiquette required good manners and courtesy, respect for seniors as well as patients and visitors.

Nurses were inducted into nursing by example and demonstration, a 'good substitute for the spoken word'.[116] This imbibed moral tradition was very much that of the community, and it did not encourage a criticism of the system itself. It was not concerned so much with individual choice; by becoming a nurse, the probationer, later student, nurse also submerged her own personality. The vocation was essentially concerned with the production of a 'role type'.[117] Hence, the person entered into the professional role of the nurse and took on the moral attributes of the profession. This could be oppressive. It was easy to lose sight of the person who inhabited the role, to forget that he or she was also a human being.[118] Yet, there was a moral case and advantage for this form of induction and role identification.

It is clear from these textbooks that Nightingale's principles of nursing as practical care prevailed as an aspiration for nursing, and in the training of nurses. Nurses worked within a living community of care. There was a common mind and unity, a result of a clearly defined purpose, and one that other professionals shared.[119] As one nurse was to remember, decades later, of her training in the early twentieth century, the constant exhortation to nurses was that they should never to forget to care.[120] All knowledge, skill and understanding was to be seen in the light of this demanding ideal, even if it was not always lived up to.

Conclusion

The undeniable weight of evidence is that nursing writers, matrons, tutors and ward sisters constantly reiterated the same message, even as their books changed through editions to recognise scientific advances: the ethical basis of nursing tradition arose from the moral character of the nurse and the moral ethos in which she trained and worked. The nurse's technical knowledge and skills, her powers of observation, and no less important, her attention to the intimate practical details of personal hygiene and comfort all depended on this framework. Order, structure, supervision and method were crucial, as were the kindness of her manner, the gentleness of her touch, and her general approach towards the patient. Activities were never menial – they were the art of nursing.

Only an apprenticeship method of training could fulfil this very practical aim. Young nurses were introduced gradually into a way of care in which they learned wisdom and sensitivity involved in touching the human body. This was a spiritual tradition which cultivated virtues and sought thereby to diminish the effect of natural human weakness inclining the nurse to the tendency of self-assertion and resentment in the face of often unattractive and unappealing humanity. As Nightingale had taught, and as nurse teachers repeated in the following decades, the human body needed the most careful, sensitive and respectful touch because it was a 'temple' of the human spirit. The physical was spiritual. This was ideally in every nurse's mind as she approached the patient. The whole system of care was envisaged as corporate and organic, nurses, sisters, matrons and doctors collaborating with a single end in view – the good of the patient. Many nursing voices from this apprenticeship have been cited, which would otherwise be unheard and consigned to oblivion. They speak with a remarkable consistency of a definite way of nursing that embodied both an 'art' and a 'science'.

Notes

[1] L.R. Seymer, 'Florence Nightingale's Writings on Nursing', *Nursing Mirror*, 1948, pp. 81–82, May 8.

[2] P. Jarvis, 'Commentary on A Case Study of a Patient-Centred Nurse', in Fulford, K.W.M., S. Ersser and T. Hope (eds), *Essential Practice in Patient-Centred Care*, pp. 193–197, Oxford, Blackwell Science, 1996.

[3] J. Croft 'Reading List' January 1875, in Seymer, L.R., *Florence Nightingale's Nurses*, Appendix 4, 1960, pp. 160–161.

[4] F.S. Lees, *Handbook for Hospital Sisters*, Acland, H.W. (ed.), London, W.S. Isbister & Co., 1874, p. 7.

[5] Ibid., p. 7.

[6] R. Williams, A. Fisher, *Hints for Hospital Nurses*, Edinburgh, MacLachlan & Stewart; London, Simpkin, Marshall & Co.; Dublin, Fannin & Co., 1877.

[7] Ibid., p. 1.

[8] Ibid., p. 2.

[9] Ibid., p. 5.

[10] Ibid., p. 12.

[11] Ibid., 15

[12] C.J. Wood, *A Handbook of Nursing for the Home and the Hospital*, preface, 8th edn, London, Cassell & Co., c. 1887.

[13] Ibid., p. v.

[14] Ibid., p. 8.

[15] Ibid., pp. 1–19.

[16] Ibid., p. 18.

[17] E.C.E. Lückes, *Lectures on General Nursing*, London, Kegan Paul, Trench, Trübner & Co., 1892, p. 6.

[18] E.C.E. Lückes, *General Nursing*, 4th edn, London, Kegan Paul, Trench, Trübner & Co., 1898, pp. ix–x.

[19] M. Mollett, 'Discipline', *Nursing Record*, 1,9 1888, pp. 99–101, May 31.

[20] A. Dannatt, 'What Constitutes an Efficient Nurse', *Nursing Record* 1, 8, 1888, pp. 87–90, May 24; *How to Become a Hospital Nurse*, London, Record Press, 1893.

[21] Ibid., p. 28.

[22] E.J.R. Landale, *Points for Probationers*, London, Record Press, 1893, p. 11.

[23] M.H.A. Voysey, *Nursing: Hints to Probationers on Practical Work*, London, Scientific Press, 1905; new and revised edn, 1911.

[24] Ibid., 1905, p. 110.

[25] M.F. May, 'The Relation of the Nurse to Doctor and Patient', in *The Science and Art of Nursing: A Guide to the Various Branches of Nursing, Theoretical and Practical*, vol. 1, pp. 109–115, London, Paris, New York, Toronto and Melbourne, Cassell & Co., 1908, p. 115.

[26] M.N. Oxford, *A Handbook of Nursing*, London, Methuen & Co., 1st edn, 1900; 8 edns 1900–1923 (7th edn revised F.A. Sheldon).

[27] Ibid., p. 1.

[28] E.M. Fox, *First Lines in Nursing*, London, Scientific Press, 1914, pp. 2–3. *First Steps in Nursing*, London, Scientific Press, 1924, pp. 14–15; 1930, pp. 14–15.

[29] M.S. Riddell, *Lectures to Nurses*, London, Scientific Press, 6 edns 1914–1936; *A First Year Nursing Manual*, London, Scientific Press, 5 edns 1931–1939.

[30] A.M. Ashdown, *A Complete System of Nursing*, London, J.M. Dent & Sons, 4 edns 1917–1943.

[31] Ibid., p. 1–2.

[32] M. Heather-Bigg, *Home Nursing*, London, St John's Gate, 1918.

[33] M. Vivian, *Lectures to Nurses in Training*, London, Scientific Press, 1920.

[34] Ibid., p. 95.

[35] E.M. Smith, *Notes on Practical Nursing*, London, Faber & Gwyer, 1929, p. 15.

[36] M. Cochrane, *Nursing*, London, Geoffrey Bles, 1930, p. 64.

[37] E. Fisher, *The Nurse's Textbook*, London, Faber & Faber, 1937, p. 1.

[38] E.C. Pearce, *A General Textbook of Nursing*, London, Faber & Faber, 18 edns 1937–1971.

[39] Ibid., 1971, p. 3.

[40] E.C. Pearce, *Nurse and Patient*, London, Faber & Faber, 3 edns 1953–1969.

[41] Ibid., 1953, p. 96; 1963, p. 97; 1963, p. 84.

[42] M. Houghton, *Aids to Practical Nursing*, London, Baillière, Tindall & Cox, 10 edns 1938–1965 (10th edn with M. Whittow).

[43] M. Clarke, *Practical Nursing*, 11th edn, London, Baillière Tindall, 1971.

[44] H.M. Gration, *The Practice of Nursing*, London, Faber & Faber, 6 edns 1944–1959 (3rd edn with D.L. Holland).

[45] L.M. Darnell, *Nursing*, London, Robert Hale, 2 edns 1959–1961.

[46] Ibid., p. 20; p. 21.

[47] W. Hector, *Modern Nursing*, London, William Heinemann Medical Books, 7 edns 1960–1982.

[48] Ibid., pp. 6–7.

[49] J.K. Watson, *A Handbook for Nurses*, 1st edn, London, Faber & Gwyer (Scientific Press), 1899; 12 edns 1899–1946.

[50] Ibid., 1899, p. vii.

[51] J.K. Watson, *A Handbook for Senior Nurses and Midwives*, 1st edn, London, Humphrey Milford, Oxford University Press, 1926; 2nd edn, 1931.

[52] J. Croft 'Reading List' January 1875, in Seymer, L.R., *Florence Nightingale's Nurses*, Appendix 4, 1960, pp. 160–161. E.J. Domville, *A Manual for Hospital Nurses*, London, J. & A. Churchill, 5th edn, 1885; 7th edn, 1891; 9th edn, 1907.

[53] L. Humphry, *A Manual of Nursing: Medical and Surgical*, London, Charles Griffin & Company, 1889.

[54] Ibid., preface.

[55] H. Morten, *Sketches of Hospital Life*, London, Sampson Low, Marston, Searle & Rivington, 1888; H. Morten, *How to Become a Nurse and How to Succeed*, London, Scientific Press, 1893; H. Morten, *The Nurse's Pronouncing Dictionary*, revised Burdett, M.L., London, Scientific Press, 8th edn, 1913.

[56] W.J. Hadley, *Nursing: General, Medical and Surgical*, 1st edn, London, J. & A. Churchill, 1902; 2nd edn, 1907.

[57] P.G. Lewis, *Nursing: Its Theory and Practice*, London, Scientific Press, 11 edns 1889–1899.

[58] W.G. Sears, *Medicine for Nurses*, 1st edn, London, Edward Arnold, 1953; 13 edns 1953–1979 (11th edn with R.S. Winwood). M. Toohey, *Medicine for Nurses*, 1st edn, Edinburgh, E. & S. Livingstone, 1953; 14 edns 1953–1986. J. Moroney, *Surgery for Nurses*, 1st edn, Edinburgh, E. & S. Livingstone, 1950; 15 edns 1950–1982. H.Bailey, *Surgery for Nurses*, 1st edn, London, H.K. Lewis, 1933; 8 edns 1933–1954.

[59] *How to Become a Hospital Nurse*, London, Record Press, 1893.

[60] C.J. Wood, *A Handbook of Nursing for the Home and the Hospital*, preface, 8th edn, London, Cassell & Co., c. 1887, p. 4.

[61] Ibid., pp. 160–161.

[62] H.O. Allen, 'A General Textbook of Nursing', *Nursing Times*, 1972, p. 639, May 25.

[63] E.C. Pearce, *A General Textbook of Nursing*, London, Faber & Faber, 16th edn, 1963, p. 7 .

[64] M.H.A. Voysey, *Nursing: Hints to Probationers on Practical Work*, London, Scientific Press, 1905, pp. 73–75.

[65] A.M. Ashdown, *A Complete System of Nursing*, London, J.M. Dent & Sons, 1st edn, 1917; 4th edn, 1943, p. v–viii.

[66] R. Williams, A. Fisher, *Hints for Hospital Nurses*, Edinburgh, MacLachlan & Stewart; London, Simpkin, Marshall & Co.; Dublin, Fannin & Co., 1877, p. 13.

[67] E.C.E. Lückes, *General Nursing*, 4th edn, London, Kegan Paul, Trench, Trübner & Co., Ltd, 1898, p. 75.

[68] A. Dannatt, *How to Become a Hospital Nurse*, London, Record Press, 1893, p. 19.

[69] Ibid., pp. 19–20.

[70] Ibid., p. 30.

[71] E.J.R. Landale, *Points for Probationers*, London, Record Press, 1893, pp. 16–31.

[72] I. Stewart, H.E. Cuff, *Practical Nursing*, Edinburgh and London, William Blackwood & Sons, 1st edn, 1899; 2nd edn, 1903; new edn, 1904; 3rd edn, 1910; 4th edn revised H.E. Cuff and W.T. Gordon Pugh, 1913.

[73] Ibid., pp. 7–8.

[74] Ibid., pp. 44–60.

[75] M.N. Oxford, *A Handbook of Nursing*, London, Methuen & Co., 1900–1923, pp. 2–3

[76] M.A. Gullan, *Theory and Practice of Nursing*, London, H.K. Lewis & Co., 1st edn, 1920; 8 edns 1920–1961 (8th edn revised by M.E. Gould).

[77] M.A. Gullan, *Theory and Practice of Nursing*, 4th edn, London, H.K. Lewis & Co., 1935, p. ix.

[78] Ibid., pp. 232–235.

[79] E.M. Smith, *Notes on Practical Nursing*, London, Faber & Gwyer, 1929, pp. 38–40.

[80] Ibid., p. 15.

[81] E.C. Pearce, *A General Textbook of Nursing*, London, Faber & Faber, 17th edn, 1967, pp. 55–56.

[82] Ibid., pp. 57–58.

[83] E.C. Pearce, *Nurse and Patient*, London, Faber & Faber Ltd., 3 edns 1953–1969.

[84] Ibid., 1st edn, 1953, pp. 88–89.

[85] H.M. Gration, D.L. Holland, *The Practice of Nursing*, London, Faber & Faber Ltd., 3nd edn, 1950, pp. 11–16.

[86] R. Wake, *The Nightingale Training School 1860–1996*, London, Haggerston Press, 1998, p. 113.

[87] F.S. Lees, *Handbook for Hospital Sisters*, Acland, H.W. (ed.), London, W.S. Isbister & Co., 1974, p. 7

[88] Ibid., p. 22.

[89] E.C.E. Lückes, *Hospital Sisters and their Duties*, 1st edn, London, J. & A. Churchill, 1886, p. 6; 4th edn, London, Scientific Press, 1912, pp. 6–7.

[90] C.J. Wood, *A Handbook of Nursing for the Home and the Hospital*, preface, 8th edn, London, Cassell & Co., c. 1887, pp. 1–19.

[91] Ibid., p. 8.

[92] Ibid., pp. 15–16.

[93] A. Dannatt, *How to Become a Hospital Nurse*, London, Record Press, 1893, p. 23.

[94] A. L. Pringle, *A Study in Nursing*, London, Macmillan & Co., 1905, p. 43.

[95] The Probationer's Page, 'Nursing Ethics I', *Nursing Times*, 1912, p. 769, July 27; 'Nursing Ethics II', *Nursing Times*, p. 862, August 24; 'Nursing Ethics III', *Nursing Times*, p. 929, September 14.

[96] Ibid., p. 769.

[97] Ibid., p. 929.

[98] M. Scales, *Handbook for Ward Sisters*, London, Baillière, Tindall & Cox, 1st edn, 1952; 2nd edn, 1958.

[99] Ibid., p. 19; 21.

[100] Ibid., pp. 44–47; 52–54.

[101] E.C. Pearce, *Nurse and Patient*, London, Faber & Faber, 1st edn, 1953, pp. 90–9; 3 edns 1953–1969.

[102] R. Williams, A. Fisher, *Hints for Hospital Nurses*, Edinburgh, MacLachlan & Stewart; London, Simpkin, Marshall and Co.; Dublin, Fannin and Co., 1877, pp. 10–11.

[103] E.J.R. Landale, *Points for Probationers*, London, Record Press, 1893, p. 29.

[104] E.M. Fox, *First Lines in Nursing*, London, Scientific Press, 1914, pp. 2–3. *First Steps in Nursing*, London, Scientific Press, 1924, pp. 14–15; 1930, pp. 14–15.

[105] E.M. Fox, 'Nursing Ethics', *Nursing Times*, 8, 366, 1912, pp. 475–478, May 4.

[106] C.J. Wood, *A Handbook of Nursing for the Home and the Hospital*, preface, 8th edn, London, Cassell & Co., c. 1887, pp. 10–11.

[107] M. Mollett, 'Discipline', *Nursing Record*, 1, 9, 1888, pp. 99–101, May 31.

[108] A. Dannatt, *How to Become a Hospital Nurse*, London, Record Press, 1893, p. 17.

[109] E.C. Pearce, *A General Textbook of Nursing*, London, Faber & Faber, 1st edn, 1937, pp. 2–4.

[110] Ibid., 10th edn, 1949, pp. 18–19.

[111] Ibid., 17th edn, 1967, p. 21.

[112] E.C. Pearce, *Nurse and Patient*, London, Faber & Faber, 1st edn, 1953; 2nd edn, 1963; 3rd edn, 1969, p. 94, 95, 83.

[113] M. Houghton, *Aids to Practical Nursing*, London, Baillière, Tindall & Cox, 9th edn, 1960, p. 16–17.

[114] D.M. Emmet, 'Professional Ethics' in Macquarrie, J. Childress, J.F. (eds), *A New Dictionary of Christian Ethics*, pp. 502–504, London, SCM Press Ltd, 1967.

[115] D.M. Emmet, *Function, Purpose and Powers*, London: Macmillan & Co., 1958, pp. 269–284.

[116] J.P. Brown, 'Faith and Nursing', *Nursing Times*, 1965, p. 1428, October 15.

[117] D.M. Emmet, *Rules Roles and Relations*, London, Macmillan & Co., 1966, pp. 151–154.

[118] R. Wake, *The Nightingale Training School 1860–1996*, London, Haggerston Press, 1998, p. 79.

[119] W. Osler, *Aequanimitas*, London, H.K. Lewis, 1904; *Counsels and Ideals*, London, Humphrey Milford, Oxford University Press, 1st edn, 1905; 2nd edn, 1921; *Man's Redemption of Man*, London, Constable & Co., 1910; *Medicine and Nursing*, London, Humphrey Milford, Oxford University Press, 1919. I.E.S., D.N. Lond., 'The Student Life: The Philosophy of Sir William Osler edited by Richard E. Verney, M.B., F.R.C.P.E., D.R.', *Nursing Times* 1958, p. 152, February 9. D. Manchèe, *Whatever Does the Almoner Do?*, London, Baillière, Tindall & Cox, 1946.

[120] M. Baker, 'Starched Collars and Starch Baths', *Nursing Times*, 92, 3, 1996, pp. 50–51, January 17.

Chapter 3

Nurse registration: rationalising the spirit, 1888–1925

Towards the end of the nineteenth century the matter of nurse registration became a contentious and divisive issue. This has been well documented,[1] but what has not been explored is the extent to which the controversy centred on the nature of nursing and the importance of its ethos. This chapter will examine hospital nursing from the end of the nineteenth century to the early twentieth century, by considering evidence presented in parliamentary debates, and analyse the attitudes and arguments that lay at the heart of the dispute. This evidence will serve as a test of the general acceptance of the Nightingale vision within nursing at the end of the century. Particularly relevant is the motivation of nurses, their values and the cultural and social backgrounds from which they came, as disclosed in the documents.

The registration debate focused on the standards of the profession. Could standards be imposed by external bureaucracy, or did they spring from the spiritual centre of the profession? Would standardisation marginalise the vocational ethos, which was the driving force of nursing care, by minimising its importance, and lead to mechanical nurses, technically trained to meet the demands of registration, but lacking a spiritual heart? Or would registration provide a necessary framework to safeguard patients, and raise the status of the profession, making it more akin to medicine? This chapter will examine these debates, the arguments adduced, and the areas of settled consensus about fundamental values.

The background and context of the debate

The issue of registration for nurses was raised as early as 1874 by Sir Henry Acland, Regius Professor of Medicine at Oxford, in the preface to Florence Lees's nursing textbook.[2] Baly has suggested that Acland, a family friend of the Nightingale family, approached Nightingale on the subject. The General Medical Council, of which Acland was a member and later chairman, had made tentative proposals in 1869 to grant certificates to occupations connected with medicine.[3] In the following decade, Sir Henry Charles Burdett, the philanthropist, hospital administrator and founder of the National Pension Fund for Nurses, sought to improve conditions of service, and to establish a register of trained nurses.[4]

The philanthropic work of Burdett led to the founding of the British Hospitals Association, and one of its members was the Matron of St Bartholomew's Hospital, Ethel Manson, later Mrs Bedford Fenwick. Mrs Bedford Fenwick disagreed with Burdett over the issue of nurse registration, and founded the British Nurses' Association in 1887, together with Catherine Wood, the Matron of Great Ormond Street Hospital. A bitter dispute over nursing registration followed. Mrs Bedford Fenwick was to publish angry editorials against Burdett in 1891 and 1892 in her journal, the *Nursing Record*.[5] Burdett believed that Mrs Bedford Fenwick was motivated by a desire for power. As he wrote decades later about the newly founded College of Nursing:

> Miss Cox-Davies' letter fails to recognise that Mrs Fenwick's first and main object is not, like that of the College, the betterment of the nursing profession and the procuring for its members a standard of shorter hours and better pay. Mrs Fenwick's party stands out because they insist on being the one and only authority which shall control nurses and nurse registration.[6]

Burdett's correspondence provides an insight into the widespread influence of the Nightingale Training School. In a letter to Sir Cooper Perry, Medical Superintendent of Guy's Hospital, he argued that he was a survivor of the few who originated the modern training of nurses, which began with Mrs Wardroper in 1869. He suggested that he had instituted lectures from honorary and resident medical staff and from specially trained and selected matrons and lady superintendents: 'There are records of the facts in minute books, correspondence and publications, together with the difficulty then experienced to get respectable, morally efficient and especially educated women to train as nurses'.[7]

Nightingale corresponded with Sir Henry Acland from 1867. In her letters, she explained why she opposed registration. She had learned from her experience of the last fifteen or sixteen years that nursing and medicine should not be mixed up, or both would be spoiled. The nurse was adequately tested by a weekly record, a system of marks recorded by training nurses, of the progress each probationer was making in each of her ward duties and in character. The training matron kept a similar monthly record under the same headings. No further recognition was needed.[8] Nursing, unlike medicine and midwifery, could not be tested primarily by written examination or 'technical verbal knowledge'. It depended more than any other occupation (except the charge of teaching children) on the moral character of the nurse.[9] Character was worth so much more than book learning, and its deficiency rendered a nurse useless. It was not possible to approve a training school by stating that the home sister or mistress of probationers had such and such ability, because the key to the whole training process was the ward sister. The ward sisters influenced the nurses and trained their qualities, capabilities and characters.[10]

Copies of Nightingale's addresses to her probationers, some of which were preserved in the collected papers of Burdett and Acland, reiterated her central theme. The morale of the training school came from the probationers. Goodness should be lived, 'by *being* it ourselves'.[11] Nightingale was adamant that nursing had to be conserved as a moral calling. She recorded her view, and her reasons, in the annual address to her probationers in 1888:

> Rules may become a dead letter. It is the spirit of them that 'giveth life'. It is the individual, inside, that counts – the level she is upon which tells. The rest is only the outward shell or envelope. She must become a "rule of thought" to herself thro' the Ruler. And on the other hand, it strikes you often, as a great man has said: if the individual finds herself afterwards in less admirable circumstances, but keeps her high level, and rises to a higher and a higher level still, if the maker of her difficulties, her opportunities – steps to ascend – she commands her circumstances; she is capable of the best Nursing work and spirit – capable of the best influence over her Patients. It is, again, what the individual Nurse *is* and can do during her *living* training and *living* work that signifies – not what she is certified for, like a steam-boiler which is certified to stand so much pressure of work.
>
> She may have gone through a first-rate course – plenty of examinations. And we may find nothing inside. It may be the difference between a Nurse Nursing, and a Nurse reading a book on Nursing. Unless it bear fruit, it is all gilding and veneering; the reality is not there, growing, growing every year. Every Nurse must grow. No nurse can stand still. She must go forward, or she will go backward, every year.
>
> And how can a Certificate or public Register show this! Rather, she ought to have a moral 'Clinical' Thermometer in herself.[12]

Despite her deep conviction, she told Acland that she was advised to remain distant from the political campaign over registration: 'I have kept *entirely* out of the fray',[13] and 'I have been particularly counselled to keep out of the "row" and have done so.'[14] But she was deeply upset by the whole issue: 'When my miserable name is mentioned as a final authority, it gives me a feeling I cannot describe. Are we not barely on the threshold of nursing? Who are we to be stereotyping? ... How is character to be tested and registered?'[15] Acland himself appreciated Nightingale's concerns, which were shared by the hospitals, but did not agree with her fears. As he wrote in 1889 to Mr Wakley, founder of the *Lancet*, about the 'hard words' being said in public:

> There are three combatants. Hospitals, who educate, Mr Burdett, who pensions, Mrs Fenwick, who registers. Personally I believe all these proposals and functions are good. In details there are many things no doubt which can be arranged best by common discussion and agreement. I have told Miss Nightingale, who is of course on the 'Hospitals' side against 'Registration' that it will certainly be done in some way. I have urged Dr Bristowe to consider whether the Hospitals cannot confer with the Nurses Association. If these unite, surely Mr Burdett can be assisted by them in his special department and object. I sympathise heartily with Miss Nightingale and the Hospitals, but I do not anticipate the evils they do from Registration *as of necessity*. [16]

Henry Bonham Carter, Secretary of the Nightingale Fund Council, took up Nightingale's cause in a pamphlet published in 1888, which employed a variety of arguments to oppose registration.[17] Firstly, nursing was different to medicine. The medical profession had a register, because of obligations in law, to certify that the candidate had passed certain examinations after a certain period of training. It guaranteed professional knowledge and skill. It dealt only with gross negligence or misconduct under the law and could not discriminate as far as character was concerned. The professional qualities by which the nurse was judged concerned her character and conduct as well as her technical skill. The important intangible qualities such as kindness, patience, trustworthiness, self-control and discretion, which were crucial to nursing, could not be registered.

Secondly, there was no consensus yet over the ideal training, and it would be premature to force nurse training schools to adopt fixed standards by legislation. In the view of many matrons and training school heads, a general register, far from safeguarding standards of nursing would actually lower them.

Thirdly, it would be extremely difficult and costly, and would involve odium in view of accusations of libel, to remove a nurse from the register, even if she were notoriously bad. Shortcomings that ought to disqualify her as a nurse would be passed over, and a really bad nurse would be 'hallmarked' as fit to be employed. The public would be lulled into a false sense of security, being led to believe that the register would protect them from incompetent and undesirable nurses.

Fourthly, the register would only include evidence of technical knowledge together with a colourless certificate of good conduct. The crucial importance attached to moral qualities would be lost. Conditions for registration would necessarily focus on the capabilities of the average nurse, and on meeting the requirements of the average training school, resulting in a general and low uniformity of qualification.

Fifthly, as an experienced hospital matron suggested, women with unsuitable motives were currently applying to become nurses because nursing had become fashionable. They did not apply because they had a 'feel' for nursing, but rather for greater social freedom as women in society once their probation was over. These women would most easily pick up the scientific part of nursing, and by virtue of their greater education would most easily pass examinations and obtain first-class certificates. This would present an injustice to less academically able, but more committed nurses and would prejudice the quality of the posts they could apply for. Only recommendation from the training institution, which knew the qualities of the individual nurse, could prevent this problem, but national registration would marginalise such individual assessments.

Lastly, registration would make it difficult to dismiss nurses, even those who were unsatisfactory. Removal from the register could only take place in cases of gross misconduct, and not for moral defects. The public was unlikely to give open evidence with reference to such defects. Acknowledged defects and weaknesses in the training and education of nurses should not be remedied by legislation but by voluntary effort and public opinion. Bonham Carter repeated these arguments in 1892.[18]

This debate about registration can be set in the context of Max Weber's thesis of the routinisation of charisma, which Nightingale's arguments can be said to have anticipated.[19] The proposal to regulate nurses by imposing a minimum standard of certifiable training, would make nurses into 'specialists without spirit', opponents argued.[20] Nurses would sink to the level of the merely mechanical, rather than rise to the spiritual demands of their calling. If the fulfilment of the calling was not related solely to the highest spiritual and moral values, the nursing ethos, which had been the strength of the profession, would irrevocably fade. To use Weber's phrase, rationalisation would impose an 'iron cage' on the spirit of the profession.

In about 1892, a petition was sent to the Privy Council, by the Council of the Nightingale Fund, petitioning against the granting of a charter to the Royal British Nurses' Association, which would enable it to set up a register.[21] The petition argued that a general register would be detrimental to the interests of nursing, for similar reasons to those given by Bonham Carter, but added that the RBNA would 'acquire a real if indirect power of controlling the education of the whole nursing profession'.[22] Moreover, the RBNA was not sufficiently representative, had not sufficient support to be entrusted with such powers, and did not have the means to carry out the responsibilities the charter would impose on it.

In the course of its argument, the petition stated how widespread the Nightingale model of nursing had become, and it provides an insight into the state of hospital nursing. Although the petitioners were no doubt keen to strengthen their case, the case was put that the systematic training of nurses had only occurred within the last thirty years.[23] Before that, hospital nurses were 'as a rule, of inferior class, and without education, who, from being menial servants of the hospital, had been promoted to the position of nurses. Their moral tone was low, and no attempt of any kind was made to improve or teach them'. The earliest training schools were at St Thomas's Hospital, the Nightingale School, and King's College Hospital, the Society of St John's House and Sisterhood. From the Nightingale School trained nurses, matrons and sisters had supplied other hospitals and established nurse training systems similar to the Nightingale School.

Nurse training schools had also been set up in many other London and provincial hospitals, for the most part modelled on the plan adopted by Nightingale. The purpose was to improve the moral qualities and character of the nurse and to give practical and scientific teaching so that she could carry out doctors' orders intelligently. To accomplish this objective, women of good character lived and trained in hospital, which became their home. They were supervised by educated matrons, scrupulously selected for good health and qualities of gentleness, tact, presence of mind, and other good qualities. At the same time a methodical system of practical and technical training by head nurses and specially appointed members of medical staff was given in hospital wards. 'It has, however, been mainly from efficiency in the measures adopted to insure the possession of and cultivate the necessary moral qualities that successful results have been obtained.'[24]

This judgement, that the Nightingale training method was widespread, is supported by a survey of training schools conducted in 1888. This survey, included in the appendix to the petition, was conducted by the Joint Committee of the Hospitals Association of thirty-four hospitals that trained nurses.[25] Nineteen replied, seventeen large hospitals and two union infirmaries. Institutions were asked questions about whether they would like a register, the length of the curriculum, the syllabus of education, and the character of the certificate they deemed necessary to qualify a nurse.

The length of the training considered necessary varied from one year (a minority view), to three years. Oral instruction by lectures and demonstrations during the probationary period was carried out by all institutions, and followed up by practical demonstrations by a female instructor in two institutions. Half the institutions who replied to the survey tested the nurse's knowledge, although it was generally considered that the cleverest nurses were often the least efficient. Opinions varied on the amount of instruction, but the majority considered lectures on medical or surgical subjects should be given once a week, apart from the practical instruction the probationer received from the head nurse. Diversity existed on the wording of certificates, whether they stated that service was completed, or gave more information as to how satisfactory the service was.

A document from that same period described the duties of the hospital matron and superintendent.[26] Her responsibilities were carefully prescribed. They included the management and supervision of staff and resources; and specified that every ward of the hospital should be visited at least four times a week to ensure that staff were strictly performing their duties, that the comfort of patients was cared for, that the ward was clean and tidy, that regulations were obeyed, and 'sobriety, good order, and decorum' prevailed. The matron or superintendent was crucial to the functioning of the whole hospital and its ethos in which training occurred and patients were cared for. Indeed, this corresponded to the view of one of the founders of the registration movement, Catherine Wood, as the last chapter has shown.[27]

The Select Committee on Hospitals 1890–1891

In 1889 a petition from a group including Mrs Bedford Fenwick's husband, a doctor at the London Hospital, led to a parliamentary Select Committee.[28] Nurses' conditions of service at the London Hospital, the group argued, were exploitative. The matron of this hospital, Eva C.E. Lückes, had written a pamphlet that year, in which she opposed the preoccupation of the BNA with professionalisation.[29] Lückes had argued that each nurse needed to strive for the highest of which she was capable, which would not be possible if the narrowness of mind shifted the focus on her work 'as a *mere* profession'. Nurses would derive no benefit, on either 'business-like grounds' or 'the more sentimental aspects', from attempts to reduce the variety of requirements 'to one dead level of crushing uniformity'.[30] It may be that Dr Bedford Fenwick had some political motive in questioning the conditions of service at the London Hospital given its matron's passionate position against registration; this after all was the agenda of both himself and his wife.

Whatever the justification for the proceedings, the evidence arising from the Select Committee shows strikingly how Nightingale's altruistic vision had become uniformly embodied. Women from all ranks of society, including the wealthy upper and middle classes, were entering nurse training schools, and undertaking concomitant demands and duties, including those that were arduous and menial. Details of the classes from which nurses came show how nursing, perhaps uniquely, bypassed the rigid class structure of the period. At St Bartholomew's Hospital in 1890, for example, of the nurses who entered training in the previous two years, 4 were daughters of architects, 7 of clergymen, 3 of farmers, 5 of manufacturers, 4 of medical men, 6 of merchants, 4 of military and naval officers, 7 of solicitors, 4 of tradesmen and 1 was the daughter of a stockbroker.[31]

The daughter of a duke was currently doing the work of an ordinary nurse in one of the wards of St Bartholomew's Hospital.[32] The daughter of a peer was working as a special probationer at the hospital, a role taken by women of education and position whereby they paid a guinea a week for the privilege of being trained for the period of three months. During this time probationers gave assistance on the wards, often 'specialling' particularly sick patients, and eventually they would put their training into practical use by visiting the sick in the community. Similarly, at the Westminster Hospital, probationers were recruited without regard to their social circumstances, and included ladies, daughters of commercial men, and officers' and doctors' daughters. The only criterion was sufficient education and goodness.[33]

Hospital work was undoubtedly very hard. Some nurses caught diseases and died. One accusation, made by several ex-probationers, was that at the London Hospital particularly, nurses were overworked, underpaid, unprotected from dismissal, illness, diseases and death, and ill-fed.[34] The criticisms were publicised in daily papers, but were refuted by several pages of extracts from letters of former probationers submitted to the committee.[35]

Long hours of standing made nurses flat-footed.[36] One nurse argued that nursing involved a sacrifice of ten years of a woman's life. This was disputed by others who argued that nursing was not a sacrifice but a pleasure.[37] Nursing was certainly not for those who were merely bored at home.[38] A former probationer at St Thomas's described the trying nature of the work: 'the harrowing scenes, the death beds, the sorrowing relatives, the atmosphere of sickness and bad smells in which you live your life'. Relatives went to the sister to ask about friends, and about their deaths. They waited at the entrance of wards while serious operations were performed, and if patients were dying it was the sister's duty to make sure relatives were there, 'they never die alone if we can possibly avoid it'.[39]

It was strongly disputed, however, that nurses' dedication was exploited. William Rathbone, a Member of Parliament, on the executive committee of both the Liverpool Infirmary and the Nightingale School, disagreed with the criticisms of the London Hospital. Daughters of his friends, as well as his own daughter, had trained for various periods of time at the London Hospital and found conditions satisfactory. They believed themselves to have been well cared for. Rathbone's daughter had written to her father that nursing was not for delicate women. It was hard work and involved the same kinds of dangers and sacrifices that soldiers incurred. But it was no more exhausting than many other trades by which women earned a living. Patients were the first objects of the hospital and, accordingly, the good of the patients was the good of the nurses. As in any trade, so in hospital work, it was expected that women of ordinary health and strength should be expected to maintain their health and earn a living.[40]

It was not only the metropolitan hospitals that benefited from the high moral quality of nurses. The same training methods in use at St Thomas's Hospital were employed by Rathbone to train nurses for the Liverpool Infirmary, once a workhouse. In fact, a Nightingale nurse, Agnes Jones, was superintendent of the infirmary, a post that brought her a premature death. As Rathbone stated, nurses were subject to authority and supervision. This was best given not by the management of the hospital, or by the medical men, but by those who trained them, the matron or lady superintendent. She recruited nurses and dismissed them, oversaw their discipline and conduct, and guided and evaluated the training of their character. Rathbone agreed with Nightingale and Bonham Carter, moral character was the essential characteristic for the good nurse. It could not be tested or examined, for nursing was practical, moral rather than intellectual. The best nurses were not those who passed examinations, but those who were known by their matrons to be trustworthy, and to have the kindness and care for patients that was so important.[41] No register could standardise this.

The chaplain and religious services, both in the wards and in the hospital chapel, were central to hospital life for both patients and nurses in the London hospitals at that period. Nurses committed themselves to compulsory regular attendance at services. Nightingale had even suggested to the House of Lords that nurses in training should take singing lessons in order to lead ward services.[42] The chaplain considered the hospital to be his parish, taking responsibility for the spiritual welfare of all his patients.[43] This does not appear to have been exclusive but was provided across the range of beliefs. Great efforts were made to use the services of the Jewish rabbi and Roman Catholic priest for Jewish and Roman Catholic patients, and kosher food was provided for Jewish patients.[44]

The vocational nature of nursing provided the motivation to undertake very demanding kinds of work. This was the essence of the anti-registration argument, which were represented in a three-part petition from nurse training schools and hospitals to the Select Committee organised by Sir Henry Burdett.[45] Four points were made in opposition to registration: that the position of the best trained nurses would be lowered; that it would be detrimental to the advancement of teaching nurses; that it would be disadvantageous to the public; that it would be injurious to the medical profession.

This was signed by medical superintendents, matrons, lady superintendents and secretaries and other senior staff of many of the United Kingdom hospitals, infirmaries and medical institutions and included signatures from St Thomas's Hospital, including those of William Rathbone, Henry Bonham Carter and Sir Harry Verney, Secretary to the Nightingale Fund Council. The second part included objections from medical men and was signed by a long list of their names. The third part was the report of a speech by Rathbone which included Nightingale's views on registration.

Rathbone repeated his evidence to the Select Committee and argued that those involved in nurse education over the last thirty years, including Nightingale herself, formed a consensus of opposition to nurse registration and the Royal British Nurses' Association, which proposed it. Registration would stereotype a lower standard in nursing and lull the public into a false sense of security. The good nurse could not be distinguished from the bad nurse by any system of testing or examination. Moral character was the pre-eminent moral qualification, a way of 'being' a nurse, demonstrated in action, but not quantifiable, measurable or standardisable.

Arguments for registration from the Select Committee 1904–1905: the position of the medical men

In 1904 and 1905 parliamentary Select Committees met to consider the registration of nurses.[46] Most nurses were women, and these were the focus of the debate. But the evidence given to the committee shows there were also male nurses, usually from the same class of person as footmen and valets, who trained as nurses and attended to men in mental asylums with medical or surgical illnesses, and against whom, it was argued, there was prejudice.[47]

Dr Bedford Fenwick, the first person to give evidence, told the committee that his concern to register nurses had begun seventeen years earlier with the formation of the British Nurses' Association (founded by Mrs Bedford Fenwick). He had first tried to persuade Parliament to constitute a Select Committee for the purpose in 1896 but failed, he alleged, because of vested pecuniary interests.[48]

Perhaps Dr Bedford Fenwick was impatient with, or even antagonistic to, Nightingale; surprisingly, he did not mention her central role when he spoke about the way nursing had developed. Before the Crimean War, he argued, nurses had tended to be aged women of the servant class. After the war there was a better class of women, while domestic work was now performed by this servant class as ward maids. There was now a demand for nurses to have a better technical education and training to meet growing demands of science and technology. He was concerned about the lack of uniformity in nurse training and diversity of training standards: individual hospitals certificated nurses as trained after varying periods, from one to three years.

According to Dr Bedford Fenwick, efficient nursing meant that the nurse should have the technical knowledge to understand and carry out the duties entrusted to her by the doctor, and to report back to the doctor symptoms she had noticed. The nurse ought to be able to take the patient's temperature and pulse correctly, know exactly how to feed the patient, how to keep him or her and his or her surroundings clean, how to manage the ventilation of the room, how to understand symptoms when they presented and be able accurately to report them to the doctor. Dr Bedford Fenwick was against nurses specialising, believing that in three years the nurse should have an adequate knowledge of both medicine, surgery as well as obstetrics to be able to nurse all cases.

There was a need, he argued, to set up a central nursing council to oversee standards of entry, training and registration and so be responsible for creating uniformity in examination and certification. This was in keeping with other professions, particularly the medical profession, which standardised training and which looked to a central body to prescribe uniform standards and regulate the profession. And although Fenwick agreed that certification of a nurse's competence from the larger hospitals demonstrated a high standard of training, his major concern was the very poor standard of badly-trained women who called themselves nurses.

Dr Bedford Fenwick was asked whether there was a true analogy between the medical profession and nursing.[49] Qualities beyond technical training, the 'bedside manner, pleasing voice and various other things', which were key for the nurse, were not so fundamental for the doctor, other than to give him a larger practice? Dr Bedford Fenwick guardedly agreed, but argued that the nurse's technical knowledge was crucial for the patient.[50] He gave an example: one of the most pleasant-mannered nurses 'who charmed every patient she had', gave a patient recovering from typhoid fever a mutton chop and he died. He had been starved as part of his recovery, but she had meant in the kindest way possible to allay the hunger that he had. According to Dr Bedford Fenwick she had killed him with kindness.

Another member of the committee thought that knowledge came with experience, and that Dr Bedford Fenwick was spoiling his case by attaching too much importance to technical knowledge. Dr Bedford Fenwick was unwavering in his belief that a General Nursing Council, through the tool of examinations leading to certificated registration, would regulate standards of nursing and by virtue of being able to bring a prosecution, prevent disreputable women forging hospital nursing certificates as was then occurring.[51]

Dr Bedford Fenwick was asked whether hospital certification would be a preferable system given that an examination could not assess the qualities of the person. Would not the possibility of seeing the nurse at work show more about her than an examiner would find out? He responded that the schedule he had drawn up, modelled on the procedure for examination and registration of doctors, met this criticism. When a medical student went up for examination at a university or other qualifying body, the student had to produce a schedule signed by the dean of his medical school to show that he had attended a certain number of lectures on particular subjects, that he had spent certain periods on hospital wards, and that his character 'is thoroughly reliable and trustworthy'.[52]

Dr Bedford Fenwick intended to follow this model for nursing and had made draft plans accordingly. At every hospital, he proposed, the matron and chairman or other officer, should sign schedules showing that the nurse had been a certain number of years in the wards, that she had passed through certain wards, that she had proved herself a trustworthy nurse, 'possessed of a good temper and other charming qualities that the opponents of registration are anxious about'. The hospital would be responsible for the answers to this schedule. It was important for the nurse to be practical, and the matron would take responsibility for assessing this. Part of the examination would need to be extremely practical, and matrons would need to be appointed. Doctors could examine technical aspects, while matrons, acting for the council, could examine the practical aspects.

To questions on funding, Dr Bedford Fenwick replied that a better status for nurses would encourage a 'better class woman' to come into the work. Hospitals would no longer need to pay salaries to nurses, working in an apprenticeship mode, rather nurses would themselves pay for their education, registration and examination, which would itself fund the regulatory body.[53] Dr Bedford Fenwick was asked whether this would exclude people from 'the poorer classes' who might like to qualify as 'perfectly useful nurses'. Furthermore: 'would not it make this calling of the nurses, I will not call it a profession, only available to those who had money to begin with?'[54] Dr Bedford Fenwick thought that present pay was so low that it would make no difference.

The chairman commented on the argument of the opponents of registration that it was impossible to examine women on the main points wanted in a nurse, namely, 'womanly qualities of sympathy, and so on'.[55] Dr Bedford Fenwick did not dispute that these qualities were needed, but believed they would be discovered during the training period by the hospital and the matron, who would then be responsible for recommendation or otherwise. The hospital would then have greater authority over the trustworthiness of those who could call themselves trained nurses.

Dr Bedford Fenwick appears to have been extremely influential. He was the first witness called, spoke of proposals as his own, and had devised the scheme for registration. Written evidence submitted to the committee, a copy of a letter written by him, in 1889, in his capacity as Honorary Secretary to the British Nurses' Association, to the chairmen of a various hospital management committees, shows how much effort he had already put in to advance his cause.[56] He had asked each hospital to appoint the matron or a member of the medical staff to discuss the issue of nurse registration. In doing so, the British

Nurses' Association hoped to gain co-operation to secure the professional reform.

Doctors generally supported the idea of registration. A Fellow of the Royal Society, Sir James Crichton-Browne, argued that it would certify a minimal standard of science, if not art. This he thought would be similar to medical registration, examination at the end of the three-year training period would exclude the incompetent and untrustworthy nurse. Testimony to the moral character of the nurse, her manner and personal traits, could be amply judged by the hospital and training school during the training period.[57] In Crichton-Browne's view, secure technical knowledge and not moral qualities were what made the nurse. Thousands of women were possessed of 'fine moral qualities' but they were not nurses.

Neither did he think that a moral character reference given at the completion of training by the training hospital was relevant. His memory of nurses working in asylums forty years before was that they were from 'a very humble class', many could not read labels on medicine bottles and needed 'lunatics' [sic] to help them. Although in his opinion many were excellent, they were largely drawn from the lower domestic servant class. Crichton-Browne agreed that nursing had made marvellous progress since he had entered the Edinburgh Royal Infirmary in 1858. Then, there were some capable nurses trained by physicians and surgeons, but many were of the 'retired charwoman type'. He believed that now there was no higher type of woman than the well-trained nurse.

But he also thought improvements had brought inefficiency.[58] There was no uniformity in training and the public was therefore unprotected. The basis of his argument was his belief that: 'All nursing is modelled upon medical science'. And he thought that registration would reinforce the nursing profession by attracting a better class of woman because of the recognised status. Finally, Crichton-Browne described the kind of examination he believed would best test nursing competency. As in the case of doctors, this needed to focus on practical duties: how the nurse managed ice applications, draw sheets, fomentations, inhalations of oxygen, hypodermic injections, taking temperature, and so on.

The physician from St Bartholomew's Hospital, Dr Norman Moore, was asked whether, from his experience, women became nurses from a love of the calling, or for more prosaic reasons, as a means of earning a living.[59] His reply was non-committal. His interest was with examination in theoretical knowledge which he felt was inadequate. Nurses could read up on subjects for examinations, but the real test was to ask nurses things that they could only learn from their training and not out of books: 'Book knowledge is very little use to them.'[60] Whatever system of registration was envisaged, responsibility for the nurse's competence lay with the doctor and should not be surrendered.[61]

Arguments for registration from the Select Committee 1904–1905: the position of the nurses

Medical men, who supported registration, emphasised the regulating of technical skill. To them the issue of moral character was secondary, but could be affirmed by a testimonial. Nurses, on the other hand, seemed to understand the indispensable importance of the virtue of care, but could not imagine that registration would endanger it.

Isla Stewart, from St Bartholomew's Hospital (Mrs Bedford Fenwick's successor and the co-author of the nursing textbook) and Margaret Huxley, who at the time had a nursing home in Ireland which cared for surgical cases, both supported the idea of registering nurses.[62] They argued that it would be a safeguard against incompetence, and also spread to all hospitals the kind and content of training now given at the best hospitals. Both matrons felt that the proposed system would not lead to the rise of nurses who were technically efficient but deficient in personal qualities.

The Secretary of the Royal British Nurses' Association, Annie J. Hobbs, thought that nurses who rejected registration were acting out of loyalty to the opinions of the matrons at their training hospitals. She argued that pro-registrationists wanted to register the fact of a 'proper training', while anti-registrationists believed that technical training counted for very little, the most important attribute of the nurse was character and this could not be registered.[63]

Hobbs did not, however, dispute the importance of character. Indeed, she argued that registration would deter frivolous careless women from applying for training. But she also admitted that the register would not prohibit technically competent nurses who were deficient in character from being registered as nurses fit to practise. This was the fear of those who opposed registration, with whom Hobbs was forced to agree. Nurses who were impatient or careless would not (could not) be able to be taken off the register, neither would a particularly quarrelsome nurse; for then one would be registering only saints.

Christina Forrest, Matron of the Victoria and Bournemouth Nursing Institute and Home Hospital, was also in favour of registration as a means of regularising standards.[64] Technical efficiency had to be measured by a practical clinical examination. She agreed that personal qualities such as sympathy, kindliness and attention could not be verified or secured by examination, but believed that this could be covered by the matron's certificate of character. She thought that technical efficiency and moral character went hand in hand. A nurse could not be called efficient unless her moral character was good. But, like Hobbs, she admitted that a name would not be removed from the register on account of moral deficiency unless a serious charge, such as theft, could be proved.

That the argument for registration did not preclude the absolute importance of vocation was made clear by Edla R. Wortabet, who had been a lady pupil at the Middlesex and London Temperance hospitals. She had paid £300 for her three-year training and subsequently worked in Beyrout [sic] where she started a training school for Syrian nurses and wrote a training book, and subsequently superintended hospitals in Bordeaux and Egypt. In her view, women who went into the nursing profession ought to feel constrained by a calling. By this, she meant not an actual call (which as her questioner suggested would not provide enough nurses), but rather 'a love for their work and a dignity over it'.[65] Although a pro-registrationist she believed in the concept of nursing as a calling, and saw no conflict with these two positions; the calling should be built on, and made into an educated profession.

Mrs Ethel Gordon Fenwick (Mrs Bedford Fenwick) gave evidence in several long speeches. These showed her to be a proactive, organised and effective political campaigner, strategically prepared to push her arguments in absolute determination to win her case.[66] Her argument rested on what she believed to be a matter of justice. She argued that the growing sense of injustice amongst the best nurses could only be remedied by placing their work on a sound basis: 'thus ensuring to them an honourable position in the estimation of the public'.

She stated that she had been intimately connected with nursing for over thirty years, a period during which thousands of women, often working in very discouraging circumstances, had taken part in raising the moral tone and practical efficiency of the care of the sick in hospitals and infirmaries.[67] The state had an obligation towards the women who had sacrificed themselves, shown such devotion to duty and so freely given their powers of organisation to accomplish the great social reform of nursing. The state could only discharge this obligation by attending to the education and working conditions of nurses.

Mrs Bedford Fenwick refuted Lückes's view that teaching nurses systematic knowledge would make them into pseudo-scientific workers, eager to assume the responsibilities of doctors.[68] Such a suggestion was 'mischievous' and not founded on fact. According to Mrs Bedford Fenwick, it was the semi-trained, untrustworthy woman who tried to hide her ignorance with pseudo-scientific pretensions. Indeed, any friction between doctors and nurses arose from deficiency in medical and nursing etiquette, by which she meant the lack in nurse training of discipline and teaching on social relations.

In order to support her case, Mrs Bedford Fenwick brought to the committee a detailed list of nursing scandals, which were also submitted as written evidence.[69] These 'typical nursing scandals' occurred from January 1898 until March 1905, and included charges such as obtaining money by false pretences, theft, forgery, fraud, judicial separation, personal injury and even murder. Details were limited to charges against individual nurses, some cases were dismissed and the result was not known of others. Despite these limitations, and the fact that these matters were not relevant to a written examination, the charges formed the basis of Mrs Bedford Fenwick's central claim that registration was essential for the protection of the public.

The fact that many of the allegations were unproven, and even dismissed, was the subject of questions.[70] Mrs Bedford Fenwick agreed that only definite allegations would be sufficient to remove the nurse from the register; neither being out of practice, or 'an unfortunate development of character' would be enough to do so. Most of the cases detailed had little relevance to the issue of registration because it would not be possible to prevent women calling themselves 'nurses' or wearing uniform. Mrs Bedford Fenwick conceded this point, but argued that registration would merely prevent such nurses calling themselves 'registered'.[71]

The arguments for registration were various. The standardising of technical competence was important, but it was also argued that registration was necessary to end the exploitation of nurses' altruism, increase the status of nursing, and thus recruitment, and to safeguard against bogus, untrained nurses. Such arguments, which at first sight appeared convincing, were called into question during proceedings. Unlike the medical men who supported registration, the nurses who were in favour of registration expressly affirmed the altruistic nature of nursing. They did not intend to bring about its undoing, but to include it.

Arguments against registration from the Select Committee 1904–1905

Yet, it was this undoing that the anti-registrationists argued would take place if registration was granted, as Nightingale and Bonham Carter had argued nearly twenty years earlier. The Chairman of the Central Hospital Council for London, the Board of the Royal Free Hospital, and Visitor for King Edward's Hospital Fund, Charles Burt, represented the opponents of registration. Their well-rehearsed arguments were set out in a document appended to the report and signed by over 300 matrons, doctors and chairmen from the major London hospitals as well as provincial hospitals, including the Edinburgh Royal Infirmary, the Radcliffe Infirmary, Oxford and Addenbrooke's, Cambridge. Signatures included those of Henry Burdett and the Secretary to the Committee of the Nightingale Fund, Sir Henry Bonham Carter.[72]

The petitioners for registration maintained that the two main arguments against registration were mistaken. These were, firstly, that the public would be protected from unskilled and competent persons, and secondly, that trained nurses would be protected from being placed at a disadvantage by imperfectly trained persons. Opponents believed that registration would be harmful to both the public and trained nurses themselves for six reasons.

Firstly, any system of registration would necessarily focus on testing technical capabilities rather than personal qualities, which were characteristics not amenable to examination or registration. It was the lack of such qualities, rather than technical incompetence, which gave rise to complaints from patients. Nursing training could not be compared to medical training. However important the personal character of the doctor, it was for his skill and knowledge that he was consulted. In nursing (unlike midwifery) the opposite was the case, although technical knowledge should not be underrated.

Secondly, far from offering security to the public, a state register of nurses would be an actual source of danger, since an unsuitable woman, merely by passing an examination, would be entitled to be on the register and hence certified as fit. Thirdly, it would be extremely difficult and costly, involving accusations of libel, to remove a nurse from the register, even if she were notoriously bad. The public would be lulled into a false sense of security, being led to believe that the register would protect them from incompetent and undesirable nurses. Fourthly, a uniform training should not be made compulsory because the needs of patients varied. A variety of knowledge and experience was required. It would be both unjust and impractical to exclude women with a more selective training, who nevertheless met patients' needs quite satisfactorily.

Fifthly, as registrationists conceded, registration would only examine and register technical abilities; technical knowledge and the passing of examinations, rather than personal qualities, would become the first essential. But the technically trained nurse, without personal qualities, was not adequate to meet the needs of patients. Lastly, a state register would lower the status of the best nurses, because of their association with nurses who had defects of character and performance, and who would not be removed from the register for the previously stated reasons. Furthermore, unduly high standards of examination would prevent perfectly adequate women giving their services; while unduly low standards would put all women on the same low level, the best qualified losing most.

Nightingale's view had not changed, the paper stated. Registration was not only misguided it was unnecessary. All hospitals gave nurses their own certificates of service at the completion of their three- or four-year training. These certificates were sufficient testimony of the nurse's technical knowledge and experience, and would not be improved upon by registration and examination by people who had no experience of the actual nurse during her period of training and service.

Sidney Holland, Chairman of the London, Poplar and Tilbury Hospitals, did not believe that any examination could demonstrate a nurse's technical proficiency because medical knowledge was constantly changing, including methods of antisepsis and sterilisation, and it was easy for a nurse to lose her skill and knowledge. More importantly, the qualities that made the good nurse, the character that enabled her to perform her duties unselfishly, could not be systematised. Nursing was unlike the medical profession, the character or goodness of the doctor was not so important for the patient as his medical skill.[73]

A significant argument of the registrationists was that registration would improve the status of nurses and therefore encourage much-needed recruitment. The majority of nurses were now from the middle rather than the upper classes, implying that educated women from the upper classes were no longer attracted to nursing. Holland, asked to comment on this argument, replied with a rhetorical question: would an educated woman who cared about nursing really be deterred from coming into nursing because of the lack of registration? No one would be stopped from going into nursing because of its status. The number of upper-class women like Florence Nightingale was severely reduced by the early twentieth century. At one time there was a great rush of such women, so that there were three to four nurses per patient. Now the average was just over two nurses per patient. Less women wanted to become nurses, and in Holland's view, registration would not add a single person. According to Holland, 'a woman who wants to become a nurse will become a nurse because she loves nursing and not because she is going to have a professional status. There is absolutely nothing in it'.[74]

Evidence to the committee showed the classes from which nurses came at that time. At a large Scottish hospital, out of 143 nurses, 13 were the daughters of clergymen, 35 of professional men, 50 of tradesmens, 6 of clerks, 32 of farmers, while 2 were in service, 5 were not known, and 54 were pupil probationers, unpaid and hence from the wealthier classes.[75]

Sidney Holland, recalled for questioning, reiterated his opinion that registration would not guarantee either up-to-date practical and technical competence or moral character, and moreover, would lead to a false sense of security among the public and among doctors. 'Registration cannot secure that a nurse has a proper nursing character or any character at all, and it cannot even secure the technical training because she may have lost her technical training during a number of years.'[76] Any examination would only be evidence of what could be crammed from a book and then forgotten, and for nursing it would be 'childishly simple' to pass. Holland suggested that Mrs Bedford Fenwick's model of registration of nurses was taken from America, where, according to her own journal, the *British Journal of Nursing*, it was not deemed a success, despite the independent spirit among New York women.

Holland was asked whether trained nurses working among poor people, going into their homes and doing housework, might find the work 'distasteful and repugnant'.[77] He replied that a 'really good woman' would do anything.

Nurses were recruited from all classes, and there was a shortage of recruits, particularly from the 'right class'.

Eva Lückes was totally supportive of Sidney Holland's position. Although she opposed registration, this did not mean she that she opposed regulation. Rather, as she stated in her pamphlet, she believed in individual training schools regulating their own nurses. This, she argued, preserved standards within the necessary moral framework. By way of example, she detailed the rigorous and organised training of nurses at the London Hospital, details which were also submitted in written evidence.[78]

After a successful examination of their health, and before meeting the patients, nurses went into a training home where they had six weeks of lectures in elementary hygiene, elementary physiology, sick cookery and practical nursing including bedmaking, bandaging, padding of splints and names of instruments. In the seventh week they were examined. If they passed and were considered suitable, the probationers were introduced into the hospital where their theoretical training began. They attended one two-hour lecture and one two-hour study period each week. During the year there were three courses of lectures given by Lückes, a member of the medical staff and a member of the surgical staff. At the end of each course of lectures written, oral and practical examinations were held. At the end of two years a certificate was completed and signed by the chairman, by Lückes, by the physician and by the surgeon; to maintain standards lecturers did not also examine. The emphasis in training was carefully planned experience. Each probationer was individually allocated to wards according to the experience she needed of different and varying illnesses, conditions and types of patients: men, women and children.

Lückes thought that uniformity among nurses was to be deprecated.[79] It was not possible to achieve uniformity of attainment, each nurse had a different personality and was suited to different work. Individual personality and character were crucial. Complaints against nurses were not usually because of incompetence but because of personality and attitude: 'She is either careless or bad tempered or selfish, or she makes mischief in the house, or her manner is objectionable.'[80] Even so, Lückes admitted that it was difficult to recruit women who were intelligent as well as good and kind. Hospital training schools could not expect perfection, but had to take women from every class and make the best of them.

A major fear of Lückes was that registration would make nurses more like doctors. This she deplored. The thrust of nurse education to meet registration would be scientific: nurses would become one step removed from doctors along the same continuum. Three years of training would register a nurse and five years a doctor. Nursing knowledge, in Lückes' opinion, was entirely different in scope and depth from medical knowledge. On this matter – what the nurse needed to know – there was some discussion.

The Chairman of the Select Committee produced some examination papers from the London Hospital Medical College, from June 16, 1904. Lückes responded that this was last years' examination paper, and that the examiner had wanted probationers to be able to go in for honours in their last examination. It was made clear to the probationers that this was voluntary, and fifteen gained honorary certificates. The Chairman read out the questions in the examination paper. Nurses were asked to give some account of special diets which might be ordered for special diseases and to explain the reasons why the diets were suitable in each case. They were also asked to give some account of the general principles upon which the modern practice of aseptic and antiseptic surgery was based and their detailed application in first, a pre-planned operation and second, an emergency compound fracture.

The Chairman approved of the stiffness of the questions. Lückes, however, thought they probably went too far. Examination questions were necessary but not sufficient. They would not remove bad nurses. The London Hospital register of nurse training provided a record of the actual work done, and being done, by each probationer.[81] With reference to supervision, Lückes said she would go further than Miss Hughes, who argued that nurses could only be certified with regards to their technical qualifications. In Lückes's opinion it would be difficult to supervise nurses and prevent them going 'rusty'.[82] A nurse's moral character was already categorised: as 'good', 'very good', 'particularly good' and 'excellent', but registration would make it more difficult to get at the kind of nurse required, and to get at her real character. It 'would be a serious blow to the nurses to stereotype mediocrity in that way'.[83]

It was Lückes's fear, echoing Nightingale, that registration would lead to 'mechanical uniformity'.[84] She did not underrate the importance of technical training, and measuring standards reached, but she strongly objected to any 'pseudo-scientific person' in the sick-room. Nurses should not think they were being developed as doctors. Nursing knowledge must be accurate and useful. Nurses needed technical knowledge, and the assurance that they possessed it at an elementary level, but the value of nurses could not be estimated by the way they passed an examination. Nursing was practical, not just theoretical. On the other hand, if a woman was too incompetent to pass an examination she was unfit for training.

The Society of Apothecaries was against registration because it feared the loosening of ties to institutions, setting nurses free from hospitals, allowing nurses to set themselves up against medical men, which would lead to antagonism between doctors and nurses.[85] This would undermine the organisation, and loyalty in relationships, which was so important to nursing tradition. The scheme of registration was an appeal for status to elevate nursing into a similar profession to that of the law, the church or medicine. As its representative argued, it was not so much knowledge but manner and personal attributes that counted: 'I mean a sympathetic nurse is everything. An unsympathetic nurse with all the knowledge in the world would not do much good, to certain cases at any rate.'[86]

Representatives from the British Medical Association, Sir Victor Horsley and Dr Langley Browne, thought there was a danger of some conflict in role responsibility between doctors and nurses, and that nurses were taking on duties that they were not qualified to carry out, so were, in a sense, competing with medical men.[87] Mrs Charles Hobhouse, previously Secretary, Treasurer and Chairman of the committee of a rural nursing association in Wiltshire, suggested that doctors feared competition and sometimes prevented nurses being employed because of that fear. She also thought it would be difficult to obtain evidence for a nurse's moral character.[88]

Sir Henry Burdett, who was vehemently criticised by Mrs Bedford Fenwick a decade earlier, now agreed that a three-year training was necessary and he, too, called for a uniformity of curriculum.[89] He commended Mrs Bedford Fenwick's determined persistence. But he also suggested that most nurses were unhappy about the idea of a registration body, such as Mrs Bedford Fenwick proposed, and were more in favour of his own proposal, that training institutions should themselves be the registering bodies.[90]

The pro-registrationists succeeded, and the Nurse Registration Act was passed in 1919. The registration debate undoubtedly aroused intense bitterness,[91] yet the need for moral character, alongside education, as a basis for nursing, was acknowledged by all.[92] What appears to have formed the basis of the dispute between the various factions was the question of emphasis. The moral arguments about the character of the nurse continued in the following years. The pro-registrationist view that standardisation would improve the status of nursing and encourage recruitment was not borne out.

Nursing ideals and Mrs Bedford Fenwick 1899–1937

The First World War had ushered in changes which affected the ethos of British society in three aspects relevant to nursing: confidence in God and religion had been dented, women were emancipated and most professions were now open to them, and there were now more diversions and attractions that people, especially women, enjoyed.[93] This observation was supported by evidence to Parliament in 1925, given by Mrs Bedford Fenwick.[94] She bemoaned the current shortage of nurses, and attributed it to the loss of altruism and increasing selfishness of young women. The shortage of nurses was not, in her opinion, due to the pay, or working conditions, but because it was difficult to get the right kind of woman in the early 1920s. There was indifference to humanitarian work, and it was, in her view, those with such commitment and altruism, like the *religieuse*, who were the best kind of nurses.[95]

According to Mrs Bedford Fenwick, this was an age of individualism, the old altruistic spirit of the *religieuse* was decreasing. There were many more distractions for young women, and as a result the minimum age for entry to the profession had been lowered from twenty-five to eighteen.[96] Even after nurse registration was obtained, Mrs Bedford Fenwick voiced the view that altruism of the kind of the religious orders, with its connotations of denial and self-sacrifice, made the best nurses. Virtuous qualities were considered essential by even the most ardent pro-registrationist.

Her evidence in 1925 was consistent with editorials in the journal she owned and edited, *Nursing Record and Hospital World*, later renamed the *British Journal of Nursing*. She repeated her belief that nursing was a sacred vocation, religiously inspired, and not merely a means of earning a living. When it became this and was dissociated from religious motives, falling into the hands of the ignorant and incapable, standards of both work and morality fell. She pointed to examples of inspiration from the past including Frederike Fliedner, Elizabeth Fry, Florence Nightingale and Agnes Jones.[97] She lamented the selfishness of the 1920s, where distractions such as bicycling were undermining commitment to patients and the unselfish devotion to duty.[98]

Mrs Bedford Fenwick pleaded, 'Nurses Keep Your Souls Alive' and called for a revival of altruism and selflessness, against a preoccupation with material concerns, 'dealing out her service to the sick in terms of pounds, shillings and pence'. People's souls needed consolation, Mrs Bedford Fenwick argued, not just their bodies, and this, the mechanical nurse was unable to give.[99] Salaries and commercialisation would not attract the humane type of woman.[100] Nursing must be maintained as a sacred vocation, for sick people were sensitive to atmosphere and would only respond to those nurses who exhibited the qualities of patience, abnegation of self and devotion to others.[101] Mrs Bedford Fenwick's view remained unchanged over the decades. In 1937, her journal carried a slightly revised repeat of her 1899 editorial.[102]

She was ardently in favour of women's suffrage,[103] and was a supporter of the more radical American feminist, Lavinia Dock, whose articles she published in her journal,[104] and who gave evidence to the Select Committee on registration, describing North American nursing where eight states had recently secured registration for nurses.[105] It may be that Dock's influences were those of evolutionary materialism. In her *A History of Nursing*,[106] written together with M.A. Nutting, caring as a basis of nursing is attributed to the animal instinct of mutual aid and support, as quoted by the revolutionary writer Peter Kropotkin.[107] This was not Mrs Bedford Fenwick's perspective. She may have been influenced by North American liberal ideas,[108] particularly as regard nursing training, but she still maintained the vocational ideal, and included articles on this theme in her journal.[109] Indeed, pressure to become politically involved with trade unionism from Labour trade unionists was resisted because of this.[110] The *Nursing Times* commented:

> From the outset we are faced by the fact that any money equivalent for services rendered, which custom may have established, is purely an artificial one, since there can be no money equivalent for ministering to the spiritual needs, giving knowledge, dispensing justice, or healing the sick; and in an ideal State these services would be available for all equally, as essential services for the State.[111]

In fact, as Bedford Fenwick's journal made clear, the statement by Mrs Sidney Webb in the Labour Party draft report: 'The only way in which nurses can deal effectively with their conditions, and exercise any sort of equality in bargaining power, is for the profession to be organised on Trade Union lines', would only be acceptable if the words 'Trade Union' were replaced by 'purely vocational'.[112]

Mrs Bedford Fenwick was not merely a feminist and careerist, as might be suggested by modern historians.[113] Whatever her complex motivations, or the influence of her medical husband upon her, the fraught debate over registration was primarily concerned with ensuring competency in nursing. For the anti-registrationist side this amounted to reducing standards, a lowest common denominator approach, which could not take account of immeasurable nursing qualities. For the pro-registrationists, the objective of registration was to set a minimum standard for public safety and at the same time create recognition and status for the training of the nurse. Both factions were agreed, however, that what might be termed 'the purely vocational' remained crucial to nursing.

Conclusion

This chapter has revealed two important pieces of historical evidence. The first is that by the late nineteenth and early twentieth century, Nightingale's principles and the ideals of nursing leaders whom these ideals influenced had become a normative living reality in hospital nursing. The second piece of evidence is that the moral significance of the nurse was regarded as quintessential to all views on registration, and was not disputed. All agreed on the vocational ethos as being fundamental to the health and well-being of the profession. The registration issue brought to light a paradox. The dependency on the vocation with its associated altruism could lead to exploitation; but by improving the status of the profession, people would be attracted who had less worthy motives. Even following the profound social changes ushered in by the First World War, this nursing ethos remained unaffected.

Nightingale's vision of the integration of nursing art and science, and the combination of theory and practice involved in the apprenticeship, was so intrinsic to the profession that it was unthinkable that it could be endangered. There was no dispute about this underlying vision, rather, the dispute lay in the emphasis given by different factions to the scientific side of nursing. Pro-registrationists focused on developing the scientific and technological side of nursing, and subjecting it to testing and registration. Anti-registrationists did not dispute that intellect and intelligence were important, but they disputed the emphasis attached to it. Doctors and nurses were seen by anti-registrationists as having different functions. Among doctors, scientific knowledge and intellect, subject to testing and registration, took precedence; moral character was a useful adjunct. For nursing, it was precisely the opposite that was true: unquantifiable, immeasurable compassion was of its essence. For the doctor the emphasis had to fall on strict scientific and technical competence, for a nurse this was necessary but not sufficient.

Notes

1 A.M. Rafferty, *The Politics of Nursing Knowledge*, London, Routledge, 1996.

2 H.W. Acland, 'Preface' in *Handbook for Hospital Sisters*, Lees, F.S. and H.W. Acland (eds), London, W.S. Isbister & Co., 1874.

3 M.E. Baly, *Florence Nightingale and the Nursing Legacy*, London, Croom Helm, 1986, pp. 77–78.

4 A.M. Rafferty, *The Politics of Nursing Knowledge*, London, Routledge, 1996.

5 E. Bedford Fenwick, 'Mr Henry Burdett again', editorial, *Nursing Record*, 6, 159, 1891, pp. 185–186, April 16; 'The History of Registration', editorial, *Nursing Record*, 8, 224, 1892, pp. 569–571, July 14.

6 Points arising out of Miss Cox-Davies' letter dated 20 February, 1919 to Sir Cooper Perry, and the Joint Report of Miss Cox-Davies and Miss Finch, MS Eng. c. 5938, *Burdett Papers*, College of Nursing Ltd., correspondence, 1916–1919, Folio 102.

7 Letter from Sir Henry Burdett to Sir Cooper Perry, MS Eng. c. 5938, 13 April, 1916, *Burdett Papers*, College of Nursing Ltd., correspondence, 1916–1919, Folio 6.

8 Letter from Florence Nightingale to Sir Henry Acland, MS Acland d.70, July 20, 1869.

9 Letter from Florence Nightingale to Sir Henry Acland, MS Acland d.70, February 27, 1872.

10 Letter from Florence Nightingale to Sir Henry Acland, MS Acland d.70, April 28, 1893.

11 F. Nightingale, *Letters and Addresses to the Probationer Nurses in the 'Nightingale Fund' School at St Thomas's Hospital and Nurses who were Formerly Trained There*, original letters and prints for private circulation held by University College, London, 1873–1900, 1886, January 1.

12 Ibid.,1888, May 16.

13 Letter from Florence Nightingale to Sir Henry Acland, MS Acland d.70, July 7, 1889.

14 Letter from Florence Nightingale to Sir Henry Acland, MS Acland d.70, July 24, 1889.

[15] Letter from Florence Nightingale to Sir Henry Acland, MS Acland do.70, April 28, 1893.

[16] Letter from Sir Henry Acland to Mr Wakley, MS Acland d.70, July 23, 1889.

[17] H. Bonham Carter, *Is a General Register of Nurses Desirable?*, London, 1888.

[18] H. Bonham Carter (ed.), *Memorandum on the Règistration of Nurses and the Royal British Nurses' Association*, London, 1892.

[19] M. Weber, *The Protestant Ethic and the Spirit of Capitalism*, Giddens, A. (intro), 2nd ed., London, George Allen & Unwin, 1930 (1976).

[20] Ibid., pp. 181–183.

[21] 'In the Privy Council', *Re The Petition for a Charter for the Incorporation of the Royal British Nurses' Association: Case in Opposition and Appendix*, signed, Finlay, R.B. and L.S. Bristowe, London, Cookson, Wainewright & Pennington, c. 1892, Ms Eng. c5934–5.

[22] Ibid., pp. 15–16.

[23] Ibid., pp. 3–4, paras 8–13.

[24] Ibid., p. 4, para. 13.

[25] J.C. Steele, J.S. Bristowe, 'Report of the Joint Sectional Committee on Registration to the Council of the Hospitals Association', March 1888, Appendix 11, pp. 44–49, in, 'In the Privy Council', *Re The Petition for a Charter for the Incorporation of the Royal British Nurses' Association: Case in Opposition to the Petition and Appendix*, signed Finlay, R.B. and L.S. Bristowe, London, Cookson, Wainewright & Pennington, c. 1892. Ms Eng. c5934–5.

[26] 'The Matron and Superintendent of Nursing', Appendix A, section i, in Hector, W., *The Work of Mrs Bedford and the Rise of Professional Nursing*, London, Royal College of Nursing, 1973, pp. 67–67.

[27] C.J. Wood, *A Handbook of Nursing for the Home and Hospital*, 8th edn, Cassell & Co., c. 1887.

[28] W. Hector, *The Work of Mrs Bedford and the Rise of Professional Nursing*, London, Royal College of Nursing, 1973, p. 42.

[29] E.C.E. Lückes, *What will Trained Nurses Gain by Joining the British Nurses' Association?*, London, J. & A. Churchill, 1889.

[30] Ibid., p. 16.

[31] *Report of the Select Committee of the House of Lords on Metropolitan Hospitals with Minutes of Evidence, Appendix and Index*, vol. 16, London, HMSO, Irish University Press Series of British Parliamentary Papers, Ford, P. and G. Ford (eds) , vol. 12, Shannon, Ireland, Irish University Press, 1890, p. 167, para. 2567.

[32] Ibid., p. 165, paras 2534–5.

[33] *Second Report of the Select Committee of the House of Lords on Metropolitan Hospitals with Minutes of Evidence, Appendix and Index*, vol. 16, London, HMSO, Irish University Press Series of British Parliamentary Papers, Ford, P. and G. Ford (eds) , vol. 13, Shannon, Ireland, Irish University Press, 1891, pp. 239–240, paras 15246–15280.

[34] *Report of the Select Committee of the House of Lords on Metropolitan Hospitals with Minutes of Evidence, Appendix and Index*, vol. 16, London, HMSO, Irish University Press Series of British Parliamentary Papers, Ford, P. and G. Ford (eds) , vol. 12, Shannon, Ireland, Irish University Press, 1890, pp. 293–345, paras 4730–5968.

[35] Ibid., pp. 587–598, Appendix H.

[36] *Second Report of the Select Committee of the House of Lords on Metropolitan Hospitals with Minutes of Evidence, Appendix and Index*, vol. 16, London, HMSO, Irish University Press Series of British Parliamentary Papers, Ford, P. and G. Ford (eds) , vol. 13, Shannon, Ireland, Irish University Press, 1891, pp. 749–759, paras 25975–25984.

[37] Ibid., p. 391, para. 18482.

[38] *Report of the Select Committee of the House of Lords on Metropolitan Hospitals with Minutes of Evidence, Appendix and Index*, vol. 16, London, HMSO, Irish University Press

Series of British Parliamentary Papers, Ford, P. and G. Ford (eds), vol.12, Shannon, Ireland, Irish University Press, 1890, pp. 330–331, para. 5711.

[39] *Second Report of the Select Committee of the House of Lords on Metropolitan Hospitals with Minutes of Evidence, Appendix and Index*, vol. 16, London, HMSO, Irish University Press Series of British Parliamentary Papers, Ford, P. and G. Ford (eds) , vol. 13, Shannon, Ireland, Irish University Press, 1891, p. 85, paras 11634–11637.

[40] Ibid., pp. 748–751, paras 25974–25998.

[41] Ibid., pp. 741–747, paras 25902–25903; *Report of the Select Committee of the House of Lords on Metropolitan Hospitals with Minutes of Evidence, Appendix and Index*, vol. 16, London, HMSO, Irish University Press Series of British Parliamentary Papers, Ford, P. and G. Ford (eds) , vol. 12, Shannon, Ireland, Irish University Press, 1890, pp. 602–616, Appendix K.

[42] Ibid., p. 604, Appendix K.

[43] Ibid., pp. 167–168, paras 2563–2575; p. 316, para. 5471; *Second Report of the Select Committee of the House of Lords on Metropolitan Hospitals with Minutes of Evidence, Appendix and Index*, vol. 16, London, HMSO, Irish University Press Series of British Parliamentary Papers, Ford, P. and G. Ford (eds) , vol. 13, Shannon, Ireland, Irish University Press, 1891: p. 87, paras 11691, 11704; p. 319, paras 16864–16886; p. 394, paras 18560–18562; p. 403, para. 188808.

[44] *Report of the Select Committee of the House of Lords on Metropolitan Hospitals with Minutes of Evidence, Appendix and Index*, vol. 16, London, HMSO, Irish University Press Series of British Parliamentary Papers, Ford, P. and G. Ford (eds) , vol. 12, Shannon, Ireland, Irish University Press, 1890, p. 452, para. 7645. *Second Report of the Select Committee of the House of Lords on Metropolitan Hospitals with Minutes of Evidence, Appendix and Index*, vol. 16, London, HMSO, Irish University Press Series of British Parliamentary Papers, Ford, P. and G. Ford (eds) , vol. 13, Shannon, Ireland, Irish University Press, 1891: p. 184, paras 14045–14050; p. 314, paras 16762–16763; p. 321, para. 16910; p. 403, paras 188813–188815.

[45] *Second Report of the Select Committee of the House of Lords on Metropolitan Hospitals with Minutes of Evidence, Appendix and Index*, vol. xvi, London, HMSO, Irish University Press Series of British Parliamentary Papers, Ford, P. and G. Ford (eds), vol. 13, Shannon, Ireland, Irish University Press, 1891, pp. 790–798, Appendix K; p. 403, para. 188808.

[46] *Report from the Select Committee on Registration of Nurses together with the Proceedings of the Committee, Minutes of Evidence and Appendix*, House of Commons, London, HMSO, 1904, 1905.

[47] *Report from the Select Committee on Registration of Nurses together with the Proceedings of the Committee, Minutes of Evidence and Appendix*, House of Commons, London, HMSO, 1904, pp. 56–57, 63, paras 905–929, 1014.

[48] *Report from the Select Committee on Registration of Nurses together with the Proceedings of the Committee, Minutes of Evidence and Appendix*, House of Commons, London, HMSO, 1904, pp. 1–7, paras 1–84.

[49] Ibid., p. 7, para. 87.

[50] Ibid., p. 7, para. 88.

[51] Ibid., p. 8, paras 90–96.

[52] Ibid., pp. 10–11, para. 139.

[53] Ibid., p. 11, para. 141.

[54] Ibid., p. 12, para. 147.

[55] Ibid., p. 12, para. 142.

[56] Ibid., p. 97, Appendix 1.

[57] *Report from the Select Committee on Registration of Nurses together with the Proceedings of the Committee, Minutes of Evidence and Appendix*, House of Commons, London, HMSO, 1905, pp. 49–53, paras 896–917.

[58] Ibid., pp. 55–60, paras 952–1029.

[59] *Report from the Select Committee on Registration of Nurses together with the Proceedings of the Committee, Minutes of Evidence and Appendix*, House of Commons, London, HMSO, 1904, p. 44, para. 621.
[60] Ibid., p. 47, para. 671.
[61] Ibid., p. 47, para. 683.
[62] Ibid., pp. 15–26, paras 179–442.
[63] Ibid., pp. 69, 72, 91, paras 1170–1174, 1264, 1622–1623.
[64] *Report from the Select Committee on Registration of Nurses together with the Proceedings of the Committee, Minutes of Evidence and Appendix*, House of Commons, London, HMSO, 1905, pp. 7–10, paras 188–263.
[65] Ibid., pp. 11–14, paras 286–339.
[66] Ibid., pp. 30–40, paras 613–776.
[67] Ibid., p. 32, para. 624.
[68] Ibid., p. 32, paras 625–626.
[69] Ibid., pp. 34–37, paras 660–719; pp. 174–180, Appendix 3.
[70] Ibid., p. 38, paras 722–724.
[71] Ibid., pp. 39–40, paras 757–759.
[72] *Report from the Select Committee on Registration of Nurses together with the Proceedings of the Committee, Minutes of Evidence and Appendix*, House of Commons, London, HMSO, 1904, pp. 98–105, Appendix 2.
[73] Ibid., pp. 29–30, para. 457.
[74] Ibid., p. 39, paras 547–550.
[75] *Report from the Select Committee on Registration of Nurses together with the Proceedings of the Committee, Minutes of Evidence and Appendix*, House of Commons, London, HMSO, 1905, p. 134, para. 2579.
[76] *Report from the Select Committee on Registration of Nurses together with the Proceedings of the Committee, Minutes of Evidence and Appendix*, House of Commons, London, HMSO, 1904, pp. 54–56, paras 805–840.
[77] Ibid., pp. 56–57, paras 853–860.
[78] *Report from the Select Committee on Registration of Nurses together with the Proceedings of the Committee, Minutes of Evidence and Appendix*, House of Commons, London, HMSO, 1905, pp. 15–16, paras 343–347; pp. 169–172, Appendix 1.
[79] Ibid., p. 16, para. 350.
[80] Ibid., p. 18, para. 379.
[81] Ibid., p. 20, paras 403–408.
[82] Ibid., p. 20, para. 417.
[83] Ibid., p. 21, paras 428–429.
[84] Ibid., p. 22–29, paras 442–606.
[85] Ibid., pp. 46–48, paras 840–889.
[86] Ibid., p. 48, para. 878.
[87] Ibid., p. 63, para. 1070.
[88] Ibid., p. 83, 85, paras 1489, 1542.
[89] *Report from the Select Committee on Registration of Nurses together with the Proceedings of the Committee, Minutes of Evidence and Appendix*, House of Commons, London, HMSO, 1905, p. 109, paras 1978–1980.
[90] Ibid., pp. 137–139, paras 2647–2686.
[91] Letter from Sir Arthur Stanley to Sir Henry Burdett, MS Eng. c. 5938, 28 February, 1917, *Burdett Papers*, College of Nursing Ltd., correspondence 1916–1919, Folio 11; Letter from Sir Henry Burdett to Sir Cooper Perry, MS Eng. c. 5938, 6 February, 1919, *Burdett Papers*, College of Nursing Ltd., correspondence 1916–1919, Folio 85; Letter from Sir Henry Burdett to Sir Arthur Stanley, 6 February 1919, MS Eng. c. 5938, *Burdett Papers*, College of Nursing Ltd., correspondence 1916–1919, Folio 87; Sir Henry Burdett, 'Points Arising out of

Miss Cox-Davies' Letter dated 20th February 1919 to Sir Cooper Perry, and the Joint Report of Miss Cox-Davies and Miss Finch', MS Eng. c. 5938, *Burdett Papers*, College of Nursing Ltd., correspondence 1916–1919, Folio 102.

[92] Letter from Sir Henry Burdett to Sir Cooper Perry, MS Eng. c. 5938, 13 April, 1916, *Burdett Papers*, College of Nursing Ltd., correspondence 1916–1919, Folio 6.

[93] A.J.P. Taylor, *English History 1914–1945*, Oxford, Oxford University Press, 1965.

[94] *Report from the Select Committee on the General Nursing Council together with the Proceedings of the Committee and Minutes of Evidence*, House of Commons, London, HMSO, 1925.

[95] Ibid., p. 26, paras 248–250.

[96] Ibid., p. 29, paras 286–289.

[97] E. Bedford Fenwick, 'Religious Liberty', editorial, *Nursing Record and Hospital World*, 1899, pp. 345–346, October 28.

[98] E. Bedford Fenwick, 'A Selfish Age', editorial, *Nursing Record and Hospital World*, 1900, p. 145 August 25.

[99] E. Bedford Fenwick, 'Nurses Keep your Souls Alive!', editorial, *British Journal of Nursing*, 1924, p. 1, January.

[100] E. Bedford Fenwick, 'Patients First: is Nursing a Profession or a Trade?', editorial, *British Journal of Nursing*, 1931, p. 57, March.

[101] E. Bedford Fenwick, 'The Sacred Vocation of Nursing', editorial, *British Journal of Nursing*, 1933, p. 149, June.

[102] E. Bedford Fenwick, 'The Life of the Spirit in Hospitals', editorial, *British Journal of Nursing*, 1937, p. 29, February.

[103] E. Bedford Fenwick, 'American Nurses', editorial, *Nursing Record and Hospital World*, 1896, pp. 205–206, March 14.

[104] L.L. Dock, 'Nurses Directories', *Nursing Record and Hospital World*, 1895, pp. 255–256, April 20; L.L. Dock, 'A National Association for Nurses and its Legal Organisation',1896, *Nursing Record and Hospital World*, p. 208–209, March 14; L.L. Dock, Letter from Miss Lavinia L. Dock, R.N., in Bedford Fenwick, E. 'A Demand for Justice for the State Registered Nurse', editorial, *British Journal of Nursing*, 1943, p. 61, June.

[105] *Report from the Select Committee on Registration of Nurses together with the Proceedings of the Committee, Minutes of Evidence and Appendix*, House of Commons, London, HMSO, 1905, pp. 40–45, paras 777–839.

[106] M.A. Nutting, L.L. Dock, *A History of Nursing in Two Volumes*, New York and London, The Knickerbocker Press, G.P. Putnam's Sons, 1907.

[107] P. Kropotkin, *Mutual Aid a Factor of Evolution*, London, William Heinemann, 1902, p. 92.

[108] E. Bedford Fenwick, 'Nursing at the World's Fair', *Nursing Record*, 1893, pp. 52–59, January 26; E. Bedford Fenwick, 'Women', *Nursing Record and Hospital World*, 1896, p. 423, May 23.

[109] E. Bedford Fenwick, 'The Sacred Vocation of Nursing', editorial, *British Journal of Nursing*, 1933, p. 149, June; M. Breay, 'Duty', *Nursing Record and Hospital World*, 1897, pp. 335–336, April 24.

[110] 'Trade Unions and the Nursing Profession', *Nursing Times*, 1926, p. 1165, December 18; 'Trade Unions and the Nursing Profession', editorial, *Nursing Times*, 1926, pp. 1165–1166, December 18; 'The Labour Conference', *British Journal of Nursing*, 1927, pp. 42–44, February.

[111] 'Trade Unions and the Nursing Profession', editorial, *Nursing Times*, 1926, pp. 1165–1166, December 18.

[112] 'The Labour Conference', *British Journal of Nursing*, 1927, pp. 42–44, February.

[113] A.M. Rafferty, *The Politics of Nursing Knowledge*, London, Routledge, 1996, pp. 28–31.

Chapter 4

From registration to the new National Health Service: the age of reports, 1923–1948

From the date of the Nurses' Registration Act, and the foundation of the General Nursing Council in 1919, it became a legal requirement that nurse training be standardised and systematised in England and Wales. This was achieved by the introduction of a national training syllabus and examination. This chapter will examine how this apprenticeship training developed, by focusing on this first syllabus, and consider to what extent Nightingale's principles still dominated. From 1923 until 1948 a variety of committees debated whether nursing and nurse training should be reconstructed, primarily in order to improve recruitment. The reports subsequently published will be discussed, with particular reference to the profession's response, the debate over the apprenticeship method of training, and the ensuing debate over nursing's art and science.

A prescribed national syllabus for state registration

The Nurses' Registration Act 1919 had vested authority in a General Nursing Council to make rules requiring candidates for admission to the register to have undergone prescribed training and possess a prescribed experience in the nursing of the sick. The draft for the first syllabus of subjects for examination was drawn up by the Education and Examination Committee of the General Nursing Council, under the chairmanship of Alicia Lloyd-Still, Matron of St Thomas's Hospital, and presented at a meeting at the Ministry of Health on March 24, 1921.[1] The recommendations from the committee, which were formally adopted, were as follows:

First, that a schedule signed by the chairman and matron of the hospital or, in the case of Poor Law infirmaries signed by the medical superintendent and matron, was required from every nurse applying to enter the state examination certifying that the applicant had passed through the educational curriculum prescribed by the council and was of good character.

Second, that the subjects for state examination should include anatomy, physiology, elementary science (including hygiene, bacteriology, sanitation), first aid, gynaecology, materia medica, dietetics, surgical nursing and medical nursing. Candidates were required to pass an examination on all these subjects included in the syllabus issued by the council. The state examination was to cover two days, the first day of two sessions would be concerned with written papers, the second day of two sessions would contain a *viva voce* examination and an examination on practical nursing.

At this meeting at the Ministry of Health it was agreed to convene an informal conference a month later, under the auspices of the General Nursing Council, in order to discuss the exact content of the first syllabus of training, and affiliation schemes, This would be what the *Nursing Times* called 'the largest, most representative and most important' informal conference of hospital matrons and sister tutors. Entitled 'Making the Future Nurse', it was held on April 28, 1921. The proceedings were published in the *British Nursing Journal*, the *Nursing Times* and the *Nursing Mirror and Midwives' Journal* the following week.[2]

Alicia Lloyd-Still introduced the discussion: 'In the past, each Training School has been a law unto itself – a condition which has resulted in a parochial interest and a widely varying standard.' In the national interest, it was now necessary to unite behind 'a fully organised body with a definite system of teaching and training', that developed the nurse's mind as well as her 'heart and hand'. The system that produced the best kind of nurse would need to avoid too theoretical a training, and pitfalls likely to produce either a clinical assistant or an efficient machine at the expense of 'the vitalising spirit'.[3]

The aim of the syllabus was to stimulate and foster the nurse's powers of development; to increase her capacity by a more extensive knowledge of subjects – scientific, social, practical – relevant to nursing; and to train her mind to a wider outlook than merely the institutional, bringing together preventative work with curative work, in order to foster the nation's health. This would allow the nurse, at the end of her training, to choose various branches of future work.

What nurse training schools had been doing individually, to a greater or lesser extent depending on the institution, was now to be systematised into one national syllabus of apprenticeship training for all to follow. The syllabus was to cover the three-year training period. The first year would commence with a preliminary school course of six to eight weeks. Tuition would ensure continuity and teach the connection of the various subjects. Anatomy, physiology, elementary science and even food values would be explained and linked with theoretical and practical nursing.

For example, all nurses, wherever they trained, would have introductory lectures on cell structure, the skeleton, joints, muscles and skin. These topics would arouse interest in clothing, personal hygiene, care of feet and hands and even methods of cleaning, and would be relevant to a lecture on the practical care of the patient. Similarly, instruction on the preparation of instruments or the dressing of wounds would be preceded by a knowledge of infecting agents, tissue reactions, methods of disinfection and sterilisation. For intelligent understanding some knowledge was needed of impurities of air, atmospheric pressure and heat, and illustrations of these principles might be sought naturally and usefully in the warming and ventilation of the ward. So, too, treatment of the alimentary canal for gavage and lavage would involve a knowledge and understanding of its structure and function as well as food values and residue, and the nature and character of water.

Explanation of the therapeutic action of drugs should be preceded by knowledge of the processes of absorption and metabolism. Correct administration of drugs meant that the nurse needed to be able to read the prescription, measure the dose accurately and know whether the measure used was imperial or metric. Instruction would be incomplete without a practical demonstration of the local application of drugs, detailing the various methods used. All these subjects were in close continuity. Hence, the widespread prevalence of venereal disease warranted knowledge and understanding of its effect on the community and its treatment and presumed an understanding of the reproductive system and of gynaecology.

Lectures and practical demonstrations would not rob the ward sister of her vital teaching role or impose a method on her that she would not necessarily have chosen. The teaching and personal approval of the ward sister was to form the basis of the nurse's practical training, guaranteed by the Nurse's Chart, a schedule of practical instruction and experience, accompanying the syllabus. Exclusively oral instruction could not replace practical teaching and ward experience. Indeed, some hospital authorities might use the ward method exclusively; they could use the syllabus as a guide to systematic teaching and subsequent examination.

The syllabus for the second and third years of training was to be in the hands of specialists for the most part. General headings rather than specification for curriculum content allowed for variation. There were diverse suggestions as to the curriculum content: some suggested materia medica, bacteriology, hospital economy; others wanted the focus to be on diseases and respective nursing care, for example the eye, ear, nose and throat or orthopaedics. The examinations had not yet been worked out but it was anticipated that they would begin in 1923 as voluntary examinations, and would become compulsory after July 1924 for all nurses desiring to register. Fourteen examination centres were approved.

According to the next speaker, Miss Dowbiggin, Matron of Edmonton Union Infirmary, and member of the GNC, the training syllabus would prepare

Poor Law hospital nurses to compete on equal terms with nurses trained in voluntary hospitals. Because of the development of more highly complex methods of diagnosis and treatment as well as the low percentage of medical staff, Poor Law hospital nurses often needed to assume more responsibility for the care and treatment of patients. The syllabus would enable nurses to learn about health as much as disease. Poor Law schools had the added bonus of preparing nurses who wanted to specialise in massage, midwifery or ante-natal work in a fourth year, as well as tuberculosis nursing, cancer, venereal disease, x-ray work, medical electricity, infant care and public health work.

Participants at the conference hoped that the proposed syllabus would raise the standard of the nursing profession and standardise nurse education. The Matron of St Luke's Hospital, Bradford, Miss Rodgers, suggested that the good theoretical nurse was almost invariably a good practical nurse. This comment evoked disagreement as well as applause.[4] Lloyd-Still herself believed that the moral ethos of service was absolutely fundamental: 'We realize that the finest, most fruitful work is done when the spirit of service is the energising force, and we would foster that spirit that we may not fall short of the great traditions of our predecessors.'[5]

Lloyd-Still's position as Matron of St Thomas's Hospital, together with her own spiritual values,[6] meant that the first national syllabus for training nurses was based on the principles instituted by Nightingale at St Thomas's. The systematic practical training developed under Lloyd-Still, and the first Sister Tutor, Marion Agnes Gullan.[7] Under Lloyd-Still, St Thomas's training had stayed true to the spirit of Florence Nightingale, the 'emphasis was throughout placed on *practical* efficiency'. The St Thomas's School 'had an indirect, albeit profound, influence on the whole of nurse training under the General Nursing Council'.[8] Indeed, State Registration was perceived to be the crystallisation of Nightingale's action.[9] It is interesting to speculate whether Nightingale's fears about registration would have been allayed by this new system. Because of the influence of leaders from the Nightingale School, whose values remained those of the tradition Nightingale herself had espoused, the training sought to maintain her ethos and synthesis of art and science. This was the Nightingale model transmitted nationally, a conversion to the principles Nightingale had preached: mind, heart and hand.

The proposed training and experience was set out by the General Nursing Council for England and Wales in 1923, and it approved a large number of institutions in which the prescribed training could be carried out. This was specified in the first *Syllabus of Lectures and Demonstrations for Education and Training in General Nursing*, issued by the GNC in 1923.[10] This syllabus of training was advisory, rather than mandatory, and was based on the subject content discussed at the 'Making the Future Nurse' conference. It included the Nurse's Chart.

The Nurse's Chart was a sheet of paper, marked into columns. The type of each ward (surgical, medical, children and gynaecology) was entered along the top. Downwards were detailed the various procedures which the nurse was expected to become proficient in. Examples of this were: domestic ward management, bedmaking and bedbathing, artificial feeding, enemas, injections, infusions, drug administration and dressings. The chart stated that it was drawn up as a suggestion by training schools. It was to be retained by the nurse, marked by the teaching sister, and deposited in the matron's office by the nurse at the conclusion of her work on each ward. As the sister taught the nursing points she was requested to mark in the column descriptive of her ward (that is, whether it was medical, surgical, children's or midwifery or gynaecology). One stroke, '/', was to signify that the nurse had been shown but was not proficient in the detail; two strokes, crossed, 'X', indicated that the nurse had been taught and was proficient. The 'X' was accompanied by the sister's initial.

Unlike the syllabus of training, the *Syllabus of Subjects for Examination for the Certificate of General Nursing*, produced the same year, was mandatory. The Nurse's Chart was appended to it.[11] The syllabus for examination was to cover three years. The table for the first year allowed for the first three sections to be linked up as a whole and taught in relationship to each other by one teacher, the sister tutor, for example. Reading downwards, headings formed the course of lectures on which the student would eventually be examined. This introduction affirmed the importance of hospital economy and ward management. District nursing, public sanitation and public health were also emphasised.

The council realised the value of lectures and demonstrations by medical practitioners and other experts on their special subjects, but attached great importance to lectures and teaching being given by fully trained nurses: matrons, sister tutors, ward sisters and so on. It was they who would bring the 'true nursing outlook' gained by personal knowledge and practical experience.[12] Also necessary were revision classes, correction of notebooks and personal supervision at all stages of training.

The examination was divided into two parts. The preliminary examination was to be taken by all probationers, at any time after the first year of training, whether training for the general nursing or the supplementary part of the register (fever nursing, mental nursing, mental defective nursing, sick children's nurses). Anatomy and physiology, hygiene and the first part of the theory and practice of nursing were covered. The final examination for general nurses contained the remainder of the syllabus, and the subjects mentioned in the attached Nurse's Chart, but with the exception of the optional column for the second and third years' training in the training schedule. Explanatory notes stated that the classification was condensed to permit free interpretation.

Scientific terms were used for convenience but were to be interpreted, especially in the first year, in an elementary way, and as much as possible in relation to practical details. Bacteriology was to be taught as part of elementary hygiene or theoretical nursing by the physician or surgeon as part of the senior course of lectures. Operating theatre technique should be taught under surgical technique and include actual theatre experience. If this was not possible, extra lectures and demonstrations should be given.

Ward management, including methods of cleaning and disinfection, could be taught under the categories of hygiene and practical nursing, while hospital economy could be taught under the categories of elementary hygiene and household science. Communicable diseases should be taught in the first year in connection with hygiene and public health, and taught again in the medical lectures in the second and third years in relation to pathology. Diseases and feeding of infants and children should have a place in the syllabus under general diseases in all three years, and not necessarily be treated as a separate subject. Public sanitation and public health would be introduced for elementary treatment under hygiene, or included in a course of chemistry or elementary science.

The syllabus was signed by the Minister of Health on March 16.[13] In the following months there was some debate over the position of existing bona fide nurses, those nurses who possessed adequate knowledge and experience of nursing the sick by reason of length of practice: how the government would make provision for them, and how they would be granted recognition by the General Nursing Council. Dr Chapple's amendment allowed previously experienced nurses who could show three years bona fide practice to register.[14]

During the 1930s and 1940s preliminary training schools became established. Minimum requirements for lectures for the preliminary examination, specified by the GNC, were: anatomy – 8 lectures; physiology – 8 lectures; hygiene – 6 lectures. Lectures for the final examination were given at set hours, which might fall on the student nurses on or off duty. For the final examination lectures were also specified: medicine – 10 lectures; surgery – 10 lectures; gynaecology – 6 lectures. Preliminary Training School, often seen as a convenient time to complete the syllabus for the preliminary state examination, increased in length and content by 1945. Study days and block study were also gradually introduced to free nurses from ward responsibilities.[15]

As the system developed the nurse's training was not merely seen as the mechanistic passing of examinations, it involved a strong personal component, and was designed for individual achievement and competence. Ward reports and records of practical experience were tools by which the nurse was individually known to ward sisters and charge nurses, and also matrons. The nurse was supervised, her report and record of instruction and practical experience was written and recorded by the ward sister and charge nurse, in the nurse's presence, and presented to the matron by the student personally. Personal interviews at regular intervals with ward sisters or charge nurses and, notably, matrons meant the work, skills, knowledge and attitudes of student nurses were closely and intimately monitored and individually known.

The nurse's learning was graduated. She started in the classroom and ward with elementary knowledge of subjects such as hygiene and anatomy and physiology. She learned the more basic tasks of bedbathing, mouth care and bedmaking first. Her experience over the three years was gradually built up, the intention being to relate what she learned theoretically in the classroom to her practical experience on the ward. As the nurse progressed she also advanced. She learned more complex diseases and their treatments and the nursing care procedures associated with them. As she was initiated into a tradition of practical care she learned to approach the human body with respect and sensitivity. The student nurse was expected to discuss and find reasons for what she was taught to do.

Nursing in the inter-war years

As the British nursing profession settled into a common training system united by a shared framework of values, concerns about nursing shortages and an increasing need for nurses in the aftermath of the First World War continued, and became the preoccupation of various committees and commissions.

The Lancet Commission was set up in 1930 to report on the shortage of candidates for hospital work, and to suggest means by which the shortage could be overcome.[16] The intention of the commission was to adapt the current system rather than recommend any fundamental reconstruction. That the commission was in sympathy with the vocational tradition was made clear in the discussion on nursing history with which the report began.[17] One of those serving on subcommittees was the textbook writer Evelyn Pearce.

By 1930 it was clear that doctors, matrons and ward sisters were deeply involved with, and committed to, the apprenticeship training. In many hospitals a sister tutor or matron gave all lectures in preparation for the preliminary state examination, while honorary medical staff lectured second- and third-year probationer nurses without fee.[18] Nursing shortages meant obsession with getting the work done, so that junior staff were not getting teaching in the individual care of patients, and senior nurses sacrificed their own leisure. Notwithstanding these pressures, it had remained 'an axiom in the nursing profession that the patient comes first'.[19]

Part of the difficulty in recruiting nurses was thought to result from a conflict of ideals.[20] Senior nurses thought the hardness of the apprenticeship was an essential part of the system which had admittedly produced nurses unsurpassed throughout the world for perception, skill and sense of responsibility. Ward sisters were convinced of the need for routine and long hours to nurture the vocational spirit, including strict discipline, uncritical obedience, punctuality, and loyalty to superiors and the institution served. This approach conflicted with the modern desire for a critical mind, a developed personality, wider interests and a normal social life. The moral ethos was often stifled by bureaucratic rules, regimented discipline and misuse of vocation:

> Ward sisters, especially those who have given their lives to hospital service without seeking administrative promotion, may be intolerant of attempts to induce them to allow to others a discipline less severe than that which they willingly impose on themselves. Their conception of vocation is high and rigid, and their attitude to the probationer is biased by their anxiety to preserve for the service of the hospital the whole of her available strength, vitality, and single-minded interest. [21]

Indeed, some witnesses suggested that the shortage of suitable applicants for nursing stemmed not from falling numbers of applicants, but from a growing need for suitable nurses, defined as: 'Some vocational impulse, a certain level of intelligence, a degree of dexterity are essential.'[22]

The commission's search for the causes of the problems in the nursing profession revealed many differences in the practices of hospitals: inequality of pay and conditions; petty restrictions; indifference to changing expectations of women; and a general failure to coordinate entry into nursing with the later stages of school life. But there were also positive findings, particularly the genuine sense of vocation which had 'so far prevented the shortage of suitable candidates from lowering at all the standards of nursing in the country'.[23]

The commission accepted the importance of the authentic vocational ethos for future recruitment and training, provided public health and administration formed part of the calling: 'It was impressed upon us by all the witnesses best qualified to speak for the profession that a sense of vocation is essential and that the standards of the profession could not be maintained merely by an economic appeal.'[24]

The *British Medical Journal*, reporting on the commission's findings, agreed wholeheartedly with this comment: 'In conclusion, the Commission makes one remark which all the time we felt needed to be made: that in nursing a sense of vocation is essential, and that the standards of the profession are not to be maintained merely by economic appeal.'[25]

A year later, an editorial in the *Lancet* found the need for change to be less pressing, because of the influx of 'suitable young women' into nursing; a possible consequence of the depression, the improvement of conditions in certain hospitals, and the publicity given to the report itself. The journal hoped that the commission would be effective still in building a nursing profession 'unencumbered by traditions which have lost their significance while retaining those which still have value'.[26]

The Interdepartmental Committee on Nursing Services, chaired by the Earl of Athlone, for the Ministry of Health Board of Education, was set up in 1937 to examine the shortage of nurses.[27] Athlone reported that the shortage of nurses was neither due to wastage in the probationer period, nor to a shortage of applicants – twice as many nurses were admitted to the register in 1937 as in 1926 – but to a demand that had outpaced supply. Hospitals had expanded, legislation in public health had increased and so had public demand for nurses. All this contributed to a growing demand for nursing services.

But vocation was no longer enough: 'in recent years the social and industrial structure of the nation has undergone such radical changes that the nursing profession can no longer rely upon the "sense of vocation" as the chief stimulus to recruitment'.[28] The status of nursing should be improved, by ameliorating remuneration and conditions of service, to enable it to compete with other careers open to women. This did not mean dismissing the vocation, rather it was to ensure vocation was not exploited:

> From the very nature of her calling there must of necessity be demands, and at times heavy demands, made on her for self sacrifice and physical and mental endurance, but it is surely wrong that in any branch of the profession her financial rewards should be even indirectly dependent upon the amount of charitable funds contributed for the relief of the sick, and that her generosity of outlook should be dimmed when she compares the conditions in her own profession with those existing in other callings.[29]

Discipline should be self-imposed, 'founded upon the conception of a nurse as a reasonable adult anxious to live up to the high traditions of service for which the nursing profession in this country is justly famous'.[30] The committee was impressed:

> by the evidence which has indirectly emerged of the high ideals of devotion to duty, self-sacrifice, and loyalty which animate the nursing profession. British nursing at its best is the admiration of the world, and it is our sincere hope that the recommendations we have made will play their part in re-establishing in the eyes of the public the dignity of a noble profession, and in assisting nurses themselves to obtain those material rewards without which happiness, contentment and *esprit de corps* cannot truly exist.[31]

The spirit of the profession, the *esprit de corps*, was not an excuse for denying material rewards. Not all nurses would have disagreed.[32]

Nursing in the war years

The Horder Committee (the Nursing Reconstruction Committee) was set up by the Royal College of Nursing in 1941, chaired by Lord Horder, and published four reports, in 1942, 1943 (two), and 1949.[33] The remit of Horder was to consider how to implement Athlone's recommendations and suggest further adjustments to the nursing services in the light of the war and post-war years. A small section of the medical profession thought that nurse training was becoming too theoretical, producing pseudo-doctors. They thought nurses needed only 'technical skill in the craft of nursing' to carry out doctors' prescribed orders.[34]

Horder rejected this. It would be wrong to lower standards and turn the nurse into a doctor's attendant. The nurse needed to know why she was treating the patient in a certain way, she also needed to be a health educator. Nursing was a profession parallel to medicine with an increasingly important role in the health of the nation.

Horder also rejected the other extreme, that the training of nurses should be similar to the training of teachers, with nurse training schools under the auspices of universities like teacher training colleges. The training of teachers was fundamentally different to the training of nurses. Not only would universities not accept candidates with lower qualifications, but teachers in training, unlike nurses, made no contribution to the service. Some members of the committee argued that 'the essentially *practical* nature of nursing might also be lost sight of'.[35]

The committee considered criticisms of the apprenticeship method of training.[36] These included suggestions that nursing involved unintelligent repetitive work; exploitation by the hospital and student overload. There was not enough time to observe or be taught and there was insufficient background knowledge to benefit from the mass of clinical material at the early stages. The questing spirit, so vital to produce the best nurses, was not encouraged by this method and technical performance was pursued without ensuring underlying knowledge and understanding.

Arguments refuted these criticisms, however. Although the profession would never be content with 'the dunce with clever hands', nursing was essentially a practical art requiring skilled technique. Continual theoretical training overlooked the supreme value to the student nurse of uninterrupted periods of supervised practical nursing, during which the student nurse was concerned exclusively with the patient's welfare. Repetitive tasks did not become routine because of the individuality of patients. During her apprenticeship the nurse became increasingly skilled in observation of both the physical and mental state of the patient, and she also became increasingly familiar with procedures.

There needed to be a middle way: to keep the apprenticeship model, but also to make the nurse a student first and an apprentice second. This could be achieved by a planned programme, a syllabus and practical work, that took account of the student nurse's learning needs first, and then secured the appropriate practical experience. The committee advocated the block system, periods when the student would be free from nursing responsibilities.[37]

The linchpin of the whole scheme was the ward sister, upon whom depended the quality and value of the nurse's training. The ward sister needed time to impart her knowledge to the student nurse, and so should not be overworked. Every ward sister should attend a course on the psychology of teaching. The inclusion of normal psychology into nursing training would help to rectify the problem of faulty methods filtering through. A case assignment method, whereby the student cared for the complete needs of a group of less severely ill patients, rather than work assignment, was recommended.[38]

Although affirming the apprenticeship method, Horder also argued for the need for an honours course in nurse training to stretch bright candidates.[39] But there was dissension: some opposed such a course, fearing from the example of American and Canadian nursing schools, where, despite precautions, the achievement of practical skill was sacrificed to the pursuit of academic knowledge.

Opinions of student nurses and potential recruits, sought by Horder, showed variation. Student nurses were prepared to give their service to the hospital in exchange for a competent training. They expected to be treated as students rather than primarily as employees, and were prepared to forego a high remuneration during training. They appreciated the need for some discipline at work, but looked for adequate off-duty time to pursue a social life.[40] The attitudes of schoolgirls, evident from their essays, argued Horder, reflected 'ignorance and prejudice' against nursing. They were not attracted by appeals to glamour or romance, and lacked enthusiasm for the historical aspect. They were, however, attracted to the scientific and community, social and public health opportunities, and were willing to study and work hard provided there were adequate rewards.[41] To find out the views of 'business girls', questionnaires were sent to forty or fifty London clerical workers. Nursing was considered by them to be 'a noble vocation' but too demanding. There was also parental prejudice, a lack of concrete information, feelings of personal unsuitability, fear of loss of social life and concerns about poor pay and conditions. Young women generally regarded work as 'dull routine, qualifying them for their weekly wage packet', unconnected to their personal lives, 'lightly undertaken and as lightly thrown over for something else'.[42]

This view found support. An editorial in the *British Journal of Nursing*, argued that children's ambitions were excited by the cinema, and the 'psychological' approach to discipline spared the rod and so spoiled the child;

as a result, nursing had become derided in the press and shunned by public opinion.[43] However, the responses to the questionnaire, published in the appendix to the report, might question this opinion. According to the responses, ordinary 'business girls' did not dismiss the concept of the nursing vocation, rather they dismissed the unjust conditions which the concept of vocation was used to justify. Respondents considered nursing to be a vocation, rather than a career. The idea of vocation itself was not off-putting, but the working conditions were: nursing was seen as 'A vocation which, if working conditions were improved, would be within the powers of many more people than is the case today.'[44]

In this respect, these findings were supported by a wartime survey about nursing recruitment, which found that many young women would be willing to become nurses if deterrents, particularly relatively long working hours and poor pay, were removed.[45] Moreover, the study of 490 student nurses found that half had become nurses because of a longstanding wish, a smaller number because of a desire to help humanity and relieve suffering, or as a career that offered opportunities for 'getting on'. The majority of respondents thought nursing was a career rather than a job. Many felt it was worthwhile; and a minority commented on the lack of freedom and the long working hours. A smaller minority mentioned poor pay as a disadvantage, a lower proportion than the earlier survey, and some nurses mentioned parental opposition on the grounds of hard work, poor pay and the necesssity for leaving home. Student nurses emphasised that recruitment publicity needed to be realistic and 'that nursing should be represented less as an easy and pleasant job and more as a job that was worthwhile and of service to the community'.[46]

To make nursing more attractive, Horder recommended student status, although this did not mean that the student should be withdrawn from practical training. The aim was to redress the balance, and counter the traditional reliance of hospitals on student nurse labour. To achieve this, Horder recommended a job analysis of nursing to find out what the work entailed and who was the best person to do it.[47] Nurse training should teach the art and practice of nursing as well as the theory needed for its intelligent execution. It should develop in the nurse a sense of mutual and personal responsibility, so that the nurse could function as both an individual and as a member of a team. Student status could not, however, be standardised.[48]

The Horder Report was generally disregarded by the profession. According to Rosemary White, the nursing historian, '[Horder] could, and possibly should, have been seen as proposing fundamental changes to the fabric of nursing, the point was missed'. In White's opinion, Athlone and later Wood were regarded as 'tablets of stone', steeped in authoritarian tradition, whereas the Horder reports were more like 'pillars of salt'.[49] They melted away. Both Athlone and Horder 'insisted on the essential need to keep nursing at all levels on a practical rather than an academic one, although Horder understood the need for theory'. For White, this reflected the educational system of the period which in the post-war period was the province of an élite, directed towards the production of graduates in the traditional professions. The emphasis was on the arts and humanities, the sciences were secondary, and the social sciences had hardly taken shape. University education was highly theoretical 'to provide knowledge for the sake of knowledge' rather than for technical or vocational application. White considers that Horder was aware of a growing technology, but 'most nurses were not aware of any level between "practical" and "academic" and considered theory to be too remote from the everyday needs of the patient to be relevant'. Yet, Horder had considered the arguments against the traditional model of education and, even so, concluded that change could be built on the existing apprenticeship system.

The question was whether the vocation might be lost in the necessary reforms. Kathleen Kitchin, a barrister-at-law, a former physician and medical psychologist, summarised the argument: nursing was, even then, a vocation, a concept which was easily degraded to mean poverty, hard work and no pay. Obedience came to mean 'bullying and petty restrictions – instead of the overriding compulsion of the clear call'. So now, nursing was to be a career – or a trade – to redress the degradations. But 'maybe, much of the baby is going to be thrown away with the bathwater – as usually happens when great reforms are afoot'.[50]

Nursing after the war: setting up the National Health Service

The end of the Second World War brought a desire from outside the profession that nursing be reconstituted after a clean break with its vocational tradition. Even in 1945 nursing had remained true to Nightingale's philosophy. A commercial attitude to recruitment and retention was now needed, and a Ministry of Health inquiry was called for.[51]

The Committee on the Recruitment and Training of Nurses was set up in 1946, under the chairmanship of Sir Robert Wood, Chancellor of the University of Southampton, with Miss E. Cockayne, Matron of the Royal Free Hospital, as a part-time member. This followed the massive impact of the Second World War and was set against the background of the impending establishment of the National Health Service and free access to health care for all. The increased demand for nurses that was likely to ensue meant there was a need for a comprehensive review of the nursing service. This was to include a survey of recruitment and training of nurses covering an examination of the proper task of the nurse and training required, the annual intake of nurses needed, from which groups of the population they should come, and how wastage could be minimised.[52]

A scientific method was used to obtain data. There was an increase of 15,000 in the total nursing force between 1938 and 1945. Recruitment problems were due to the increased demand for nurses. Interviews and statements from unselected nurses, student nurses and ex-student nurses, showed that there was an atmosphere of dissatisfaction and discontent in many nurse training schools: 'Generally speaking, there is a considerable sense of frustration, and discipline is felt to be harsh and cramping and quite out of accord with modern notions of personal freedom.' This criticism did not apply to 'disciplinary requirements in periods of duty, but more to the restraints imposed upon a nurse's freedom in her personal life when she is not on duty'.[53]

The contract that most student nurses were compelled to sign at the beginning of their training, 'with all its vague but ominous legal implications', prejudiced nurses against their future career. Senior nursing staff seemed to be out of touch with the outlook of the young. Both student nurses and qualified nurses held similar opinions, the only difference being one of degree. Those who stayed in nursing, stayed because of direct pressure from parents 'or their own sense of vocation'. It was not nursing itself that caused such dissatisfaction, but the conditions of training. Selective interviews of ex-student nurses who had left nursing found that the 'crux of the whole problem of wastage seemed to lie in the sphere of human relationships'.

A common complaint was the lack of help, cooperation, encouragement or sympathy from senior staff. Many senior staff were described as 'narrow-minded', 'old-fashioned', 'sour' and 'bad-tempered', humiliating students in the presence of colleagues and patients, and making the student's life 'a misery'. Several senior staff were described as 'hard-hearted' and 'inhuman', refusing requests without explanation. Complaints concerned the amount of cleaning, being treated as inferiors, petty restrictions, taking blame for what had not been taught, and a resulting atmosphere of evasiveness and dishonesty. Rigid conformity made it difficult to preserve individuality.[54]

The type of discipline pervading training schools was the most important cause of wastage. It was derived from the self-abnegation of 'a conventual tradition', an insularity that was 'preserved more or less unaltered by the profound changes in social outlook which have affected the community as a whole'.[55]

Wood rejected this tradition. To reduce wastage, nurses should no longer be regarded as junior employees subject to an outworn system of discipline. They should be accorded student status 'with the conditions such status implies, so far as the intrinsic requirements of nurse training permit'. There should be a new selection procedure for student nurses, and a method of selection to senior posts which would ensure that only those who had the capacity to develop satisfactory human relationships were appointed. There should be improvements in diet, amenities and accommodation, and the training day should be reduced to a more 'normal' working day by the introduction of a three-shift system.[56]

Wood questioned the prevailing objective of nurse training, to prepare nurses for bedside nursing: 'This system is rooted in a tradition which knew little of preventative medicine or positive service for maintaining the health of the community.' The state policy of full employment meant that it was vital to minimise the incidence and after-effects of ill-health. This might involve a complete reorientation in primary nurse training as a preparation for work in all health fields, social, industrial and educational, as well as institutional.

The student nurse was a student in name only. Training was incidental to her daily activities: 'A substantial proportion of her time is spent on non-nursing duties which could be properly performed without any nurse-training at all.' Time spent on nursing practice, including some theory, was repetitive, and a reduction of the training period from three years to two years was recommended. The apprenticeship model was considered redundant as a way of inducting nurses into the science and art of nursing.[57]

Health nursing and sick nursing should be considered side by side, and the approach should be from the normal to the abnormal. The broader conception of health – health preservation and health prevention – should have a higher profile: 'that the individual must be regarded as a complete entity, body and mind: that the social as well as physical environment must be considered, and that positive health must be secured for families and communities as well as for individuals'. Hence, the preventative aspects of health care were to be integrated with the curative through the whole course of nurse training.[58]

But it was also recognised that there were an increasing number of chronic sick people and aged infirm in institutions and hospitals, suffering from the disabilities of old age. Wood suggested that nurses who worked in this 'disheartening' branch of nursing 'with a devotion inconceivable in any other profession' were to be respected. In Wood's view, there was little economic value in such work: nursing the chronic sick 'is now wholly "humanitarian", for patients do not recover and go back to work, so a reduction in the patient's stay yields no economic return'. The assumption was that if the patient's stay could be made to yield economic return there would be an economic inducement to endow medical and nursing treatment more generously.[59]

Wastage was not due merely to the unsuitability of the individual, but to the individual's interaction with the total environment. Better techniques needed to be implemented to disclose instability or unsuitability of temperament, as well as educational and intellectual inadequacy. Selection tests were proposed, based on accumulated knowledge in comparable fields, and devised by psychologists, through interview, questionnaire and standardised intelligence tests.[60]

Wood's positivist and scientific outlook, which was impatient of what were considered to be outdated and irrelevant values, sought a radical modernisation of nursing; the nursing profession, however, clung to its traditional values. In the view of nursing leaders, the virtuous character of the nurse remained essential. A total of 132 report forms, completed and sent to the working party by ward sisters, assistant matrons and matrons of London County Council general hospitals, showed what nurses considered to be important qualities, and were analysed by the report. Qualities mentioned repeatedly, in descending order, were: kind to patients; interest in work; reliable; keen, or keen to learn; neat and tidy; capable or intelligent; conscientious; 'good' worker; willing or anxious to please; trustworthy. Although recognising the importance of 'nurse quality', the working party believed it was possible to devise tests to assess such characteristics, and claimed to have carried out several experiments to throw further light on 'nurse quality'.[61]

Wood considered the apprenticeship model, with its routine and repetitive duties, was low in status. The assistant nurse role (which came into being in 1943) should not be perpetuated and nursing orderlies should replace the assistant nurse. This raised the question of the nature of nursing. The correct ratio of nursing orderlies to trained nurses could only be determined if nursing work was subjected to a job-analysis and definition, or rather, redefinition: 'Such definition would be required in order to specify exactly what routine and repetitive nursing duties and techniques in hospitals and elsewhere could properly be undertaken by such an auxiliary grade.'[62]

Despite these radical recommendations, and notwithstanding criticism of some authoritarian discipline, Wood also recognised the key function of the traditional role of the ward sister in setting the tone of the hospital, and acknowledged that this depended on her personal qualities:

> On her ultimately depends the efficient administration of the institution, and on her falls the burden of cultivating friendly and co-operative relationships between students, staff and patients. The tone and atmosphere of the ward or department and, therefore, the welfare of the patients are set by her personality and outlook. If she lacks the qualities needed for the sympathetic management of others in her charge, the entire organisation of the hospital will suffer.[63]

Wood's analysis was not scientific enough for one member of the committee, John Cohen, who sent a minority report to the Minister of Health.[64] The Minister asked for responses from interested parties; these were generally critical.[65]

E.E.P. MacManus, Matron of Guy's Hospital, made an immediate response in the *Nursing Times*.[66] She welcomed the work done, and saw the central issue as: 'how to control the incidence of sickness; how to give the right type of care to every type of patient and how to produce the right type of persons, nursing aids, orderlies, and domestics to carry out these tasks'. She accepted without question that doctors carried the ultimate responsibility for the sick.

MacManus believed that Wood confirmed Horder's view that more nurses were entering training every year, but there were factors underlying nursing shortages which Wood had not acknowledged: the enormous increase in hospital beds throughout Britain caused by the war-time expansion of hospitals; the increasing number of people seeking hospital care rather than care in their own homes, attributable to the break-up of homes, housing shortage, and shortage of domestic help. Misleading statistics aggregated figures and included the heavy wastage from mental hospitals and special hospitals in comparison to a much lower wastage from general hospitals, where the general nurse trained.

MacManus thought that there was too little mention of the abnormal times of the war period in the Wood Report. Not only were girls entering training from difficult home situations, but many were under eighteen: 'Seventeen years or even sixteen years is too early an age at which to introduce a girl to the sad and often hopeless side of the life of the sick. Her character has had no time to mature.' The shortage of trained nurses during the war years led not only to staffing levels below that of pre-war years, but also to 'trained staff' who were elderly returners through the civil nursing reserve. Although some had been experienced ward sisters some had not and their lack of knowledge increased the difficulties under which student nurses gained their training.

Added to this, the shortage of domestic staff meant that student nurses had to perform domestic duties which had been taken from them fifteen or twenty years before. Although the report had stated that a quarter of the nurse's time was spent on domestic tasks, this was not the fault of the student nurse or the employing hospital but of the government, failing to provide domestic labour despite representations from nursing leaders.

MacManus thought that the job analysis was crucial. It 'raises a vital question which must be decided, and the colour of the decision will paint the whole picture of British nursing for the next decade'. Wood was critical of 'sheer repetition' of ward work, but this was how student nurses learned their skills, by constant practising of them. As MacManus asked:

> Is our young nurse only learning to pass examinations, and to become a trained nurse, and not being a nurse during her training? Let us beware of the example of those countries that, in former years, over-developed the student aspect of the nurses' training, almost to the exclusion of the art of bedside nursing and the gain of

> a daily increasing sense of responsibility. Some of them have seen their error and are now rectifying it.

MacManus disliked the idea of the two-year basic training, fearing that it would lead to a 'Jack of all trades and master of none'. She also believed that training should widen, but if nurses were turned into students it would narrow. Horder sought to improve the profession and make a better nurse, while Wood sought merely to increase the number of nurses. This was setting up quantity over quality, and she did not believe a quality nurse could be produced without adequate experience: 'Medicine and surgery and medical and surgical nursing skill are the rock bottom of all sick nursing.'

The block system of training, advocated by Horder, which alternated periods set aside for academic study with 'long untroubled periods of regulated practical nursing training in the wards', and which was now in place, had been an effective reform. This too-short training period advocated by Wood was a fundamental weakness. Although public health nurses were important, ultimately the need would always be for the bedside nurse: 'let us not forget that at the last, to bed will all flesh come, and may there be a good nurse at the bedside', McManus concluded.

The King Edward's Hospital Fund for London sent comments to the minister.[67] The Wood Report had drawn conclusions, however innocently, about nurse wastage from evidence that was itself unreliable.[68] Displaced grievances meant that nurses who left might have given reasons such as poor food, inadequate social life, and difficult superiors, when they may, in fact, have not found satisfaction in their work; nurses who had a clearly defined reason for leaving, such as marriage or the home, did not mention other causes of dissatisfaction. The love of care for sick people had always been the main incentive to take up nursing and its rigours. It was right to temper the rigours, but the incentive should remain untouched. Wood did not achieve this:

> A test which should be applied to any proposed reorientation of training is the extent to which it allows the student nurse the deep satisfaction of feeling that she is becoming responsible for the well-being of her patients, with some degree of continuity and with steadily increasing skill. We do not find provision for this in the scheme outlined in the Report.[69]

According to the *Nursing Times*, the King's Fund had answered the question 'What is the proper task of the nurse?' with the reply 'that her primary task is to care for the sick and helpless under medical direction'.[70] The King's Fund did not agree that preventative measures and preparation for public health nursing would meet the urgent need for nurses. Neither did it support the suggestion that the primary nurse training would have to become preparatory to professional work in all health fields. It was a wasteful and mistaken policy to give full training in the skilled care of the sick to all engaged in social or educational work in the health fields: 'They maintain that reforms in nurse training should tend towards greater skill in actual bedside nursing, though with the ability also to educate the patient for healthy living after recovery.'

The King's Fund suggested that the real underlying causes of wastage were to do with impersonal ward routines and ill-related theoretical syllabuses.[71] The high wastage rate in the first year of training, and immediately after preliminary training school, was due to the protracted method of selection. The main deficiency in the system of training was the inadequate number of trained nurses compared to those in training. More reasonable hours and conditions as well as the possibility of regular bedside teaching and supervision were the only remedies. The main cause of the faulty human relations between some ward sisters and student nurses was due to shortage of trained staff and the subsequent strain on them induced by responsibilities and pressure of work and inadequate help.

There should be more appointments for those newly trained nurses who wanted to continue in practical nursing. The major wastage was the loss of the newly trained nurse from the hospital because she was induced, by grants and training opportunities, to move away from bedside nursing. There was a place for the untrained nursing auxiliary or assistant as a good bedside nurse, but she should not take full responsibility for the patient.

The King's Fund was in favour of student status if it meant that the training experience was arranged according to the student's educational needs and not dictated by the staffing needs of the hospital. However, it would not support the idea if it meant less involvement in the ward work and care of the patient, because this would not produce the good bedside nurse for which Britain had such a good reputation.

The Royal College of Nursing appreciated the modern scientific methods used by the Wood working party but believed that it had made insufficient allowance for the war. Some deductions were based on inadequate data: for example, causes of dissatisfaction and wastage should have considered opinions not only from ex-students but also the administrative nursing staff under whom they worked.[72]

There would be a continuing shortage of nurses because of a decrease in a number of women available, and an intensive job analysis of nursing from the perspective of the requirements of the patient was required. Preventative medicine together with advances in psychology, although important, should not take precedence over curative medicine. The demands for bedside care among the elderly would increase. Satisfactory staff relationships should become the subject of a study, and modern methods of work simplification should be introduced. The position of the student nurse as a learner should be recognised, and her practical work be designed for her benefit, but it would be more appropriate to use the term 'student nurse status' rather than 'student status'. The student nurse was primarily an employee of the hospital, controlled and supervised by the ward sister and administrative staff, rather than teaching staff, although close cooperation was required.[73]

The RCN did not agree with Wood that student nurses were more concerned with employee relations to superiors than training methods or examinations; neither did it agree that repetitive nursing tasks were for the sake of the organisation rather than the learning needs of the student. A distinction should be drawn between repetitive tasks that were for the sake of the hospital and repetition at different levels which was of educational value: 'Nursing by "case assignment" should ensure that this repetition was carried out in the interests of the student'. A three-year training leading to one register and including experimental methods, block and study day systems was needed, and nurse teacher training (the training of sister tutors, ward and departmental sisters) both in quality and numbers, should be reviewed.

The General Nursing Council Memorandum was 'no less disapproving'.[74] Statistics on wastage used by Wood were misleading because they related to the abnormal situation of the war period when many girls entered nursing not from a genuine desire to nurse but to avoid other forms of work. Wood did not mention 'dislike of contact with sick people' as a cause of wastage, a cause that only came to light after the student nurse had started training and which would occur regardless of conditions of training. The reinstitution of tests for intelligence, English and arithmetic, together with the personal interview with the matron of the training school, would ensure the suitability and aptitude of the candidate:

> Proper selection of candidates at the outset would reduce considerably the adverse propaganda spread by unsuitable candidates who fail to complete training and who are anxious that the blame for their failures should rest, not upon themselves but upon the hospital.[75]

The GNC agreed unanimously that student nurses should not be subjected to an outworn (it underlined 'outworn') system of discipline, although a certain degree of discipline was essential for the good of patients and the smooth running of the hospital, and necessary in the Nurses' Home for the welfare and comfort of all residents.

Nurses should not be burdened with domestic work, but this was due to the shortage of domestic labour during and after the war: 'This fact is greatly to be deplored and has without doubt been the cause of much wastage during training.' The student nurse should be responsible solely for the care of nursing equipment and such domestic duties that were part of the training during the preliminary course.

The GNC disagreed that the training should be shortened. Repetitive duties were an essential part of nurse training because they enabled a gradual acclimatisation. Every patient reacted differently to illness, and nursing procedures and treatments needed to reflect this. Nurse training was a progressive build-up of theoretical knowledge and practical duties: 'The elimination of so-called "repetitive duties" on which the reduced training is based would result in robbing the student nurse not only of the ability to nurse but of satisfaction in nursing.'[76]

The content of training outlined by Wood was broadly approved of by the GNC. The period of training should be laid down by the council, affiliated and associated schemes should cease, and examinations should remain. The basic nature of training was emphasised, the nurse's knowledge and skill would need to be established in the period following the three-year training. In the three-year training the nurse would be given the status of a student nurse, she would not undertake domestic duties, and a block or study system would be in operation. There would need to be adequate domestic staff and trained nurses. The student nurse would have a greater degree of supervision over the first eighteen months of training after which she would take more responsibility. The student's schedule of practical ward work, to be filled in and initialled by the ward sister, was a supervisory safeguard. In future more detailed records of the student nurse's experience during training should be kept.

The GNC argued that it was essential that the student nurse 'be allowed to *nurse* and to realise her own individual responsibility towards the patients in her care'.[77] Provided there were sufficient teaching staff to correlate theory and practice, and sufficient trained staff to ensure proper supervision, the GNC thought the system would produce a good nurse. The GNC agreed that training should be dictated by the needs of students rather than staffing arrangements. Nevertheless, training should not be under the control of independent directors, but remain with the matron of the principal hospital in each training unit: this relationship was proven. And the practical teaching of the student nurse while in the wards should continue to be undertaken by the ward sister.

Experimental centres, or external advisors on nurse education and research, were not wanted by the GNC. It was responsible for education and training, examination, registration, discipline, and inspection of training schools: 'Confusion would be created throughout the country unless national standards for the admission and training of student nurses continue to be laid down by the General Nursing Council.'[78] Yet the council agreed that university representatives could be elected under the existing constitution.

As to the proposal for the assistant nurse, the council disagreed that this level of second-grade nurse, although chiefly intended to nurse the chronic sick, was debarred from wider activities. The chief recruitment problem of these nurses, according to the GNC, was low pay. The GNC was quite clear that the assistant nurse should supplement the work of the registered nurse, but not absolve the student nurse or registered nurse from 'so-called "repetitive work" '. The GNC was concerned that closure of the roll for assistant nurses, and discontinuing the recruitment of pupil nurses, would mean that the chronic sick would be cared for by untrained people. The Wood Committee had given too little consideration to the important role of the assistant nurse. In response to Wood's question about whether to employ ancillary staff, the GNC suggested that '*ward* orderlies but not *nursing* orderlies' should be employed.[79]

White's analysis of the responses to Wood omits much of these detailed GNC arguments, but argues that the GNC, primarily composed of matrons, wanted matrons to remain in charge of schools of nursing, and wanted also to retain its functions in approving and inspecting training schools: 'There is an inescapable feeling of disapproval emanating from this memorandum, a primness and a preference for the maintenance of the status quo.'[80] But the GNC's concerns were supported by most of the organisations and individuals who responded, and reflected a similar concern with the needs of the patient. The GNC concluded the memorandum by stressing to the minister their view that Wood had not taken sufficient thought of the needs of the patient, 'which in fact must form the basis on which any conclusions relating to nurse training must be built'.[81]

The British Hospitals Association thought Wood was utopian and disregarded limiting factors.[82] Figures for wastage were directly related to the abnormality of the war emergency and were therefore artificial. The extent of the discipline and harshness of senior staff was exaggerated, although, admittedly, unnecessary harshness and petty restrictions did exist, and nurses' employment terms and conditions and working relationships needed improvement.

The association also disagreed that repetitive work was not in the interests of the student, and that her training was incidental to her duties. Unnecessary repetition should be eliminated but many aspects of nursing training could only be learned by intelligent repetition, particularly the capacity for observation. If the student did not understand this in training, she would still have much repetitive work to do when trained so that the issue would not then be student nurse wastage but newly-trained nurse wastage.[83]

In addition, the association questioned how student status would meet the nurse's need for practical training. The nurse who attended the ward as an observer would interfere with the work of the ward, and would not gain responsibility by gradual acquisition, which was an integral and continuous part of the training of the student. The aim of training was to 'produce a first-class and sympathetic practical bedside nurse and that the student should throughout her training acquire the fullest sense of responsibility to her patient'. This could only be acquired as a member of the ward team, at the bedside and through responsibility to the ward sister: 'To acquire her arts and skills the student in nursing must be as much apprentice as she is student.' Full student status would only bring the trainee misconceptions about the nature of her role. The report's lack of emphasis on the apprentice side as an essential of nurse training was 'disquieting and our apprehensions in this respect will, we believe, be very widely shared'. Revision of nurse training should build on the present system but take account of needs and limitations.[84]

The Nuffield Provincial Hospitals Trust welcomed the scientific methods used by the Wood working party as tools of a precise investigation resting on verifiable facts rather than opinion.[85] However, the members of the group (consisting of the principal of a large teacher training college, an educational psychologist, a medical practitioner, and two experienced nurses) had a fundamental criticism: 'the absence of the necessary data for an adequate answer to the first of the main questions which the working party was asked to examine, namely, "What is the proper task of a nurse?".'[86] The solution to nursing problems must be derived from verifiable data and required a precise definition of the essential duties of a nurse:

> for example, what type of man or woman is suited for nursing training; what training do they need; how can the professional life of a nurse be moulded to a form acceptable to modern young people and in harmony with their attitude to service; how can more efficient use be made of existing nurses, or how many more nurses may be required?[87]

According to the Nuffield Provincial Hospitals Trust, the value of Wood's work was limited because it failed to carry out a careful job analysis. Wood's 'rather naïve psychological analysis of nurse qualities' was no substitute. And, while the Nuffield Trust concurred with the proposal for 'student status', this did not imply that nurse training should become more theoretical. It should be practical, in hospitals and public health services. Only then could the student acquire skill, experience and maturity of judgement and personality: 'Just as a student of a teachers' training college, when doing practice teaching in a school, co-operates with the school staff and shares with them the life of a school teacher, so a student nurse during her practical training must live the life of a nurse.'[88]

Nurse wastage could be reduced by 'harmonising hospital discipline with modern ideas' by removing unnecessary 'class' distinction between the various strata of the hospital hierarchy, and giving nurses themselves a more effective voice in their institution.[89]

A report was also presented to the Minister of Health by ten leading but anonymous nurses.[90] The foreword explained that the group members were all experienced nurses with special opportunities for observation of the problems associated with nursing: 'Between them they possess a unique knowledge of nursing in Great Britain and abroad.' Their anonymity was because most of the members held official posts, and several had contributed to the commentaries of other groups.

The names, qualifications and positions were known to ministers, as letters exchanged between civil servants reveal.[91] They were G.B. Carter, of the Wellcome Museum; O. Baggallay, of the Florence Nightingale Foundation; L.M. Darnell, assistant at the Nursing Recruitment Centre; J. Eyre, Senior Assistant Tutor at Yardley Green Sanatorium, Birmingham; O.P. Griffiths, Inspector of Training Schools from the General Nursing Council; A.M.D. Leslie, Matron of West Middlesex County Hospital; E.C. Pearce, member of the General Nursing Council and author of nursing text-books; and M.B. Powell, Matron of St George's Hospital. Two members – B.A. Bennett and O.F. Griffith – did not have their job titles given.

Although changes in the nature of illness and patient needs warranted changes in the composition, duties and training of the health team, the role of the nurse was unchanging. In a statement reminiscent of Pearce's writings, the group wrote:

> The nurse is first and foremost an interpreter and so must explain and reassure not only the patient but also his relatives and friends. She is the hostess in ward or department and must be personally satisfied that her guests are at ease, well fed, well housed and happily occupied. It is her duty to care for, or to oversee the care of all the mental and bodily needs of the patients entrusted to her, observing and reporting accurately on their conditions. As a member of the therapeutic team she will be personally responsible for treatments allotted to her and will give the skilled assistance required by the doctor and other members of the team. She must be prepared for emergency, foreseen or unforeseen, and tackle it until the doctor comes. She must be a teacher of health so that patients know how to maintain health regained.[92]

The Ten were concerned that Wood did not acknowledge these fundamental arts and skills of nursing: 'Qualities and functions ... understood and practised by many nurses', were in danger of being lost. Wood gave no guarantee that they would be taught and practised by students. A definition of nursing was needed that encompassed the safeguarding and building up of the life-forces of the individual and the society. It was unnecessary to differentiate between the nurse caring for the sick and the public health nurse: 'because the whole idea of prevention and of health promotion is contained in the one word "nurse" ... There is a great need for a statement of the basic requirements of patients as a foundation for the practice as well as for the training of nurses.'

Basic bedside training was vital: 'From another point of view the basic training might be looked at as the period spent in the ranks before officer status is attained.'[93] A case assignment method for training and flexibility in the hours spent in learning experiences was commended. Perhaps influenced by Carter, and her writings,[94] the Ten argued that hospitals should no longer depend for their functioning on cheap probationer labour, but on trained women who, like other workers, should have good conditions, pay and prospects. Teachers trained in modern educational methods were needed. Some nurses should be able to be selected for degree courses in science, sociology or the arts in preparation for undertaking research in order to help the progression of the profession. Alternatively, the Ten suggested, young graduates should be attracted into the profession.

The Ten were agnostic about the precise mix of theory and practice, and were in favour of experiment over shortened training. They acknowledged the need not only to accommodate the majority of candidates drawn to nursing by a motivation 'first and foremost to care for patients', but also those 'attracted by the sociological aspects of the health service and whose interest in bedside nursing is secondary'.

Nursing needed to have a place for both kinds of candidate, and in doing so make room even for those with a small capacity for theoretical leaning who could be excellent practical nurses. Yet, the group was clear about the importance of examination, suggesting that the system of examination for admission to the register be revised, that a practical examination, assessed by external examiners, be introduced. At the end of the training period the nurse should be competent to practise.

There should be special training courses for senior posts, but these should be associated with a hospital and patients: 'Nurses would be less tempted to underrate practical nursing and overrate theoretical instruction if their course of post-certificate study were associated with a hospital and patients.' The Ten sought to retain married nurses and recruit more male nurses.[95]

Evaluating the comments, the Minister of Health acknowledged that few bodies accepted the training proposals outlined in the report.[96] Some bodies, notably those representing nurses, challenged the statistics on wastage during training, and there were criticisms of the report's emphasis on preventative nursing. While the principle of student status was broadly acceptable, and the necessity to reduce and eliminate domestic duties was admitted, there was general agreement that repetitive duties were essential. Some bodies insisted on apprenticeship as being more satisfactory than student status.

The nursing journals printed extracts of these comments.[97] Miss E. Cockayne found herself having to defend the report because of what she considered to be its inaccurate reporting in the press, from which she concluded 'that "freedom of the press" has its drawbacks!'[98] On May 15, the *Nursing Mirror* reported, with great approval, that the Nuffield Trust was undertaking an investigation into the proper task of the nurse, an inquiry to be chaired by H.A. Goddard.[99] The report welcomed the 'vision' and 'common-sense' of the Nuffield Provincial Hospitals Trust in setting up its own investigation. It found great similarities between the viewpoint of the Nuffield Trust and the memorandum on the Wood working party report presented to the Minister of Health by the Group of Ten. This memorandum was also welcomed by the *Nursing Mirror*: 'Excellent memorandum all should read'.[100]

In January 1948 the *Nursing Mirror* suggested in its editorial that the current problems besetting nursing could only be solved if two courses of action were taken. First, the restoration into nurse training 'of the simple, compassionate, bedside nursing skills – the real *basic* nursing training, which expresses the soul of nursing, not merely its brain'. This was quite different from a comprehensive training (excellent as that may be in addition). And second, 'the development of freedom of life, and thought, then only partly understood in the hospital world'.[101]

White notes how little reaction there was from ordinary nurses in the nursing press on the momentous reports of Horder and Wood.[102] Preoccupations centred on the spirit of service, and concerns that the vocational ideal was being lost, although some thought the vocational ideal was too much stressed.[103] One correspondent argued that more nurses did not mean better nurses, who treated the patient not as an object or case 'but a living human being, body, mind, soul, with hopes and fears beyond the scope of our imagination'. The new NHS would relieve financial strain but the nurse would always be central to the patient. Patients should be put first. It was feared that 'in an age of reports, councils, committees and boards' which aimed to make nursing more attractive in order to recruit the increased number of nurses necessary, the patient, as the purpose of nursing, was being forgotten.[104]

Conclusion

The practical spirit of service to the patient was the central preoccupation of nursing organisations from 1932 to 1948, although commissions and committees were concerned to raise the status of nursing, improve conditions of service and aid recruitment and retention. Criticisms of nursing apprenticeship made by Horder and Wood, for example, no doubt reflected certain mores in post-war society, impatient with traditional values,[105] which assumed that the high standards of nursing commitment to patients was natural, and did not need inculcation. These criticisms were harbingers of the kind of debate to come later.

The paradox of improving pay, conditions and status, while preserving vocation, remained. Herein lay the potential for conflict, and a clouding of the nature and purpose of the nurse's role. These tensions were reconcilable, however. As a nurse tutor wrote at the close of this period, it was important to attract the right type of candidate by making clear what nursing demanded: 'At the same time every effort should be made to improve conditions where indicated and, because the best nurses are self-sacrificing by nature, especial care should be taken to avoid exploitation of this characteristic ... Nursing is, and always will be, a Christian duty – nothing less than the highest standards should content us in so great a work.'[106] This comment sums up what was felt to be the essence of nursing, and why the apprenticeship method of training was considered, by the profession at least, to be so important in maintaining the integrity of nursing.

Notes

1 'The General Nursing Council for England and Wales', *British Journal of Nursing*, 1921, pp. 187–189, April 2.

2 'Conference on Nursing Education', *British Journal of Nursing*, pp. 266–272, May 7; 'The General Nursing Council of England and Wales', *Nursing Mirror and Midwives' Journal*, 1921, pp. 90–92, May 7; 'Making the Future Nurse: Great Conference on the Syllabus of Training and Affiliation Schemes', *Nursing Times*, 1921, pp. 498–512, May 7.

3 Ibid., p. 266; p. 498.

4 Ibid., p. 271; p. 502; p. 91.

5 Ibid., pp. 266–267; p. 498.

6 L.R. Seymer, *Dame Alicia Lloyd Still 1869–1944*, London, Nightingale Fellowship, St Thomas's Hospital, for private circulation only, 1953.

7 R. Wake, *The Nightingale Training School 1860–1996*, London, Haggerston, 1998, p. 94, 100–101.

8 L.R. Seymer, *Florence Nightingale's Nurses*, London: Pitman Medical, 1960, pp. 126,129.

9 J. Barclay, *Why No Nurses?*, London, Faber & Faber, 1946, p. 14.

10 General Nursing Council for England and Wales, *Syllabus of Lectures and Demonstrations for Education and Training in General Nursing*, London, General Nursing Council for England and Wales, 1923.

11 General Nursing Council for England and Wales, *Syllabus of Subjects for Examination for the Certificate of General Nursing*, London, General Nursing Council for England and Wales, 1923.

12 Ibid., p. 2.

13 'The General Nursing Council for England and Wales', *Nursing Times*, 1923, pp. 271–276, March 24.

14 ' "Existing" Nurses: A Settlement at Last', *Nursing Times*, 1923, pp. 665–666, July 14.

15 E.R.D. Bendall, E. Raybould, *A History of the General Nursing Council for England and Wales 1919–1969*, London, H.K. Lewis & Co., 1969, pp. 180–181.

[16] *The Lancet Commission on Nursing: Final Report*, London, Lancet, 1932.
[17] Ibid., pp. 11–26, paras 2–28.
[18] Ibid.,p. 61, para. 107.
[19] Ibid., p. 12, para. 4.
[20] Ibid., pp. 28–29, paras 32–36.
[21] Ibid., p. 30, para. 37.
[22] Ibid., p. 35, para. 50.
[23] Ibid., p. 166, para. 349.
[24] Ibid., p. 166, para. 350.
[25] 'The Hospital Nursing Service', editorial, *British Medical Journal*, 1932, pp. 344–346, February 20.
[26] 'The Lancet Commission on Nursing', editorial, *Lancet*, 1933, pp. 369–370, February 18.
[27] Ministry of Health Board of Education, *Interdepartmental Committee on Nursing Services: Interim Report*, the Rt. Hon. The Earl of Athlone, Chairman, London, HMSO, 1939.
[28] Ibid., p. 8, para. 10.
[29] Ibid., p. 9, para. 12.
[30] Ibid., p. 55, para. 138.
[31] Ibid., p. 77, para. 170.
[32] G.B. Carter, *A New Deal for Nurses*, London, Victor Gollancz, 1939.
[33] The Royal College of Nursing, *Nursing Reconstruction Committee Report and Supplements*, Lord Horder, Chairman, London, The Royal College of Nursing; Section I, The Assistant Nurse, 1942; Section II, Education and Training, 1943; Section III, Recruitment, 1943; Section IV, The Social and Economic Conditions of the Nurse, 1949.
[34] Ibid., section II, 1943, p. 10, para. 12.
[35] Ibid., p. 11, para. 14.
[36] Ibid., pp. 11–12, paras 15–16.
[37] Ibid., pp. 12–18, paras 17–37.
[38] Ibid., pp. 20–21, paras 47–48.
[39] Ibid., pp. 22–23, paras 52–53.
[40] The Royal College of Nursing, *Nursing Reconstruction Committee Report and Supplements*, Lord Horder, Chairman, London, The Royal College of Nursing; Section III, Recruitment, 1943, pp. 56–57, para. 6.
[41] Ibid., p. 63, para. 28.
[42] Ibid., p. 66–67, para. 35–37.
[43] 'The Decline in Nursing', *British Journal of Nursing*, editorial, G.M.H., 94, 2140, 1946, pp. 121–122, November.
[44] The Royal College of Nursing, *Nursing Reconstruction Committee Report and Supplements*, Lord Horder, Chairman, London, The Royal College of Nursing; Section III, Recruitment, 1943, p. 83, Appendix II.
[45] K. Box, E. Croft-White, *Recruitment to Nursing: an Inquiry into the Attitudes of Student Nurses to their Profession with Special Reference to the Present Recruiting Campaign*, Regional S.7 London, Wartime Social Survey for Campaigns Division of the Ministry of Information, Appendix, October, 1943.
[46] Ibid., pp. 2–4.
[47] The Royal College of Nursing, *Nursing Reconstruction Committee Report and Supplements*, Lord Horder, Chairman, London, The Royal College of Nursing; Section IV, The Social and Economic Conditions of the Nurse, 1949, p. 7–8, Foreword.
[48] Ibid., p. 9, para. 3.
[49] R. White, *The Effects of the National Health Service on the Nursing Profession 1948–1961*, London, King Edward's Hospital Fund for London, 1985, pp. 18–19.
[50] K.F. Kitchin, 'Nursing the Individual', *Nursing Times*, 1943, pp. 772–773, October 16.

[51] J. Barclay, *Why No Nurses?*, London, Faber & Faber, 1946.

[52] Ministry of Health, Department of Health for Scotland, Ministry of Labour and National Service, *Report of the Working Party on the Recruitment and Training of Nurses*, Sir Robert Wood, Chairman, London, HMSO, 1947, p. iii.

[53] Ibid., pp. 35–36, paras 90–92.

[54] Ibid., p. 36, para. 94.

[55] Ibid., p. 41, para. 105.

[56] Ibid., pp. 42–43, paras 108–110.

[57] Ibid., pp. 45–48, paras 119–126.

[58] Ibid., p. 50, para. 130.

[59] Ibid., pp. 105–109, paras 2–17.

[60] Ibid., pp. 58–60, paras 164–174.

[61] Ibid., pp. 61–63, para. 177–181.

[62] Ibid., pp. 77–78, paras 247–251.

[63] Ibid., p. 93, paras 4–5.

[64] J. Cohen, *Working Party on the Recruitment and Training of Nurses, Minority Report*, London, HMSO, 1948.

[65] R. White, *The Effects of the National Health Service on the Nursing Profession 1948–1961*, London, King Edward's Hospital Fund for London, 1985, pp. 18–19.

[66] E.E.P. MacManus, 'The Working Party Report – a Critical Survey', *Nursing Times*, 1947, pp. 834, 839, November 29.

[67] King Edward's Hospital Fund for London, *Comments on the Report of the Working Party on the Recruitment and Training of Nurses Submitted to the Minister of Health*, London, King Edward's Hospital Fund, November, 1947.

[68] Ibid., p. 2 para. 6.

[69] Ibid., p. 3, para. 7.

[70] 'New Comments for Consideration', editorial, *Nursing Times*, 1948, pp. 1–2, January 3.

[71] King Edward's Hospital Fund for London, *Comments on the Report of the Working Party on the Recruitment and Training of Nurses Submitted to the Minister of Health*, London, King Edward's Hospital Fund, November, 1947.

[72] 'The Royal College of Nursing, Memorandum on the Report of the Working Party on the Recruitment and Training of Nurses', *Nursing Times*, 1948, pp. 260–262, April 10.

The Royal College of Nursing, *Memorandum on the Report of the Working Party on the Recruitment and Training of Nurses,* London, Royal College of Nursing, 1948.

[73] Ibid., p. 8.

[74] 'G.N.C. (England and Wales) Report on W.P.R.', *Nursing Mirror*, 1948, p. 201, June 26. The General Nursing Council for England and Wales, *Memorandum of the General Nursing Council for England and Wales on the Report of the Working Party on the Recruitment and Training of Nurse*, London, GNC, Public Record Office, MH 55/2070, January, 1948. R. White, *The Effects of the National Health Service on the Nursing Profession 1948–1961*, London, King Edward's Hospital Fund for London, 1985, p. 26.

[75] The General Nursing Council for England and Wales, *Memorandum of the General Nursing Council for England and Wales on the Report of the Working Party on the Recruitment and Training of Nurses*, London, GNC, Public Record Office MH 55/2070, January, 1948, pp. 1–2.

[76] Ibid., p. 3.

[77] Ibid., p. 5.

[78] Ibid., p. 7.

[79] Ibid., p. 10

[80] R. White, *The Effects of the National Health Service on the Nursing Profession 1948–1961*, London, King Edward's Hospital Fund for London, 1985, p. 27.

[81] The General Nursing Council for England and Wales, *Memorandum of the General Nursing Council for England and Wales on the Report of the Working Party on the Recruitment and Training of Nurses*, London, GNC, Public Record Office, MH 55/2070, January, 1948, p. 11.

[82] The British Hospitals Association, *Memorandum of Comment on the Report of the Working Party on the Recruitment and Training of Nurses Submitted to the Minister of Health*, Wettenhall J.P., Secretary, London, The British Hospitals Association, February, 1948.

[83] Ibid., p. 6, section II, para. 10.

[84] Ibid., p. 7, section III, paras 12–13.

[85] Nuffield Provincial Hospitals Trust, *Observations Submitted to the Ministry of Health on the Ministry's Working Party on the Recruitment and Training of Nurses*, Oxford, Oxford University Press, 1948.

[86] Ibid., p. 3, para. 3.

[87] Ibid. p. 4, para. 3.

[88] Ibid. pp. 4–6, paras 4–10.

[89] Ibid., p. 11, para. 18.

[90] The Ten Group, *Working Party Report on the Recruitment and Training of Nurses: Comments Submitted to the Minister of Health by the Ten Group*, Croyden, Surrey, H.R. Grubb, February, 1948.

[91] Letter from N.D. Walker to J. McCree Esq., Ministry of Health, Whitehall, London, S.W.1., 9 April 1948; Letter from J. McCree to N.D. Walker, Department of Health for Scotland, St Andrew's House, Edinburgh 1., 12 April, 1948, Public Record Office, MH 55/2063.

[92] The Ten Group, *Working Party Report on the Recruitment and Training of Nurses: Comments submitted to the Minister of Health by the Ten Group*, Croyden, Surrey, H.R. Grubb, February, 1948, p. 4.

[93] Ibid., p. 6.

[94] G.B. Carter, *A New Deal for Nurses*, London, Victor Gollancz, 1939.

[95] The Ten Group, *Working Party Report on the Recruitment and Training of Nurses: Comments submitted to the Minister of Health by the Ten Group*, Croyden, Surrey, H.R. Grubb, February, 1948, p. 7.

[96] Minister of Health, 'Summary of Comments by Interested Organisations to the Minister of State for Scotland', London, Public Record Office, MH 55/2063, 1948.

[97] 'New Comments for Consideration', editorial, *Nursing Times*, 1948, pp. 1–2, January 3; 'The Royal College of Nursing Memorandum on the Report of the Working Party on the Recruitment and Training of Nurses', *Nursing Times*, 1948, pp. 260–262, April 10; 'More Ado about Working Party's Report', *Nursing Mirror*, 1948, pp. 390–391. February 28; 'British Hospitals Association on Working Party's Report', *Nursing Mirror*, 1948, p. 418, March 13; 'Nurses Comment on W.P. Report', editorial, *Nursing Mirror*, 1948, pp. 17–18, April 10; 'Notable memorandum on W.P. Report', *Nursing Mirror*, 1948, pp. 25–26, April 10; 'G.N.C. (England and Wales) Report on W.P.R.', *Nursing Mirror*, 1948, p. 201, June 26.

[98] 'Discussing the Working Party Report: A Talk by Miss E. Cockayne, Matron, Royal Free Hospital', *Nursing Times*, 1947, pp. 910–911, December 27.

[99] 'Job analysis', editorial, *Nursing Mirror*, 1948, pp. 97–98, May 15.

[100] 'Nurses Comment on W.P.Report', editorial, *Nursing Mirror*, 1948, pp. 17–18, April 10.

[101] 'Facts for 1948', editorial, *Nursing Mirror*, 1948, pp. 271–272, January 17.

[102] R. White, *The Effects of the National Health Service on the Nursing Profession 1948–1961*, London, King Edward's Hospital Fund for London, 1985.

[103] 'Gone are the Days', letter, M.C.S., *Nursing Mirror*, 1948, p. 46, October 16; 'Realism and Idealism', letter, Two S.R.N.s, *Nursing Mirror*, p. 79, October 30.

[104] D. Whittaker, 'Patients First', letter, *Nursing Mirror*, 1948, p. 238, July 10.

[105] A.J.P. Taylor, *English History 1914–1945*, Oxford, Oxford University Press, 1965.
[106] E.H. Hodsoll, 'The Assistant Nurse', *Nursing Times*, 1950, p. 733–734, July 15.

Chapter 5

British nursing tradition and the North American influence, 1948–1960

The Nurses Act 1949 implemented some of the less contentious issues of the Wood Report, widening the remit of the GNC and establishing Area Nurse Training Committees.[1] However, the 'brave new world' envisaged by the Wood Report did not come to pass: 'Powerful elements in the profession were opposed to the separation of training schools from the hospitals.' Hospitals could not afford to grant student status to nurses and thereby lose their workforce.[2] The profession was unmoved by outside criticisms from its traditional values, the deep-seated belief that apprenticeship made the 'proper' bedside nurse. The 1950s saw a major affirmation of the profession's stand, in a report from an external body. Paradoxically, this period also saw the start of the North American nursing influence, which challenged the confidence of this tradition. This chapter will examine the paradox, and bring to light the different views, their underlying presuppositions, and their crucial effects on the development of nursing.

The ethos of British nursing: vocation or career?

Although concerns were expressed in the House of Lords in 1948 concerning the shortage of nurses, the peers agreed that statistics indicated that the shortfall was due to expanding need.[3] As Lord Crook said: 'The truth is that to-day we have more nurses and more trainees in the hospitals than ever we had before ... 7,000 more employed than a year ago, and in fact 31,000 more employed than in 1938.' There were 51,000 trainees compared to 43,000 in 1938.[4] Several of the peers who spoke appeared keen for the government to follow the Wood recommendations, and move nursing away from its restrictive tradition.

The nursing profession differed, however. There was general agreement that practical nursing, with its underlying values, was best taught at the bedside by the most experienced and most qualified nurse, the ward sister. But ward sisters had ward and patient responsibilities and often did not have time for teaching. A remedy was sought in the role of the practical instructor. In 1948, a practical instructor working at a London Hospital reported on such a scheme.[5] Its purpose was to provide nurses with more practical teaching, by augmenting the ward sister and working with her, but not to replace her: 'In this way a team spirit prevails, the nurse realizes that theory and practical work is closely allied and a high standard of training is maintained.'

M. Scales, probably the writer of the textbook published two years later, was concerned about this development.[6] She argued that to preserve British nursing it was vital to adhere to 'the essence of our teaching which has produced such wonderful nurses'.[7] The increasing belief that the learning of skills could be divorced from learning how to nurse was a deep concern to many ward sisters. But, as White suggests, the 1950s saw a shift in professional values, as the emphasis on altruism and service began to wane, and the educational theme grew in strength. Although in the 1950s 'Nurses had plenty of altruism',[8] their training outside the educational system lacked legitimacy, its educational or training standard could not be measured. Being registered meant nothing.

White argues from this that nursing became a pluralist social system. Generalist nurses, with their identity as semi-skilled workers, were concerned with their social or functional status in the hospital, and had instrumental and material values. The specialists sought to gain professional authority by emphasising the intellectual meaning of nursing. They sought improved educational standards and even a move into higher education. Nurse administrators, on the other hand, held bureaucratic values. If they were to win arguments with bureaucrats they had to learn to play the game: 'Altruism, they noticed, meant little in the fight for resources, or power in policy making'. According to White, it was little wonder that so many nurses perceived a significant loss of status. Nursing lacked professional authority and many began to look elsewhere for an improved status.[9]

Whether many ordinary nurses actively wanted an increased status for nursing is questionable, but dissatisfaction may have been stimulated by outside academics who had little sympathy for the traditional ethic of service. A study by Farnworth raised just such questions.[10] Farnworth found that, except for those who felt a particular vocation to nursing, there were many other career options, and this had adversely affected nursing recruitment. Nurses themselves thought that nursing was low in prestige and lacked status in the mind of society: 'the Cinderella of the Health Team'. Among non-nurses there was evidence of an attitude which held nursing to be an inferior career for a well-educated girl.[11]

This study, extracts of which were also published in *Nursing Times*,[12] was conducted between 1948 and 1951, and compared nursing to teaching, clerical work, saleswomanship [sic] and light factory work. Nursing was found to be second only to teaching for its prestige level with the exception of 'the use of initiative at work' where nurses were rated lower than saleswomen. The public was also questioned about the advantages and disadvantages of three occupations: teaching, nursing and secretarial work.

Out of the three occupations, nursing disadvantages were the most emphasised by the public, and hence Farnworth concluded that public opinion was, to an extent, more biased against nursing than either teaching or secretarial work.[13] The public thought that the limitation on recreation and encroachment on personal freedom were the main disadvantages for nurses as against the other occupational groups. The disadvantages of nursing were perceived to be those of long hours, low pay and out-of-date discipline both off and on duty.[14] As one social science student responded, nursing was a vocation and to the right type, pay and conditions were unimportant.[15]

In her introduction, Farnworth commented on the low status of nursing before Nightingale's reforms, but did not discuss the part moral values played in the change. She thought psychological research would explain why secular nursing was not highly valued.[16] The editorial writer of the *Nursing Times* did appreciate the significance of moral principles to the value of nursing, and was moved to comment on this argument. Despite the need for nurses in those early years of the profession, Nightingale was adamant in demanding and maintaining a high standard 'rather than saying, as many do now, that the need is so great we cannot afford to be selective'. Nursing was a service and appealed to those whose background had taught them that service to the community was of the highest not the lowest value'. Recognition of the value of such service should also be demonstrated by the public in improved pay and conditions for nurses, and in giving them positions of responsibility within the community.[17]

The moral quality of the nurse continued to be fundamental. This was elaborated in 1953 by M. Simson, a student nurse, in a prizewinning essay in the British Medical Association Competition, published in the *Nursing Times*. The essential quality and the nucleus of the nursing vocation was to possess a love of humanity:

> for in this attitude self is never spared for the beloved, the chores involved are not drudgery; the dirty and less pleasant jobs for the patients which can cause them so much discomfort, are not avoided or sketchily done ... none of this becomes too heavy a burden to the nurse with a vocation.[18]

Nursing, according to Simson was not a vocation for girls without perception or perseverance, or who disliked restrictions. Only the nurse with a genuine regard for her patient, no matter how awkward or demanding he or she might be, who had tact, patience and perseverance, could establish the right atmosphere by creating trust in her patient and promote team spirit among her colleagues:

> How easily and unobtrusively an angry nurse can give an unkind tweak to a stuck dressing, carelessly rip off a piece of sticking plaster, give an unnecessarily hard rubbing to a sore back, suddenly jerk a mattress or roughly comb a patient's hair; oh! there are so many ways of annoying an annoying patient.

Simson appreciated that not all nurses did have such a vocation, and yet, even so, they could be useful. Careerist nurses might have a determination and ambition that enabled them to fulfil their creativity through personal attentions to the patient. But she believed that often this was insufficient, because the creative careerist nurse often did not have the sensitivity and temperament to allow her to be patient and enduring. The nursing profession needed to have people with a vocation, for only this would produce the 'perfect nurse'. Indeed, nursing made the person.

Simson's essay reflected traditional teaching. For example, Catherine Wood, a half-century earlier, had similarly cautioned against the temptation to selfishness: 'cold, unloving hands', hurrying over an offensive dressing with 'ill-concealed expressions of disgust'; handling a limb 'in a hasty, cross manner'; refusing the patient's requests to move his pillow or change his position, 'or to comply so hastily that the sick man regrets having asked you'.[19]

Much of the contention during the 1950s concerned the nature of the nurse's role, and the essence of nursing. In 1953 the *Nursing Mirror* published a series of three anonymous articles under the heading 'The Basic Things of Nursing'.[20] Nursing was a personal but unequal relationship, aided by religious faith; a vocation in the sense of fitness for care; and a service: 'a spiritual business ... the complete fulfilment of their capacities, physical, mental and spiritual'.[21]

Letters from ordinary nurses to the nursing journals reflected concerns about what the values of vocation implied for the nurse. George Lance argued that the war exploded 'the fallacy of the vocational nurse'. Nursing was a job like any other requiring aptitude. While the general public thought of nurses as 'ministering angels', more than a dearth of nurses was needed to 'alter the psychology of the masses'; overbearing matrons and browbeating sisters were responsible for the present unrest.[22] Responses argued that 'aptitude' was not enough, vocation was crucial. Kindness, sympathy and understanding, the basis of the vocation, were vital to the smooth running of the ward, but were currently being lost as nurses treated their work as just another job.[23]

Bedside care: the proper task of British nursing

In 1953 the Nuffield Provincial Hospitals Trust investigation, *The Work of Nurses in Hospital Wards*, chaired by H.A. Goddard, was published.[24] This had taken up the challenge which the Wood Report had failed to do: to determine the proper task of the nurse. The investigation examined the 'present' task of the nurse, and compared it to what was considered to be the 'proper' task of the nurse. The report appreciated the changing and increasing demands on nurses: complex hospital administration; development of medical science; rise in standards of living and the change in social class of patients. Yet, with reference to Nightingale's writing, the report argued that there was continuity in the needs of human beings in health and sickness, and the meeting of these was the nurse's especial province: 'There is no escaping the conclusion that this view is not generally held today; or, if it is, that circumstances prevent its being put into practice.'[25] Although in theory the trained nurse's sphere of work covered all tasks of patient care, in practice she could no longer undertake them all, and many were devolved to student nurses and orderlies. This reflected the division of functions occurring in the United States between graduate and practical nurses which had led to a hierarchical division of labour: the administration of medicines and poultices were the proper task of the skilled nurses while the routine tasks of care were delegated to less trained people.

Nearly three-quarters of nursing in a general ward was concerned with the physical needs common to all patients, and although such needs varied over time and between individuals, basic nursing determined the outline of ward routine. Despite this, technical nursing was given a priority, so that during the student nurse's training over the three years, technical nursing played a larger part in her training while basic nursing played a lesser part. Technical nursing procedures were detailed, and included such tasks as recording temperature, administration of drugs, bandaging, irrigation and catheterisation.[26]

Because of the priority attached to technical nursing, the patient's medical needs were seen as more important than his or her physical needs, so mealtimes were interrupted by doctors' rounds, for example, and patients were often fearful of using a bedpan or going to the bathroom during the consultant's rounds. Furthermore, basic nursing suffered because of an inadequacy of staff which resulted in a complete lack of any provision for bedfast patients to wash their hands after using bedpans, or at any other time outside the washing routine (mostly twice a day).

Two alternative approaches for the future development of the nursing role were suggested: either the nursing role could develop into that of a medical technician, or the nurse could insist that the basic and technical aspects of nursing were indivisible. The first approach was the route taken by the nursing profession in the United States where the graduate nurse, the practical nurse and the nursing aide were each responsible for different aspects of patient care. This approach was in line with Horder, section IV; it would fit into the age of specialisation, and it would also facilitate student status, which was then not possible because of the need to staff wards. This approach would also suit those nurses more fitted to technical knowledge than others. The division of function would neatly fall into 'technical' and 'basic'.[27]

This approach was not recommended by Goddard, however. Firstly, it would not be in the best interests of the patient; secondly, because the nurse needed to observe the patient's condition and report to the doctor, she needed to spend more rather than less time with individual patients; and thirdly, although technical skill was now an essential requirement of nursing, if it became the basis of nursing it would destroy the original ethos of nursing and turn the nurse into a medical technician. Human needs were inseparable. Medical, emotional and physical needs were interrelated. A junior student nurse (or auxiliary) making a bed might be able to carry out that task, but may not notice facts about the patient's condition which the trained nurse would notice immediately: 'Understanding and meeting a patient's emotional needs is a peculiarly delicate task.'[28]

Observers had noted how little time both trained and student nurses spent in personal conversation with patients. Even during visiting times nurses were tidying cupboards or spending time 'making stock'[sic] rather than talking to patients without visitors. The explanation usually given was either lack of time or fear of admonishment. An alternative explanation sometimes put forward was that by doing things for the patient, rather than merely talking to him, it was often possible to get him to talk and so find out about him, and 'the good nurse will find opportunity for this in the course of ordinary nursing duties'.[29]

Of crucial importance to the investigation was its recognition of the fundamental worth of Nightingale's ideal, the care of the individual patient, and not merely as a medical or surgical case. The report repeated her statement that the nurse was not merely there to spare the patient physical exertion, 'I would rather say that she ought to be there to spare him from taking thought for himself.' The investigation believed that this was still the ideal of the majority of nurses:

> It is significant that it probably comes nearest to realisation in private wards where nursing is often in the hands of trained or senior student nurses working under some form of patient-assignment. *It is submitted that this ideal of the unity of nursing as a service for patients should not be sacrificed until the alternative has been tried.* This requires acceptance of the principle that bedside nursing is the proper task of the state registered nurse.[30]

Goddard was definite: the ideal of the unity of nursing as a service for patients should not be sacrificed until the alternative had been tried. Bedside nursing was the proper task of the State Registered Nurse. This referred to direct care, whether basic or technical nursing, given to all patients, not simply the bedfast. The people who were at present giving personal care to patients, according to the definition of what constituted 'real' or 'proper' nursing were not trained nurses but student nurses. This was because the normal complement of trained nurses, whatever the size of the ward, was limited to two – the ward sister and the staff nurse. And many of these trained nurses sought to move into administration; the end result of nurse training for the hospital service was not nursing but administration.

The implications of this shortage of trained nurses were that ward sisters were overburdened with administration, and preoccupied with the business of the ward, constantly interrupted, and unable to give much time either to bedside nursing or to teaching. The staff nurse was the sister's deputy, seen by many as a temporary position, a step on the ladder, unsatisfying because it offered neither direct patient care nor executive responsibility. Goddard proposed that direct patient care should be the province of the staff nurse. Already occurring in some hospitals, it needed to be spread more widely. Consideration needed to be given to the optimum size of the nursing unit, a critical examination of nursing procedures, the application of method studies to nursing duties, the need to relieve strain on ward staff and peak periods of the day and the use of auxiliary nursing staff as a 'second pair of hands'.[31]

Goddard thought that despite providing the main nursing workforce, student nurse training was inadequate. This was because ward sisters and staff nurses were involved in ward management rather than bedside nursing. Student nurses were students in name only, and then in attitude of mind rather than reality. The ideal situation, in which the student could choose tasks which would build up her knowledge and skill, did not exist, because students were essential to the service needs of the hospital; their learning needs were subordinated to this. But if the trained nurse assumed her proper role, then the needs of students could be seen in their proper perspective, because she would no longer be the mainstay.

This did not mean that student nurse training should be entirely theoretical or 'divorced from that element of practical responsibility which is such an important feature of the tradition of nursing in this country'. Placing the responsibility for the student's practical training on the ward sister was the guarantee against this happening.[32] So long as the minimum of nursing care was already provided, student nurses could still be entrusted with practical work, carried out in conjunction with trained staff and planned in accordance with the student's training.

And, in a diagrammatic representation, the report pictured the sister as central to the functioning of the ward, responsible for trained staff exercising their function of direct patient care, overseeing the domestic staff, and with responsibility for the practical training of student nurses.[33] On the basis of this systematic job analysis the report found that trained nurses were becoming increasingly preoccupied with technical and administrative duties and relegating the basic care of patients to the untrained student nurses.

Goddard described the conclusion and recommendation of his report as 'a renaissance of nursing thought'.[34] He explained his own presuppositions further at the RCN conference held to discuss the report. He had come from the industrial sphere, and imagined the job analysis would provide only temporary interest, but as the work proceeded, and his understanding of nursing increased: 'I began to experience that sense of vocation which turns a job of work into a crusade, and I determined that what knowledge or skill I did possess could not better be employed than in the service of the nursing profession.'[35]

The publication of the report preoccupied the nursing journals, which included extracts, editorials, reports and comments.[36] The *Nursing Mirror* welcomed the report, agreed with its emphasis on the key position of the ward sister who had an impossible load, and strongly stated its own view that the development of nursing should not follow the North American path:

> We have never felt happy about the 'specialisation' developments in nursing that have been so much seen in the U.S.A., and the idea and practice of two grades of nurse have never been a great success here – as witness the comparative failure of Assistant Nurse enrolment. We are certain that to put the *bedside* back into nursing is psychologically wise, as well as being administratively desirable.[37]

The current focus of nurse training was administration rather than nursing, and this in turn led nurses to abandon hospital work and move into private nursing. This was the crucial issue, for it was 'real' or 'basic' care that brought people into nursing, and if they were not able to practise it, they were eventually driven away. Basic training in bedside nursing (better described as 'basic care' to distinguish it from merely physical care), was the conviction of 'many of the deepest thinkers in nursing', and the only solution to the problem of diminishing interest in hospital nursing.

These views were repeated. Bedside care was crucial because caring for the sick was the primary motivation for girls to become nurses. But nurses in training were progressively moved away from it. If this urge was stifled by insisting that technical skill should be the basis of nursing, rather than an important aspect, and the nurse turned into a medical technician, there would be wastage. Nurses who remained would be the cold-hearted, super-efficient, unsympathetic individuals; clever people perhaps, but without comfort for the patient.[38]

The *Lancet* welcomed Goddard and its evidence, and agreed its recommendations.[39] The Royal College of Nursing was more critical. Its initial response, published in an editorial in its journal, the *Nursing Times*, welcomed the scientific analysis, but forewarned of 'comments, criticisms and suggestions'.[40]

In its more detailed comments, the RCN accepted the distinction drawn in the report between basic and technical nursing but did not accept the conclusions.[41] Nursing procedures could not be divided by a hard and fast line from the patient's disease. Administration should not be seen as separate from bedside nursing: the idea that 'unless the nurse is standing beside the bed she is not nursing'.[42] What the report called 'administration' was in fact 'ward organisation' and was actually an important deployment of resources for 'total nursing care'.[43] The RCN disagreed with Goddard about what constituted the proper task of the nurse, and rejected its view that the trained nurse was 'forsaking her true vocation, the personal care of the patient, for something which does not touch him at all – "administration"'. The RCN also repudiated the corollary: 'the plea in the Report for a re-statement of the theory of nursing which will emphasise that the proper task of the State registered nurse is bedside care'. Nightingale did not in fact provide the imagined support, the RCN suggested.

In the light of what it perceived to be the ongoing problem of recruiting nurses, the RCN proposed a completely different pattern for nursing. The care of the hospital patient was the responsibility of a team. The State Registered Nurse should head this team, with student nurses gradually taking over more organisational and supervisory tasks, so that by the end of her training she could, with her team, be responsible for the care of a group of patients under the ward sister's direction, and eventually, become responsible for the whole ward. The ward sister's main function was as a manager of resources. This, the RCN believed, would offer maximum care by ensuring that not only the patient's physical needs were met, but also that his or her sense of confidence and security were built up: 'This can be nursing at its very best, and in this sense the ward sister can be the provider *par excellence* of bedside care.'[44]

The RCN believed that problems of recruitment of trained nurses warranted a new method of staffing hospitals. Because so many student nurses were leaving before qualifying, or even after qualifying, their training was not cost-effective. The number of student nurse training schools should be reduced, students should be more rigorously selected, and a much greater share of the hospitals' nursing service should be carried out by assistant nurses and auxiliary personnel. The assistant nurse should be seen as one of the most stable elements of the national nursing service, an integral part of the profession.

The RCN thought that Goddard was not numerically, financially or socially justifiable. Instead it proposed a reorganisation of ward personnel into a team of varying expertise and qualities, organised by a team leader who would ensure care was focused on the patient, but would not herself give that care, although she would be available to the patient if requested. North American influence was discernible in the proposal for 'group or patient assignment' as a way of enabling newly qualified nurses to focus on personal care of their patients, and so reduce dissatisfaction: 'The concept of patient-centred care by a team composed of both nursing and auxiliary staff, and working under the leadership of a trained nurse has, as far as the college is aware, not been tried in this country.'[45]

With reference to the *Lancet*,[46] the RCN called for a new fourfold structure in nursing: women of high academic, technical and administrative ability with clinical and teaching skills and management expertise; 'comfortable competent bedside nurses with no academic pretensions'; intelligent orderlies attracted by an interesting job; and students in training. This was both a vertical and a horizontal expansion.[47]

The Royal College of Nursing totally misunderstood Goddard's theme, the preservation of the unity of nursing. It did not accept that the distinction between basic and technical tasks could be maintained at all stages of the patient's illness. What might be basic for one patient could become technical for another patient: 'This was a tragic misunderstanding of Goddard's thesis, as the result of which patient care continued to be more and more fragmented and nursing became more and more hierarchical.'[48]

The Goddard Report made no such hierarchical distinction. Both basic and technical nursing were equal because they revolved around the patient. The RCN, however, thought Goddard was proposing the division of nursing into technical tasks, basic nursing and non-nursing duties, tasks carried out by senior nurses, junior nurses and untrained staff respectively. According to White, Goddard was 'the most misunderstood and misread study of any made during the period 1948–61, with the possible exception of the Wood Report itself ... in its misunderstood form, it survived and had more influence than most others. Its misrepresentation was even perpetuated in the Royal Commission on the National Health Service, 1979.'[49]

Goddard's approach was, in fact, affirming the British nursing tradition. The *Nursing Mirror* discussed the House of Lords debate on Goddard which followed its publication.[50] Lord Moran had said that bedside nursing was the only place to learn accuracy of observation, and keep that knowledge alive. He was opposed to the American system where the graduate nurse, who could do technical procedures, was really a junior doctor, and disliked the 'menial' duties of bedside care. These were left to the practical nurse: 'If you have been ill in America, as I have, you will realise that you do not get anything of what we mean by nursing.' Even in England, more and more time was devoted to technical training and examination, at the expense of basic training, and Lord

Moran believed this was a negative development.[51] Lord Haden-Guest also disapproved of the entirely different American system.[52]

The objectivity and factual nature of the Goddard Report was viewed as a great strength.[53] But it was also confirmed by experience. A year later, Goddard spoke about his own recent stay as a hospital patient, which had born out the job analysis report to such an extent that if he had to write it again he would not change a word of it.[54] Goddard's approach found further anecdotal support. Having left the Services, after the war, a trained nurse wrote that she could not get a job nursing the sick. She would only be considered for an administrative ward sister's post and there were no vacancies. As a probationer, 'I wished to become a nurse to help people who were sick and suffering to get better'; eventually she became a sister but was not actually expected to nurse: 'That year nearly broke my heart.' Nurses had to choose between two entirely different professions: the nurse or the administrator.[55]

Preparing the bedside nurse

The proper role and purpose of the nurse defined the preparation of the nurse. The first *Syllabus of Subjects for Examination for the Certificate of General Nursing* published by the General Nursing Council in 1923, was revised in 1925, 1933 and 1929 and reprinted in 1952 and 1955.[56] Until 1951 the syllabus appeared as a schedule to the Nurses Rules. In 1951 the Minister of Health agreed that detailed syllabuses no longer needed to appear as schedules provided the content followed the broad outlines that appeared in the schedules. This allowed the education committee of the General Nursing Council the chance to revise syllabuses without the necessity of legislation. In 1950 a section entitled 'Introduction to Psychology', which included two parts: outline of general psychology, and applied psychology, was typewritten and appended to the syllabus for part 2 of the preliminary examination. These subjects became compulsory from October 1951. In 1950 the oral examination in anatomy, physiology, hygiene, medicine and surgery was discontinued and the practical examination increased: for the preliminary examination from thirty to forty minutes, and for the final examination from forty minutes to one hour.[57]

In 1952 a new syllabus was approved with an updated layout, but it was little changed, appearing with the same headings as before, except for the amount of detail specified, and the addition of human behaviour in illness and social aspects of disease. Some categories were revised.[58] The syllabus differed slightly for male and female nurses; emergency care replaced obstetrics and gynaecology. For the first time, in 1952, The Nurse's Chart, originally a folded piece of paper attached to the syllabus, became a separate, more detailed, hardback book, the *Record of Practical Instruction and Experience for the Certificate of General Nursing.*[59]

The Guide[60] accompanying the syllabus stressed the importance of formal lectures, professional cooperation, ethical conduct, method and orderliness and supervision of practice:

> It is at this early stage that good foundations of the true art of nursing as distinct from, and in addition to, dexterity in 'carrying out procedures' can be laid. If the student realises the part she can play in the ward team and the value of her powers of observation, her thoroughness and her accuracy, she will be eager to enter upon her first ward experience with the confidence that a good preparation has been given her.[61]

Training was to ensure that nurses knew the reasons for their practice. The 1923 syllabus was thus updated and perpetuated in 1952 and again in the 1958 revision, having a similar biomedical content. The Guide was specific that the nurse was to learn to 'visualise her professional heritage'.[62]

The GNC specified the number of class hours as 300.[63] Prior to 1950 there was little pure knowledge input in the classroom. From the late 1940s, following the Horder Report, the block system developed, and nurses were taken out of clinical experience for blocks of theory of four, five or six weeks a year in a School of Nursing and then went back into the clinical situation.[64]

Nursing preparation was the transmission of a culture. A talk by an educationalist described how one of the functions of the professional group was 'the handing on of those skills and techniques and values and beliefs which characterize what we know as the group pattern or way of life'. This pattern was the obligation of duty, by which the nurse learned her attitudes and her practical skill as a craft which she was obliged to hand on to the next generation of nurses.[65]

The ward sister was still crucial, but the nurse tutor also had a role in the transmission of this culture of nursing. Perhaps this was why a study in 1954, by Janet Aitken, found the role of the nurse tutor to be somewhat nebulous.[66] Ward sisters were reluctant to become tutors because it would mean losing their bedside role. Nurse tutors themselves were dissatisfied, not only because of teaching pressures, but also because they did not have enough patient contact. The study recommended increased cooperation between the tutor and ward sister to give the tutor closer contact with the nursing of the patient. Although Aitken's study was based on the premise that the nurse tutor role was important, it affirmed the ward sister as the person crucial to the education and training of nurses: 'We are of the opinion that ward sisters should continue by precept and example to undertake a major share of practical instruction and the teaching of basic skills and the supervision of their practices.'[67]

A similar view was expressed by a ward sister from St Thomas's Hospital, Miss L. Le Quesne. Having been to the United States she had seen how unsatisfactory it was for ward sisters not to feel responsible for the development of nurses. The ward sister needed to have some influence on the nurse's developing maturity, capability and growth as a person.[68]

The North American influence

An insistent questioning of the vocational ethos was beginning to occur as British nursing began to fall under the charm of the North American system, which had already adopted educationalist ideals. In 1927 this had been a cause of concern to the North American physician, Alfred Worcester, whose writing influenced Cicely Saunders.[69] While there was much that was commendable in developments in nursing, Worcester wrote, there was a danger that mental and technical education were encouraging intelligence and dexterity, while the nurse's heart was left undeveloped: 'Undoubtedly one great defect in modern nursing is the lack of this heart service. And certainly in some part this is due to the fact that the high inheritance belonging to the nurse's calling is so often forgotten.'[70]

By the 1950s the North American influence began to have an overt effect on the British nursing ideal. Articles on North American nurse education and organisation were published in the nursing press. American nurses visiting Britain, as well as British nurses who had visited the United States, were enthusiastic about the North American nursing system. Doris Kremsdorf, US Fulbright Scholar, was impressed by the dedication and devotion of the British nursing profession, and found the most striking difference between British and American nursing to be in the method of approach. In Britain, she was told, 'all are welcome who will come to nurse the sick', and although there was natural wastage, it was hoped that a large proportion would remain in hospital service in some subordinate or related position. In the United States entry to the profession was a finely devised, selective process, involving a physical, educational, psychological and emotional screening procedure. This was cheaper, less wasteful, and less of a shock to the individual, and 'is much safer for the patient and is contributing towards maintaining the high standards of the profession'.

Even so, Kremsdorf admitted that each state established its own individual requirements for entrance to basic nursing as well as the organisation of the school, so there was no universal standard or uniformity. Those individuals who were not admitted to recognised training schools might enter 'the school of practical nursing' which prepared assistant nurses with a less theoretical and less intensive course of instruction: 'These same people would undoubtedly have failed under the stresses of technical expertness, intellectual achievement, and growing responsibility which characterises nursing in the United States today.'[71]

In the same year, Gladys Carter reviewed the book of a North American writer on the contribution of university education to the training of nurses.[72] Carter argued that if nursing was to be accorded university status it would need to demonstrate that it could be regarded as a discipline in its own right. Carter stopped short of advocating university education in Britain but did argue that the 'book breaks new ground' and should be closely studied.

Carter, a Canadian, who had previously taught at the University of Toronto School of Nursing, was awarded the first research fellowship in nursing, which was attached to the Department of Social Medicine at the University of Edinburgh. Her first project was to review the work of the sister tutor and to survey university courses for the sister tutor certificate. She was sympathetic to the North American system. She suggested that the Windsor, Ontario, experimental nurse training school, which separated education from service requirements, and educated nurses in two years, was a bold initiative worth emulating.[73]

The *Nursing Times*, the official journal of the Royal College of Nursing, reflected this growing interest in North American nursing in the 1950s, and its different attitude towards theory and practice, art and science. For example, Canadian education for nurses at McMaster University was the subject of an article in 1953.[74] Gladys Carter, the following year, argued for experimental training for nurses in Britain, reminding her readers of the scheme in Ontario.[75] And a British nurse tutor, who had studied advanced nursing in Toronto, wrote on trends in nursing education in Canada and the United States, impressed by the view that nursing education should ultimately be under the aegis of the university.[76]

North American nursing differed fundamentally from British nursing. One of a series of American letters by the American nurse E.D. Stevens Fisher noted that nursing duties were often performed by 'non-professional staff' because of the shortage of nurses, and although untrained, these 'non-professionals' were intelligent and kind. Graduate nurses tended to be drawn away from the bedside and hence from their vital relationship to patients, often built while performing simple practical duties. There was much talk of 'team nursing', where a mixed skill team, including a graduate nurse, orderly and aide, cared for the individual patient.[77]

The North American influence began to permeate British nursing thinking, albeit minimally. Vivien Jenkinson, a ward sister at St George's Hospital, studied at Toronto University School of Nursing, and had introduced patient assignment to a small ward in 1948.[78] Barbara Fawkes, Principal Tutor at the Middlesex hospital, described her year at Teachers College, Columbia

University, New York, and referred to the emphasis on psychological, sociological and cultural studies in the curricula.[79]

A *Nursing Times* editorial described the profound impression on British nursing visitors created by North American graduate and postgraduate nursing programmes.[80] Reports of investigations and studies of nursing in the United States were strongly in favour of degree courses as the future basic preparation of the professional nurse. The prevailing view from North America was that the university course should not be narrowly vocational, but professional subjects should be integrated into a more liberal programme. Opinion in Britain was divided on the value of a basic nursing degree. Universities would not welcome the idea, because of difficulty with accommodation as well as conflicts with educational policy. Under the chairmanship of Marjorie Houghton, the education committee of the Royal College of Nursing was considering the question of introducing a nursing degree course, because of the increasing scope and responsibility of nurses in both hospital and public health; but also to tap 'a numerically small but valuable source of recruits who would not otherwise be attracted to nursing'.

The debate surrounding North American ideas on nursing preoccupied the annual conference of the Sister Tutor Section of the Royal College of Nursing, chaired by Gladys Carter.[81] The subject chosen for the conference: 'The Function of the Training School is not only to Teach the Mind but to Form the Character', suggests prevailing values remained. Indeed, traditionalist nursing leaders defended passionately the vocational tradition of nurse education against modernist nursing leaders, impressed with the North American model and its psycho-social emphasis.

Speaking at the conference, in defence of the traditional Nightingale concept of nurse apprenticeship as a moral training, was the historian Lucy Seymer. Her view was supported by M.E. Gould, Principal Tutor at St Thomas's Hospital. Gould commemorated the centenary of the foundation of modern nursing, and sought to re-articulate the precepts of the 'leader' of the nursing profession as a measure of the success or failure of the individual nurse: 'Miss Nightingale has told us one way in which we could strive to do this, by example rather than precept, by striving after these things ourselves, by *being* what we would seem, not seeming what we would like to be.'

Gould argued that this model was similar to that of Thomas Arnold, who advocated the importance of the communal life, the life of the community, and religious worship 'in a country that sets store by religious worship and teaching'. Character training for Arnold involved religious principles, gentlemanly conduct and intellectual ability. For Nightingale such principles were vital in imbuing probationers with a spirit that would 'raise them above the mere scramble for remunerative posts'. The need was to prevent gossip, self-concern and preoccupation with personal slights 'that our first thoughts in the morning will not be of God ... They must all realise that their responsibility was not only to tend sick bodies, but to guide sick minds and to help sick souls.' Statutory examinations enforced a certain minimum standard, but the main role of nursing training was character training: 'The British nurse would remain one of whom her country could be proud, and of whom our founders could say "she has a well-trained mind and a sound and gracious character".'

The next speaker, M.M. Springer, Principal Tutor at Hull Royal Infirmary, had been to America. Before her visit, she had heard positive comments of American nursing education from American writers, and disparaging comments from returning British visitors. But Springer thought that the North American approach reflected Nightingale's belief that training should equip nurses for teaching and leadership. The foundation of Columbia University Teachers College, and the work of the National League of Nursing corresponded with Nightingale's belief in progress. Springer's interpretation, however, may be questioned by Nightingale's own words. In her paper, delivered in Chicago in 1893, Nightingale had listed the dangers of what she called 'stereotyping, not progressing'. These dangers included fashion and lack of earnestness; mere 'money-getting'; making nursing a profession and not a calling and so failing to keep up the moral tone, and here she added a footnote: 'In the United States it is probable that private nurses are of higher education than in England. On the other hand, they have the doubtful dignity of graduates.'[82]

Springer, however, was much more impressed by the North American system.[83] North American nursing education relied on evaluators who 'sit down together and decide on the qualities they regard as desirable in their trained nurses'. This was documented on a form and shown to the student at the beginning of her training to indicate which qualities she was expected to develop. Forms varied from hospital to hospital, but they broadly concerned the application of principles, quality of nursing care, manner and attitudes towards patients, colleagues and superiors, instruction to patients, interest in learning, appearance, dependability and adaptability. These factors were assessed with the evaluator (usually a head nurse). The student made her own comments, discussed them with the evaluator and then signed the form. Assessment was graded but was intended for encouragement as well as constructive criticism.

The notion of 'character' appeared to pose the major difference in the two systems. Seymer and Gould held the nurse's character to be developed by induction into moral and religious precepts. According to Springer, in North America, character development was self-directed through psychological insight. Trainee nurses individually researched case studies in the hospital library. They focused on the social circumstances of the patient as well as health promotion. This method trained powers of observation and resourcefulness and gave students practice in organising ideas and planning patient care. Nurses met once a week with presentations and discussions of their case studies. As a result of these 'ordeals', students acquired not only information but also 'an enviable' poise and confidence. Initiative was encouraged by the setting of individual and group assignments, and a sense of responsibility was developed through student government. In many hospitals rules and regulations were prescribed by students, faculty members might collaborate with them or merely act in a consultative capacity. Student nurses mixed socially in the university, and studied subjects beyond the nursing curriculum, broadening their outlook.

Character formation was also part of 'the guidance and counselling service'. The counsellor, usually a member of the faculty, interviewed the nursing student, helped her resolve difficulties and assessed 'her personality and potentialities'. Education was the art of developing the physical, the intellectual, the aesthetic and the moral faculties, the formation of manners and improvement of the mind, especially in youth. The time of 'adolescence' was a time of turbulent youthful idealism which the Americans, Springer said, frankly exploited. And at the end of training was 'the capping ceremony', and the training school greatly influenced the formation of nurses' characters and influenced their destiny.

B.N. Fawkes, Principal Tutor of the Middlesex Hospital, recently returned from the United States, Canada, New Zealand and Australia, opened the discussion which folowed the speeches. She suggested that North America was aiming to produce 'a good nurse, a health teacher and a good citizen'. Although comparisons reflected different cultures, historically, geographically and climatically, nevertheless the model of nurse training in the United States was impressive: in the pre-clinical course, for example, students studied sociology and went out to work amongst people of different racial and cultural backgrounds. Reporting on this diversity (Italians, Jews, Germans, English and French), they learnt tolerance, initiative and consideration for others. Group work and the presentation of case studies encouraged a sense of responsibility and prevented selfishness. Panels had been set up to discuss the integration of nurses' training, each panel consisting of three teachers and a student. There was an emphasis on teaching health by precept as well as example. The students were also involved in their own curriculum development committees, planning their own training, which helped develop their ideas and a more mature outlook.

In the question and answer session that followed, Springer and Fawkes admitted that in North America there was a tension because practical nurses, who remained on one ward, were often more knowledgeable and experienced than student nurses. Practical nurses carried out the work of the ward and did not feel happy about the student nurses who were fee-paying and able to have teaching and a training. There were no practical examinations. The nurse was tested and evaluated prior to registration by her training school. One questioner, Miss Smith, observed that character training in Britain was largely taught in the wards where unselfishness, observation and the capacity for teamwork were developed under the examples of the ward sister and staff nurse. How, she wondered, did such character training arise in the American system.

Fawkes thought that student nurses in North America had adequate practical experience even though they did not do so much of the routine nursing care, because they learnt about the 'cases' they were nursing. Carter added, from her experience in Toronto, that the broadening effect of the university education was followed by a period of gradually increasing nursing experience, in which students had the time necessary for good nursing.

Later that year, at a conference on ward teaching, Fawkes again expounded North American ideas, including the involvement of the ward orderly and team nursing.[84] She also suggested the introduction of the North American concept of the clinical instructor into ward teaching. She was challenged by a ward sister, Miss M.L. Leavesley, from The Hospital for Sick Children at Great Ormond Street, who argued that, despite all changes necessitated by increasing technology and the need for classroom-based theory, the core of nursing should still be taught in the wards and departments. Nursing was a craft, and no craft could be learned away from its material. Similarly, the Principal Tutor of the Royal Free Hospital, E.J. Bocock argued, with reference to Nightingale that education involved both a general and professional education (in which the individual made her own effort), but it also involved a sound moral training.[85]

This view was reflected in the arguments of Rosemary Murray, Tutor in Charge of New Hall, Cambridge, in her address to a conference at the Royal College of Nursing in 1956. The education of the nurse was different to that of a student, she maintained. The acquisition of technical skills of nursing, best accomplished on the wards, depended on the character and personality of the teacher. In the education of the nurse the art of nursing should be taught alongside the theory. The reverse of this meant that the student was emphasised too much at the expense of the nurse trainee. This was happening in America: 'One feels that in America there is a tendency this way and that some of the courses for training nurses result in the formation of a technician and not of a nurse.' The education of the student nurse should enable the nurse to heal – sometimes, to relieve – often, and to comfort – always.[86]

Nurse training was to become a recurring theme. The 1954 meeting of the Royal College of Nursing Council, for example, discussed the development of a nursing degree course, and suggested that this needed a course content more closely approaching that of university departments of sociology rather than university departments of medicine.[87]

In 1955 the *Nursing Times* published several articles concerned with this issue. Joyce Akester called for university education in order to improve the status of nursing. She disputed the argument that the diminishing pool of grammar school girls would mean that nursing should focus on a predominantly practical training, and believed that the danger of sacrificing practice to theory in a university course would need to be faced. The argument that such education would lower the standards of bedside care was 'prejudice', as were the deep-rooted objections to the 'educated' nurse prevalent in both nursing and medicine. There should be a two-tiered system. The unacademic secondary modern school girl would be trained in the basic nursing duties essential to the patient's comfort in which sympathy and kindness were more important than high intelligence, while the smaller number of academic grammar school girls would be a university-educated élite who would become nursing leaders. Akester foresaw the main objection: that some excellent nurses might be excluded because of their educational background. This was inevitable if regrettable.[88]

The Times took up Akester's comment in its editorial, which agreed with the idea of university-trained grammar school nursing leaders, as well as the shortened two-year practical training for secondary modern school girls: 'Assistant nurses have often in full measure a sense of vocation, together with patience, kindness, and sympathy and the ability to make patients comfortable.'[89] This editorial was followed by a letter which criticised the General Nursing Council for expecting too much of human nature by relying on the sense of vocation for an adequate supply of nurses.[90]

Akester's approach was criticised by Lilian Darnell,[91] the nursing textbook writer, and Ione Spalding.[92] Both Darnell and Spalding believed that Akester, in seeking to raise the status of nursing, was influenced by a false set of values. Darnell thought that the main consideration of nursing should be the qualities of character and personality of the nurse, even though these were difficult to assess. The essence of nursing was based on human understanding, and 'the spirit' of the nurse was essential to nursing work, which needed to be distilled and refined in all forms of education and training. Spalding argued similarly that there was a great danger in nursing losing its vocational ideals of service amid concern for rights and status and a preoccupation with the material and scientific.

A letter in the *Nursing Times* summarised the contemporary situation. Akester and Spalding reflected two poles of thought that were prevalent in the nursing world in the mid-1950s: 'In the one, no mention of ideals, in the other no mention of "higher" or "further" education.' Yet, the correspondent did 'not believe for a moment that the authors are unconscious of those aspects about which they are silent'. Rather 'they are not sufficiently in the forefront if their minds to be mentioned'. Ideals and education were both fundamental. Since the title 'profession' could not have been won by a university education, it must have been won by nursing's ideals: 'Therefore don't let us cast them off, or allow them to fade away.' This was happening because of the embarrassment of talking about ideals to 'present-day youngsters', and such ideals and attitudes needed to be inculcated in new nurses by the practical example and teaching of understanding older nurses.[93]

That vocational ideals still predominated in the 1950s may be seen by the publication of the Royal College of Nursing prayer in its professional journal, *Nursing Times*.[94] Nursing art was taught by apprenticeship practically. At the RCN Ethics and Public Health Conference, Edna Jackson, Deputy Chief Nursing Officer at the Ministry of Health, referred to the ethics of nursing forming 'a precise part of our early training as nurses, and old and new textbooks on nursing refer to it in wise but brief paragraphs in the first chapters but seldom refer to it again'. Loyalty, obedience, sympathy, accuracy, appeared in nearly all textbooks and had stood the test of time of thirty years, but training could only strengthen those qualities, it could not produce them. At the same conference, Mercy Wilmhurst, formerly General Superintendent of the Queen's Institute of District Nursing, suggested that nursing ethics were built on Christian morality.[95]

Change at the Royal College of Nursing

According to White, 1956 was a year of a profound change in the philosophy of the Royal College of Nursing.[96] That year the RCN thought it necessary to re-examine some established principles in the light of social change, and particularly with regard to the National Health Service, and it published a statement of nursing policy.[97] Yet, the chairman was clear in the foreword that this examination, 'like the Horder Reports before it, assumes that a sense of vocation is fundamental to nursing and will remain so whatever adaptations of policy may be necessary'. A new pattern of organisation in all branches of nursing was proposed, to include a wide range of personnel with varying qualifications and capacities. The hospital team, under the supervision of the ward sister, should be directed by a State Registered Nurse and include State Enrolled Assistant Nurses and auxiliary helpers.

In line with the comment on Goddard, the RCN suggested that the ward sister would be the provider *par excellence* of bedside care. Care would be delegated by the trained nurses to those beneath them in the hierarchy. They would not themselves practise 'basic' bedside care. Student and pupil nurses should be attached to hospitals only according to training needs. The whole nursing service, not only the nursing team, should be led by first-class leaders, who had knowledge, skill and understanding, as well as a wise and humane outlook and professional integrity.

The ward sister and team leaders should be responsible for teaching and ensuring that all workers were 'imbued with a sense of vocation and loyalty'. Personnel relationships were crucial, 'the team is not a machine but a group of people co-operating to a common end'. [98] Not only 'horizontal expansion', but also 'vertical expansion', was required. University education was seen to be the future trend in nursing, and with it came the desire to build up a body of nursing knowledge through engaging in research activity. There should be more discrimination in selection of candidates as students for the State Register, and students should have student status in basic training and no longer be regarded as 'pairs of hands'. Post-certificate education, which prepared nursing leaders, might also include cultural elements and a 'liberal approach'.

Although advocating a university degree course as a strategy for vertical expansion, with the aspiration of bringing into the profession more trained minds with a broad outlook, the report emphasised that it was not suggesting all nurses should have university training. It did not believe 'that this is necessary to develop the true nursing qualities of practical skill, human understanding and the all-important sense of vocation'.[99] These 'essentials' should be nurtured by training at all levels. Nevertheless, the report argued that the development of a university degree course would attract people into the profession who currently found it 'intellectually unsatisfying' and so took up other careers.

The report also called for a change in teaching methods: a 'situation approach' case study method, as recommended by the World Health Organization,[100] which related clinical teaching to individual patients, focusing on human and nursing relationships rather than isolated nursing procedures. So, for example, the nursing student should be taught to bathe a patient, not give a bed bath, that what counted was the person rather than the task.

Two further sections in the report called for improved conditions of service, both financially and in terms of hours of work, and an increased contribution to policy-making by taking part in professional organisations.[101] This last, included a call for nurse training to give the nurse an insight 'into the wider potentialities of her calling', and suggested that the General Nursing Council revised syllabus of 1952 pointed the way to this, but needed to be interpreted with imagination and skill as well as augmented by discussions on 'professional adjustment'. These two sections were followed by a final section headed 'The Case for Research'.[102] The RCN resolved to establish an authoritative research body to examine problems of the nursing profession, sponsor operational research as appropriate, and test the application of its findings.

White argues that until 1956 the RCN had taken a Nightingale approach to the nursing profession. It upheld the image of the nurse as generalist controlled by a nursing hierarchy. After 1956, the college followed the model upheld by Bedford Fenwick, with the nurse as specialist, undergoing a similar educational process as the doctor, and within a professional monopoly: 'Instead of subordinating nurses to the service ethic, for the first time a College document spelt out the needs of the profession as being equal to and supportive of the needs of the patient.'[103] By implication, the report was assuming 'menial' nursing work to be of lesser value.

The medical profession seemed to agree and broadly supported the report. The *Lancet* published a comment entitled 'The nursing team', which commended the idea of 'horizontal expansion' in which the State Registered Nurse would lead a team where most of the basic nursing care would be given by the assistant nurses.[104] Not all doctors shared this view, however. Letters in the *Lancet* expressed worries that the nursing profession was changing in such a way that it was in danger of losing its original ethos. W. Ritchie Russell argued that the desire to improve the status of nursing was misplaced.[105] C. Wilfred Vilning described the urgency of the recruitment situation and the need for more highly trained nurses. He believed that the inferior status of the assistant nurse needed to be redressed. University training would improve the status of nursing by attracting educated school-leavers, who were currently being lost to the profession.[106] Brian Watkin disagreed with Russell, although expressed sympathy with his approach. He argued that nurses needed to be prepared for administrative and leadership roles.[107]

Ritchie Russell's letter was also responded to in the *Lancet* by Thomas Anderson. He had originally written to the *Lancet* in 1953, and was disappointed by the lack of response. In this earlier letter he had argued that changes in nursing were proceeding without regard to the needs of the community. Now he thought there was a need for a two-tier system of nursing. Basic training should provide the fundamental training for all, and those with special interests or aptitudes would undertake further training. This was not analogous to the recently introduced 'assistant nurse', because it should not be inferred that basic nursing was somehow inferior, an inference that would lead to lower standards. Anderson disputed the nursing profession's desire to create an officer class of nurse, delegating the real care of the patient to the 'auxiliary' or 'aide', who would be *de facto* the real 'nurse': 'One might wonder whether it would not be proper to retain the word "nurse" for the person who really nurses and find some new title for this officer grade?'[108]

The *Lancet* published several more letters on this subject. Ronald Macbeth supported Ritchie Russell, quoting his experience of North American nursing:

> Anyone who has recently visited hospitals in the United States will have noticed the *reductio ad absurdum* which the craving of nurses for academic status has created in that country. In hospitals other than those staffed by nuns, the graduate nurses in charge of beds tend to sit majestically at desks outside their wards, doing the 'office work' and making critical (though often pertinent) comments on such matters as the blood chemistry of their patients. The real nursing is done either by orderlies or by the patients.[109]

Akester endorsed Vilning and Watkin.[110] Disagreeing with Russell, she argued that there was a need for different tiers of nurses in nursing, with different types of training, and she affirmed the need for a grade of nurse administrator prepared by university training. G.M. Wauchope and C.M. Ottley supported Russell's view and deplored the fact that the 'ordinary nurse' taught the basic technique of nursing should be considered to be downgraded: 'Nursing, in our view, is a subject totally inappropriate to a university curriculum leading to a degree.'[111] A letter by D.J. Rose followed, which supported Anderson, arguing for more 'ordinary nurses' trained for the 'routine' care of patients.[112]

The RCN affirmation of vocation in its statement of policy provoked correspondence in the *Nursing Times*.[113] Sally Harvey was uneasy about this reference.[114] Anne MacDougall disagreed: 'This spirit of service is surely the sense of vocation fundamental to nursing'.[115] The following month a letter was published which thought vocational nursing to be 'humbug'.[116] These letters in 1958 were expressions of the changes already afoot in British society which would come to fruition in the 1960s.

That year, at the Royal College of Nursing Founders Lecture, Sir John Wolfenden, Vice-Chancellor of Reading University, spoke of the profound change occuring in moral values, as a result of increased global communications and the philosophy of humanism. Although he himself had sympathy with humanistic aspirations he could not see 'why, on strictly and simply human grounds, loyalty and self-sacrifice and kindliness should be more valuable than their opposites'.[117]

Dr R. Fletcher, Lecturer in Sociology at Bedford College, London, speaking at the RCN, also reflected on changing values in society. He believed that there was a gloomy view of mid-twentieth-century society, characterised by industrialism, the overwhelming power of the state, the predominance of science and the decline of traditional beliefs, and the dangers of war. Yet he also argued for the 'vocational element of nursing' which had its outlet 'in dealing with the sick and their relatives in a sympathetic and sensitive manner. Sickness is often the most distressing period of a man's experience, when he needs human treatment. By giving him this a great contribution to human happiness is being made.'[118]

In the discussion that followed, the possibility of a shortened university course was suggested for nurses as part of their training. Fletcher believed it doubtful that vocational studies could be so integrated, and he doubted the overall value of a degree course for nurses.[119] This was echoed by another writer in the *Nursing Times* of that year. E.M. Meir, an English graduate, who went into nurse training, argued that it was a disadvantage to the student nurse, mainly because it did not help in learning practical skills. This writer saw the main advantages of a degree as coming later in a nurse's career, and for personal fulfilment.[120]

The wife of the Minister of Housing, H. Brooke, visited North America, and described the nursing situation there for the *Nursing Times*. She noted the two-tier system of nursing: the degree nurse, who graduated from college or university with a degree as well as a nursing diploma, and the practical nurse, with only an elementary education, common sense and a love for people, who assisted professional nurses by providing practical care. Yet, even in the United States recruitment was a problem, and Brooke noted the doubts of many senior nurses as to whether such training methods would produce reliable nurses 'though they would be the first to say that nurse training must advance with the times and not be hidebound by loyalty to the past to the detriment of progress in the future.'[121]

Conclusion

The 1950s was a period of intense debate about nurse education, the nature of the nurse as generalist or specialist, and whether nurses should continue to be trained according to the British system, or be developed through a supernumerary college-based, degree programme, as in North America. As Goddard realised, what was at stake was the proper task of the nurse and the very identity of nursing.

Despite Goddard's affirmation of the Nightingale tradition, by the turn of the half-century there was a perceptible loss of confidence in the traditions generally, and in the traditional apprenticeship model of nursing in particular. Perhaps it was this time of societal and moral change, including increased communications, that encouraged a search for new ideas, particularly North American ideas; educational philosophy differed fundamentally between Britain and North America.

As shown elsewhere, North American nursing was influenced by the liberal educational ideal of self-actualisation, and the philosophy of John Dewey's American pragmatism.[122] North American nursing was optimistic about the intrinsic potential of human nature, reflecting the prevailing philosophy of education as a creative, liberating process of personal self-development. The

British concept of education was perhaps more realistic. Human nature had to be nurtured and disciplined in order to shape the capacity for moral virtue. American nursing education was therefore nurse-centred, whereas the British nursing tradition sought to make the nurse patient-centred. As a modern British educationalist has recognised, for the nurse to learn to be responsive to patient needs entails an introduction into the practices of a corporate tradition.[123]

Notes

1 G. Rivett, *From Cradle to Grave: Fifty Years of the NHS*, London, King's Fund, 1998, p. 109.

2 B. Watkin, *The National Health Service: the First Phase*, London, George Allen & Unwin, 1978, p. 49.

3 House of Lords Parliamentary Debates (Hansard), *Shortage of Nurses*, London, HMSO, 1948, c.283–313, November 9.

4 Ibid., c.384–385.

5 M.G. Shout, 'Teaching Practical Nursing', *Nursing Times*, 1948, pp. 761, 764, October 16.

6 M. Scales, *Handbook for Ward Sisters*, London: Baillière, Tindall and Cox, 1st edn, 1952; 2nd edn, 1958.

7 M. Scales, 'A Ward Sister's View', correspondence, *Nursing Times*, 1948, p. 804, October 30.

8 R. White, *The Effects of the National Health Service on the Nursing Profession 1948–1961*, London, King Edward's Hospital Fund for London, 1985, p. 256.

9 Ibid., p. 257.

10 M. Farnworth, *A Study of the Social Prestige of Nursing*, London, report submitted to the Medical Research Council, 1952.

11 Ibid., p. 1.

12 M. Farnworth, 'The Social Prestige of Nursing', *Nursing Times*, 1952, pp. 604–605, June 21; pp. 628–631, June 28; pp. 688–690, July 12.

13 Ibid., p. 631.

14 Ibid., p. 690.

15 M. Farnworth, *A Study of the Social Prestige of Nursing*, London, report submitted to the Medical Research Council, 1952, Appendix 4, i.

16 Ibid., p. 1.

17 'Recruitment – a Social Problem', editorial, *Nursing Times*, 1952, pp. 601–602, June 21.

18 M. Simson, 'Is Nursing a Vocation?', *Nursing Times*, 1953, pp. 899–900, September 5.

19 C. J. Wood, *A Handbook of Nursing for the Home and the Hospital*, 8th edn, London, Cassell & Co., c. 1887, pp. 18–19.

20 'The Basic Things of Nursing 1: A Relationship between two People', *Nursing Mirror*, 1953, p. 1598, September 18; 'The Basic Things of Nursing 2: Profession or Vocation?', *Nursing Mirror*, 1953, p. 1662, September 25; 'The Basic Things of Nursing 3: Service and Satisfaction', *Nursing Mirror*, 1953, p. 28, October 2.

21 Ibid., p. 28.

22 G. Lance, 'Staff Shortage has not Affected the Modern Training of the Nurse', Point of View, *Nursing Mirror*, 1953, p. 1216, August 7.

[23] E. Pooley, 'Wanted – Nurse with a Vocation', letter, *Nursing Mirror*, 1953, p. 38, October 2; F. Bell, 'Nursing is a vocation', letter, *Nursing Mirror*, 1953, p. 244, October 23.

[24] The Nuffield Provincial Hospitals Trust, *The Work of Nurses in Hospital Wards: Report of a Job-analysis*, Goddard, H.A., Director, London, Nuffield Lodge, Regent's Park, 1953.

[25] Ibid., p. 127.

[26] Ibid., pp. 38–39.

[27] Ibid., p. 131.

[28] Ibid., p. 132.

[29] Ibid., p. 132.

[30] Ibid., 132–133, report's emphasis.

[31] Ibid., p. 142.

[32] Ibid., p. 146.

[33] Ibid., p. 147.

[34] 'Study Conference – "The First Step" ', editorial, *Nursing Times*, 1953, pp. 479–480, May 16.

[35] 'The Job Analysis Study Conference', *Nursing Times*, 1953, pp. 482–484, May 16.

[36] 'The Work of Nurses in Hospital Wards: Report of a Job Analysis Undertaken by the Nuffield Provincial Hospital Trust, *Nursing Times*, 1953, pp. 176–177, February 21; 'Extracts of the Report will be Published in this and Subsequent Issues of this Journal: Introduction', *Nursing Times*, 1953, pp. 177–178, February 21; 'The Work of Nurses in Hospital Wards: Abstract of the Report of a Job Analysis Undertaken by the Nuffield Provincial Hospital Trust', *Nursing Times*, 1953, pp. 203–206, 211, February 28; 'Allocation of Ward Duties', editorial, *Nursing Times*, 1953, p. 225, March 7; 'The Work of Nurses in Hospital Wards: Abstract of the Report of a Job Analysis Undertaken by the Nuffield Provincial Hospital Trust, concluded', *Nursing Times*, 1953, pp. 233–237, March 7; 'Change of Direction?', editorial, *Nursing Times*, 1953, p. 253, March 14; 'The Work of Nurses in Hospital Wards: Abstract of a Job Analysis Undertaken by the Nuffield Provincial Hospital Trust, continued', *Nursing Times*, 1953, pp. 259–264, March 14; 'Job Analysis Study Conference', editorial, *Nursing Times*, 1953, p. 455, May 9; 'Study Conference – "The First Step"', editorial, *Nursing Times*, 1953, pp. 479–480, May 16; 'The Job Analysis Study Conference', *Nursing Times*, 1953, pp. 482–484, May 16; 'The Job Analysis Study Conference', *Nursing Times*, 1953, p. 506–508, May 23; 'Recruitment – a Social Problem', editorial, *Nursing Times*, 1952, pp. 601–602, June 21; 'The Work of Nurses in Hospital Wards', *Nursing Times*, 1953, pp. 750–755, July 25; 'College Conference on the Job Analysis', editorial, *Nursing Times*, 1953, pp. 1233–1234, December 5; 'The Job Analysis Report', *Nursing Times*, 1953, pp. 1238–1240, December 5; 'The Job Analysis Report', *Nursing Times*, 1953, pp. 1273–1275, December 12; 'Job Analysis on Nursing: "The Work of Nurses in Hospital Wards"', *Nursing Mirror*, 1953, pp. 456–458, February 20; 'The Proper Task of a Hospital Nurse', editorial, *Nursing Mirror*, 1953, pp. 480, 496, February 27; 'The Proper Task of the Nursing Profession', editorial, *Nursing Mirror*, 1953, p. 512, March 13; 'Job Analysis Report', *Nursing Mirror*, 1953, pp. 163–162 (concluded opposite page), April 17; 'Job Analysis Report', *Nursing Mirror*, 1953, pp. 502, 522, May 22; 'House of Lords Debate on Nursing, Job Analysis Theme', *Nursing Mirror*, 1953, pp. 503–504, 522, May 22.

[37] 'The Proper Task of a Hospital Nurse', editorial, *Nursing Mirror*, 1953, pp. 480, 496, February 27.

[38] 'The Proper Task of the Nursing Profession', editorial, *Nursing Mirror*, 1953, p. 512, March 13.

[39] 'Facts about Nursing', leading article, *The Lancet*, 1953, pp. 379–380, February 21.

[40] 'Hospital Job Analysis', editorial, *Nursing Times*, 1953, p. 173, February 21.

[41] The Royal College of Nursing, *Comment on the Nuffield Provincial Hospitals Trust Job Analysis of the Work of Nurses in Hospital Wards*, London, Royal College of Nursing, 1953, November.

[42] Ibid., p. 8, para. 5.
[43] Ibid., p. 9, paras 6–7.
[44] Ibid., p. 10, para. 8.
[45] Ibid., pp. 13–14, para. 20.
[46] 'Nursing Problems in the Provinces', leading article, *Lancet*, 1953, p. 1292, June 27.
[47] The Royal College of Nursing, *Comment on the Nuffield Provincial Hospitals Trust Job Analysis of the Work of Nurses in Hospital Wards*, London, Royal College of Nursing, 1953, November, p. 20, para. 34.
[48] R. White, *The Effects of the National Health Service on the Nursing Profession 1948–1961*, London, King Edward's Hospital Fund for London, 1985, p. 203.
[49] Ibid., p. 197.
[50] 'House of Lords Debate on Nursing, Job Analysis Theme', *Nursing Mirror*, 1953, pp. 503–504, 522, May 22.
House of Lords Parliamentary Debates (Hansard), *Hospital Nursing Services*, London, HMSO, 1953, c.421–450, May 12.
[51] Ibid., c.436–437.
[52] Ibid., c.441.
[53] 'Facts about Nursing', leading article, *The Lancet*, 1953, pp. 379–380, February 21.
[54] 'The Means at our Disposal', *Nursing Times*, 1954, pp. 1230–1231, November 5.
[55] C.A. Russell, 'The Nurse Must Choose Whether She Wants to be Nurse or Administrator', Point of View, *Nursing Mirror*, 1953, p. iv, August 21.
[56] General Nursing Council for England and Wales, *Syllabus of Subjects for Examination for the Certificate of General Nursing*, London, General Nursing Council for England and Wales, 1923; revised 1925, 1933, 1939, 1952, 1955.
[57] E.R.D. Bendall, E. Raybould, *A History of the General Nursing Council for England and Wales 1919–1969*, London, H.K. Lewis & Co., 1969, p. 149.
[58] General Nursing Council for England and Wales, *Syllabus of Subjects for Examination for the Certificate of General Nursing*, London, General Nursing Council for England and Wales, 1952, revised 1952; General Nursing Council for England and Wales, *Syllabus of Subjects for Examination for the Certificate of General Nursing for Male nurses*, London, General Nursing Council for England and Wales, 1952, revised 1958.
[59] General Nursing Council for England and Wales, *Record of Practical Instruction and Experience for the Certificate of General Nursing*, London, General Nursing Council for England and Wales, undated.
[60] General Nursing Council for England and Wales, *Guide to the Syllabus of Examination for the General Register*, London, General Nursing Council for England and Wales, undated.
[61] Ibid., p. 10.
[62] Ibid., p. 8.
[63] E.R.D. Bendall, E. Raybould, *A History of the General Nursing Council for England and Wales 1919–1969*, London, H.K. Lewis & Co., 1969, p. 181.
[64] E.E.P. MacManus, 'The Working Party Report – a Critical Survey', *Nursing Times*, 1947, pp. 834, 839, November 29. E.R.D. Bendall, 'Commitment to What?', in *A Time for Commitment*, Baroness Cox of Queensbury, Chairman, pp. 35–42, London, ENB, November 15, 1983.
[65] N. Mackenzie, 'Needs and Resources in the Nursing Profession I: The Means to the End', *Nursing Times*, 1953, pp. 1236–1237, December 5; 'Needs and Resources in the Nursing Profession II: The Pattern of Ward Life', *Nursing Times*, 1953, pp. 1267–1268, December 12; 'Needs and Resources in the Nursing Profession III: The Pattern of the Classroom, *Nursing Times*, 1953, pp. 1288–1290, December 19.
[66] Ministry of Health, Department of Health for Scotland, *Report of the Committee Set Up to Consider the Function, Status and Training of Nurse Tutors*, Janet K. Aitken, Chairman, London, HMSO, 1954.

[67] Ibid., p. 13, para. 26.
[68] 'Function, Status and Training of Nurse Tutors', *Nursing Times*, 1955, pp. 145–149 February 11.
[69] C. Saunders, 'The Modern Hospice', in *In Quest of the Spiritual Component of Care for the Terminally Ill: Proceedings of a Colloquium*, Wald, F.S. (ed.), pp. 41–48, Yale University School of Nursing, 1986, May 3–4.
[70] A. Worcester, *Nurses and Nursing*, Cambridge, Harvard University Press, 1927 p. 172.
[71] D. Kremsdorf, 'An American Nurse Looks at British Nursing', *Nursing Mirror*, 1953, p. 145, May 15.
[72] G.B. Carter, 'Collegiate Education for Nursing: A Review of Dr. Margaret Bridgeman's Book', *Nursing Times*, 1953, pp. 812–813, August 15.
[73] 'Edinburgh University – the First Research Fellowship in Nursing', *Nursing Times*, 1953, p. 311, March 28; G.B. Carter, 'Windsor, Ontario, Experimental School: A Review of Dr. Lord's Evaluation', *Nursing Times*, 1953, pp. 316–318, March 28.
[74] G. Sharpe, 'New Trends in Curricula for Schools of Nursing 1: In Canada', *Nursing Times*, 1953, pp. 814–815, August 15.
[75] G.B. Carter, 'Experimental Training for Nurses', *Nursing Times*, 1954, pp. 6–8, January 2.
[76] S.M. Burkinshaw, 'Trends in Nursing Education', *Nursing Times*, 1954, pp. 204–205, February 20.
[77] E.D. Stevens Fisher, 'American letter – 13: A Series of Personal Views and Comments on Life in America', *Nursing Times*, 1954, p. 286, March 18.
[78] 'Working Conference at St Andrew's University for Trained Nurses in any Field Organized by the Scottish Board of the Royal College of Nursing', *Nursing Times*, 1954, pp. 421–422, 430–431, April 17.
[79] B.N. Fawkes, 'A Year at Teachers College, Columbia University, New York 1: Introduction', *Nursing Times*, 1954, pp. 1017–1019, September 18; 'A Year at Teachers College, Columbia University, New York 2: Public Health in Basic Training', *Nursing Times*, 1954, pp. 1075–1076, October 1; 'A Year at Teachers College, Columbia University, New York 3: Personnel and Counselling Problems', *Nursing Times*, 1954, pp. 1140–1141, October 15.
[80] 'University Co-operation', editorial, *Nursing Times*, 1954, pp. 1085–1086, October 8.
[81] 'The Function of the Training School is not only to Teach the Mind but to Form the Character', *Nursing Times*, 1954, pp. 871–876, August 14.
[82] F. Nightingale, 'Sick Nursing and Health Nursing', in Hampton, I.A. (ed.), *Nursing of the Sick*, pp. 24–37, New York, McGraw-Hill, 1893.
[83] 'The Function of the Training School is not only to Teach the Mind but to Form the Character', *Nursing Times*, 1954, pp. 871–876, August 14.
[84] 'Ward Teaching', *Nursing Times*, 1954, pp. 1283–1285, November 19.
[85] E.J. Bocock, 'The Education of Nurses', *Nursing Times*, 1954, p. 601, June 5.
[86] R. Murray, 'Looking Ahead – The Education of the Student Nurse', *Nursing Times*, 1956, pp. 362–366, May 4.
[87] 'The College Council Meets', *Nursing Times*, 1954, pp. 1044–1045, September 25.
[88] J. Akester, 'The Education of the Nurse', *Nursing Times*, 1954, pp. 918–200, August 19.
[89] 'Training Nurses', editorial, *The Times*, 1955, p. 7, August 22.
[90] J.H. Chillman, 'Training Nurses', letter, *The Times*, 1955, p. 9, August 25.
[91] L. Darnell, 'The Education of the Nurse: Further Considerations', *Nursing Times*, 1955, pp. 1056–1058, September 23.
[92] I. Spalding, 'Professional Ideals,' *Nursing Times*, 1955, pp. 1198–1200, October 21.
[93] J.E. Home, 'Ideals and Education', letter, *Nursing Times*, 1955, p. 1259, November 4.
[94] 'The College Prayer', *Nursing Times*, 1954, p. 750, July 10.

[95] 'Ethics and Public Health Nursing', *Nursing Times*, 1954, pp. 264–267, March 11, pp. 294–295, March 18.

[96] R. White, *The Effects of the National Health Service on the Nursing Profession 1948–1961*, London, King Edward's Hospital Fund for London, 1985, p. 262.

[97] The Royal College of Nursing, *Observations and Objectives: A Statement on Nursing Policy*, London, Royal College of Nursing, 1956.

[98] Ibid., p. 5.

[99] Ibid., p. 11.

[100] 'Pattern of Nursing Education: Report of W.H.O. Working Conference', *Nursing Mirror*, 1954, pp. 426,434, May 15.

[101] The Royal College of Nursing, *Observations and Objectives: A Statement on Nursing Policy*, London, Royal College of Nursing, 1956, pp. 22.

[102] Ibid., p. 23.

[103] R. White, *The Effects of the National Health Service on the Nursing Profession 1948–1961*, London, King Edward's Hospital Fund for London, 1985, p. 264.

[104] 'The Nursing Team', Annotations, *Lancet*, 1956, p. 1090, November 24.

[105] W. Ritchie Russell, 'The Future of Nursing', letter, *Lancet*, 1956, p. 1261, December 15.

[106] C. Wilfred Vilning, 'The Future of Nursing', letter, *Lancet*, 1956, pp. 1353–1354, December 29.

[107] B. Watkin, 'The Future of Nursing', letter, *Lancet*, 1956, p. 1354, December 29.

[108] T. Anderson, 'The Training of Nurses', letter, *Lancet*, 1953, pp. 1047–1048, May 23; T. Anderson, 'The Future of Nursing', letter, *Lancet*, 1957, p. 45, January 5.

[109] R. Macbeth, 'Future of Nursing', letter, *Lancet*, 1957, p. 96, January 12.

[110] J.M. Akester, 'Future of Nursing', letter, *Lancet*, 1957, p. 96, January 12.

[111] G.M Wauchope, C.M. Ottley, 'Future of Nursing', letter, *Lancet*, 1957, p. 96–97, January 12.

[112] D.J. Rose, 'Future of Nursing', letter, *Lancet*, 1957, p. 97, January 12.

[113] Royal College of Nursing, *Observations and Objectives: A Statement on Nursing Policy*, London, Royal College of Nursing, 1956.

[114] S. Harvey, 'Vocation', letter, *Nursing Times*, 1958, p. 816, July 11.

[115] A. MacDougall, 'Vocation', letter, *Nursing Times*, 1958, p. 870, July 25.

[116] D.D. Stalford, 'Vocation' letter, *Nursing Times*, 1958, p. 932, August 8.

[117] J. Wolfenden, 'Moral Values in a Changing Society', *Nursing Times*, 1958, pp. 794–797, July 11.

[118] R. Fletcher, 'A Changed Society and its Effects on Nursing', *Nursing Times*, 1958, pp. 530–532, May 9.

[119] 'Staff Nurses Conference', *Nursing Times*, 1958, pp. 500–502, May 2.

[120] E.M. Meir, 'Nurses with Degrees', *Nursing Times*, 1958, p. 629, May 30.

[121] H. Brooke, 'In Search of Ideas', *Nursing Times*, 1958, pp. 680–681, June 13.

[122] A. Bradshaw, *Lighting the Lamp*, London, Scutari Press, 1994.

[123] P. Jarvis, 'Commentary on A Case Study of a Patient-Centred Nurse', in Fulford, K.W.M., S. Ersser, and T. Hope (eds), *Essential Practice in Patient-Centred Care*, pp. 193–197, Oxford, Blackwell Science, 1996.

Chapter 6

The turn of the tide, 1960–1972

The 1960s, the period in which the values of British society were radically altered, was also the period for nursing in which the apprenticeship system and its ethos came under sustained attack. This culminated in the Briggs Report of 1972 which set in train the break with the tradition. As previous chapters have shown, although the apprenticeship system of nursing, its principles and values, had been subject to scrutiny and criticism in previous decades, the profession itself was united in its defence. Gradually this unity fractured so that by the 1960s the self-understanding of nursing's tradition was increasingly fragmented. This chapter will examine the sociological and psychological influences on change, and review the evidence and arguments used in its support. Previously unexamined evidence will raise the central question, the extent to which the sea-change in nursing was justified.

The context of patient care

A hundred years after nurse training began at the Nightingale School, there is every indication that Nightingale's principles still dominated British nursing.[1] The ward sister controlled the ward in which student nurses learned. Consultants were classified as visitors; they and house officers and registrars had appointed times to conduct their rounds. At other times the ward was closed to them, specifically to enable patients to rest. The ward sister's influence was not only with respect to medical staff, but also with respect to her nursing superiors, and naturally, also with respect to all staff and student nurses.

Specified nursing work included giving bowls and mouthwashes, attention to pressure areas, feeding seriously ill patients, charting fluids, recording observations, and performing nursing treatments. Each task had a prescribed time, which included a time for ward prayers. Nursing administrators had a daily round. Aspects of care that might be very important to the patient, but which he may be unwilling or unable to ask for – commodes, cups of tea, wound dressings, drugs, even newspapers – had an appointed time.

By the early 1960s rigorous routines, the safeguard of patient care, and the basis of apprenticeship training, were argued to have become rigid and restrictive. The report of a group of senior nurses, chaired by the Matron of St

George's Hospital, Muriel Powell, sought to bring reform.[2] The timetable of the ward was to be revised, so that patients would no longer be woken unnecessarily early. Hospital life was to be as near to home life as possible, so that patients could sleep longer in the morning and rest more during the day.

North American nursing revisited, 1960–1961

Debate over the apprenticeship continued into the 1960s. L.R.C. Haward, an occupational psychologist, argued that nurses in the future would either be university-trained technicians or bedside attendants, much as in the United States.[3] Moreover, a new approach to the selection and training of nurses was needed. The *Nursing Times* disagreed: the example of the ward sister and matron was crucial in the formation of character, 'that cornerstone of Miss Nightingale's philosophy'.[4] Through apprenticeship the nurse learned endurance, patience, tolerance and fortitude. A similar, anonymous response to Haward's article argued that it was a rather detached and mechanical psychological analysis; the writer thought that the essence of nursing must remain the vocation.[5] Other writers argued that the most important characteristic of the nurse remained the unmeasurable quality of kindness. Academic cleverness was quantifiable, and although it was important it was no substitute for kindness.[6] Even though modern society was obsessed with status it still expected the traditional nurse.[7]

The *Nursing Mirror* also asked 'What is Wrong with Apprenticeship?' Nursing was essentially a skill and a craft, not an academic subject learned from books: 'all "head" knowledge is the servant of the hands and the understanding heart'. It was derived from the medieval craft guilds which sought the highest possible standards of workmanship in the particular craft. In order to become a master the apprentice had to go through stages of training and testing, rather like the nurse. Through these stages the apprentice, like the nurse, entered into a hierarchy and a tradition.[8]

Beatrice Brysson Whyte, Sister Tutor at Guy's Hospital, and co-author of the textbook, *Bedside Nursing*,[9] was a leading nurse in the 1960s and 1970s.[10] She studied in America in 1959 as the result of a Florence Nightingale Memorial Committee Scholarship, and joined the General Nursing Council as a member in 1965. Whyte played a significant part in the work of the Education Committee, becoming chair of the council's *ad hoc* Committee on Examinations and Assessments in 1975. Her contribution after this period seems to have been at post-registration level as a member of the Joint Board of Clinical Studies. She pioneered the use of objective tests and structured examination questions, and initiated processes that linked theory with practice and developed schemes of continuous assessment. The Guy's Practical Workbook became a template for other schools of nursing.

However, unlike many of her colleagues during this period, Whyte was not so enamoured with American nursing systems. In two articles in the *Nursing Times* in 1960 and 1961 she analysed the differences between the North American and British systems of nursing, with particular regard to nurse preparation. North American hospitals were staffed by student nurses, practical nurses and nursing aides, who performed bedside care, while graduate nurses, trained at colleges, preferred not to remain at the bedside but turned instead to teaching and research.[11]

According to Whyte, aides took temperatures, made beds, bathed patients and assisted with serving meals. For them, nursing was 'just another job', and hence evening shifts were often not covered, so that, for example, patients did not have evening washes, or have their beds made. Graduate nurses gave medicines, took blood pressures, bathed patients and carried out simple treatments. The head nurse sat at the nurses' station with the ward secretary.

While equipment was plentiful in comparison with Britain, cleanliness was poor. A patient's spilled ginger ale remained sticky on the floor all day, dead flowers littered window sills, locker tops remained undusted, waste-paper baskets were unemptied, often with dirty dressings thrown in them by doctors. Doctors were aloof, they communicated with nurses in writing, leaving messages in books. They performed many tasks such as dressings, removal of sutures, passing oesophageal tubes, that would have been performed by nurses in Britain. Young interns worked harder and longer hours than their British counterparts, but did not expect the same help or cooperation from their nursing colleagues as British doctors did. Unlike American nurses, British nurses developed nursing judgement through their bedside experience. American doctors had no such resource from their nursing colleagues.

Whyte thought that North American health care had positive aspects: medical attention, the importance attached to communicating with patients, the food, the limitless supply of equipment and the friendly, easy-going atmosphere of the wards. But there was a deficiency in the actual bodily care. There were staff shortages and a lack of integration of ancillary staff. This had resulted in an untidy nurse, who by best British standards 'lacks forethought and finish; she preaches total patient care but does not know how to practise it'. The patient's care was fragmented. After an operation, for example, recovery from anaesthesia was in the recovery room, medicines were given by the 'medicine nurse', intravenous infusions set up by the 'intravenous unit nurse', breathing exercises given by the 'medicine unit nurse', temperature taken by the aide, meals served by the dietician, then the patient would be brought back to the ward by the helper, have his wounds dressed by the intern, and his back 'rubbed' by his wife.

The American system was economically driven, suspicious of alternative systems, such as the British system, that might deemed to be charitable. North American nurses assumed a superiority to British nursing, perhaps because British nurses were enthusiastically bringing home North American ideas. Whyte, however, preferred the British system.

In her second article, Whyte took a perspicacious look at this contrast between the British and American philosophy of nurse education.[12] The different ethos was summed up by a remark from an American clinical tutor: 'Our nurses must not be used for service, they are here to learn.' The degree was a pathway to status and, in order to combat the problem of differences in intelligence, standards were lowered to make a degree attainable by everyone. The American nurse had to pay for her degree course and work her way through college as any other student. She was taught to consider herself primarily as a student, and was apt to see the patient in relation to her own needs rather than his.

The ward was a place where she spent a few hours only, to gain experience of patients suffering from the particular condition she was studying. She did not have the chance to see how her contribution fitted into the total pattern, and her loyalties were divided between her instructor and the head nurse. The student was constantly told that she had to be a leader, but the current status of the American head nurse was not such as would inspire nurses to take on that job. British nurses assumed responsibility immediately, whereas North American nurses were supported for three years and then expected to assume immediate responsibility. Neither method was entirely satisfactory, but the British system produced more able nurses.

Although there were many more nurse teachers in North America than there were in Britain, they were often inexperienced. Told that they were capable of teaching immediately following their degree in nursing, teachers were often keenly aware of their limitations and could actually be afraid of their nurses. The presence of a clinical instructor removed the responsibility of teaching from the head nurse. Class teaching was often poor because of the lack of practical experience by the teacher. The emphasis on class hours rather than achievement of nursing skill meant that the nurse finished her course almost completely lacking in clinical judgement. This may not be such a problem in America, where the nurse worked under the direction of the doctor, 'but in England where the nurse and doctor work as colleagues, theoretical as opposed to practical training would eventually mean the end of the art of nursing as we know and practise it'. Experience was vital and should not be forgotten or dismissed as 'repetitive tasks'.

Whyte argued that the American nurse, although descended from a long line of bedside nurses, now had no resemblance to any of them: 'In raising the "standard" of nurse training they have succeeded in raising it too high for bedside nurses and leaving the patients worse off at this moment than they ever were.' Instead, American nursing has produced an administrator, a research worker, and, to a lesser degree, a teacher. In some hospitals it was a case of 'never have so few been supervised by so many'. Nevertheless, there was great administrative efficiency in such an enormous country, research uncovered and dealt with problems long before British nurses had thought of them, and the American teacher had much more time to prepare for, experiment in, and evaluate her teaching than overloaded British nurse tutors.

Whyte concluded that British nursing could learn lessons from the United States but should not 'follow them blindly down the slope for the wrong reasons'. British publicity, rather than methods, was at fault for not identifying what gave the British nurse her unique ability at the bedside. Perhaps uniqueness lay in the role of the ward sister, the focal point of the ward; or else, in that nurses were taught to feel responsible for their patients from very early in their training. Whatever made British nursing unique should be identified before it was thrown away.

Two letters in the *Nursing Times* supported Whyte's analysis. M.L. Campbell, writing from New York, congratulated Whyte 'on her vivid, entertaining and devastatingly accurate account of nursing as it is over here'.[13] Isabel G. Duncan was also disappointed at American standards.[14] But another correspondent refuted deprecations of the North American system as the result of 'old-fashioned' values.[15] Insights from psychology expressed in concepts such as 'nurse–patient relationship, group therapy, supportive theory, therapeutic environment and a host of others', were a great force for good in American nursing.

Here was the dichotomy between British and North American nursing. In Britain still, at the start of the 1960s, the nurse was accorded status by the general public precisely because she was a practical bedside carer. The 'bedpan round', for example, was considered to be of supreme importance in nurturing the nurse–patient relationship.[16] In North America practical nurses had a lesser status than graduate nurses; bedside nursing had less prestige than research and teaching.

Many did not agree with Whyte. A report on an exchange of nurse teachers between Belfast, Toronto and Boston, (*Nicusane – Northern Ireland, Canada, United States of America Nurse-Teacher Exchange*), found the North American system of nurse education impressive, with advantages over the UK apprenticeship method, even though the strengths of the UK system and the weaknesses of North American nursing were acknowledged.[17] The vocational apprenticeship, with its clear-cut objectives of care and cure, was held by those in the UK to be 'real nursing'; but the conformity and conservatism it produced was deprecated.[18] UK nurses embraced bedside care and placed teaching, technical skill, supervision and administration secondary to it. In North America the opposite applied.

Yet the Nicusane Report also noted that this was a minority view in 1963: 'The idea that practical training is vastly superior to theoretical training is dying hard in Great Britain.'[19] Tutors in Belfast were experienced nurses, with practical experience, whereas in Toronto and Boston the contrary was true. In Belfast students were taught more formally than in North America and examinations were both written and oral, in school and in State Registration, whereas in North America examination was written only. Practical experience and apprenticeship in Belfast was compared to the more theoretical approach and student status of both Boston and Toronto. Confidence in the British tradition was about to be seriously attacked and undermined.

Professional unanimity breaks down

In 1960 Brian Abel-Smith, Professor of Social Administration at the London School of Economics, published his seminal work, *A History of the Nursing Profession*, which became the inspiration for most modern nursing history writing and teaching. Covering the period 1800 to the late 1950s, the book relied heavily on secondary sources, particularly for its views on Nightingale. Abel-Smith did not seek to give an impartial account of nursing history, but rather to apply analyses from social policy to the development of nursing. As the book noted on its cover, Abel-Smith's perspective was that of 'a sociologist who discards the myopic sentimentality of nurses as dedicated heroines upon whose selfless service the community was entitled to rely'.[20]

This was a political history, focusing on structures and rivalries, and as such was intentionally selective in the material used:

> Facts do not speak for themselves. By their selection and presentation the reader is influenced to accept the viewpoint of the writer. For this reason an author should at some point come into the open and expose his values to the criticism of the reader. This is the purpose of the final chapter.[21]

Abel-Smith believed that the history of nursing was no different to the history of any other occupation. What was exceptional, he argued, was the difficult and demanding nature of the work, the emotional demands and psychological stress nursing engendered, the retreat into group loyalty, the discipline and the search for perfection which it entailed and which not everyone could handle. The result was a widespread public admiration for those who took on the work. As he concluded: 'In this sense, nursing is a vocation.'[22]

But in Abel-Smith's opinion, this ideal exploited nurses. Standards for nurses on pay, hours and management attitude were different to those of the outside world; but nurses were deterred from vehement protest by the discipline imposed by matrons, and loyalty to group and hospital:

> and by the spirit of uncomplaining service which was taken to be the heritage of their profession. Underfed, overworked, and underpaid, they struggled on rather than break a 'professional' code of honour. Activism was unprofessional, worse still it would have undermined the cherished spirit of vocation: it smelt of hard bargaining and the pursuit of selfish material interests. It was also unfeminine.[23]

The book provoked disagreement. The Principal Nursing Officer at the Ministry of Labour, and Chairman of the International Council of Nurses, B.A. Bennett, reviewed it with concern. She suggested that the title of the book was a misnomer, because the book was a history not of the nursing profession, but of the politics of general hospital nursing: 'It makes much – probably far too much to be of any value today – of the rivalries between the professional organisations in the early part of the century.'[24]

Abel-Smith had used many reports and documents, according to Bennett, but his consultations may have influenced his selection. She thought it a valuable book, which needed to be read in context, alongside other books, and with a wider knowledge of the actual situation. She thought that those who read it would be knowledgeable enough to 'sort it out for themselves'. Bennett was particularly critical of one passage in the book: Abel-Smith had argued that Nightingale popularised nursing for ladies, who then wrenched control from Nightingale, and 'kicked down the ladder'. According to Bennett: 'This does not tell the whole story and is a distorted and almost mischievous use of words.'

Bennett criticised Abel-Smith's conclusion and underlying thesis, that salaries, conditions of service, standards of training, and delegation of duties, needed to be resolved in order to improve recruitment. On the contrary, Bennett argued, most people would not agree. Furthermore, it was inaccurate, in that it was not the case that nursing was suffering from a recruitment crisis: 'The number of persons employed in nursing and who have taken up training has increased enormously (at a guess 100,000 in the last thirty years if we include *all* who contribute to nursing care).' Problems of recruitment were because of the enormously increased demands. So Bennett concluded that improvements in nursing structures and methods could occur without radical upheavals. Despite such misgivings, Abel-Smith's history became an influential classic, a 'major work' which commanded 'respect if not always agreement'.[25]

Another important piece of work to influence the future of nursing was the Freudian analysis of Isabel Menzies, who worked at the Tavistock Institute of Human Relations, and whose approach was derivative of the psychoanalysis of Freud's pupil, Melanie Klein.[26] Menzies's research observed facts similar to those adduced by Goddard in 1953, but interpreted them vastly differently. As she wrote in the *Nursing Times*, Menzies hoped to encourage nurses to become self-conscious and emotionally aware. She believed this would counter the stress that nurses experienced.

The two approaches of Goddard and Menzies were very different, although their criticisms, that nursing was task-orientated and hierarchical, were similar. For Goddard the patient was central; for Menzies, effectively, the nurse's emotional repertoire was central. According to Menzies, the organisation militated against closeness of patient and nurse, which nurses wanted, and despite the fact that 'teaching emphasizes its importance'.[27] Menzies, however, rejected the traditional nurse–patient relationship. In Freudian terms, it was a defence mechanism that inhibited personal 'growth' of the nurse.

When Menzies's report was published in the journal *Human Relations*, a review appeared in the *Nursing Times* that was severely critical of both the method and analysis of her study.[28] The reviewer disagreed with Menzies's analysis. Her work had originated from a general hospital which had called in the author to help work out a duty rota for student nurses. But neither the system, the study, nor the changes, were described in full. Instead, a theory was proposed to explain the findings. The only data given by which to judge the theory was the data chosen to support it.

The theory was Kleinian theory, which had attracted a considerable following, 'but is hotly debated even among psychoanalysts'. This theory, following from Freud, proposed that infants' strong feelings gave rise to fantasies about other people and themselves which in turn led to anxiety. Anxiety was controlled by projecting feelings on to others, or by sublimating them. In Menzies's view, this was precisely what nurses did when they controlled their strong feelings by defence mechanisms that sublimated primitive urges of love and hate for patients. The hospital provided nurses with defence mechanisms by preventing nurses from becoming too intimate with patients. This was achieved by task assignment, by uniforms which minimised individuality, by ignoring nurses' feelings, by treating all grades of nurses alike and by failing to provide nurses with personal counselling. Defence mechanisms displaced responsibility upwards through a nursing hierarchy, so that nurses carried out their tasks in ritualistic and unthinking ways. Hence, personal satisfaction was not achieved.

The reviewer was critical of Menzies's work. While not wishing to deny the fact of neurotic anxiety, or the 'silly things that Miss Menzies has shown up', the reviewer could not accept the main theory of neurotic anxiety underlying individual behaviour. If this were so, then periods of greatest carnage, death and disaster, would lead to a breakdown of the nursing services. In fact the contrary was the case: 'When death and disaster are greatest, as in war, nursing is most adaptable and successful.'

There were four main criticisms of Menzies's report. Firstly, standardisation was a method of economy and order, rather than a defence mechanism. Organisation, for example the tidiness of equipment, reduced stress because the nurse knew where to find her equipment, and job assignment was efficient. Secondly, Menzies's theory relied on a weak analogy. A theory developed from individual human behaviour could not be generalised to a ward, a hospital, or indeed, British nursing as a whole. Thirdly, the study was biased. Data was collected within a socio-therapeutic relationship. But, according to the reviewer, facts should be collected in a neutral way and a theory developed from the facts, rather than using a frame of reference that assumed a pathological state. If facts were fitted to suit an underlying theory, it would not be surprising if a diagnosis of pathology resulted. Finally, the study method was not fully described. Although it was stated that seventy nurses, 10 per cent, were interviewed, there was no suggestion that this was a random sample, and no discussion about how many interviewees showed the kind of anxiety described: 'As a rule great pains are taken to make sure that the staff understand and are not threatened by the study itself.' This was not the case in Menzies's study.

The reviewer proposed another explanation from the data of Menzies's study. The hospital had incompetent leadership:

> Poor administration made it difficult to carry out the primary task of caring for the sick. The staff were worried about this. Those who had a pride in their work, who could not stand the muddle and the unhappy atmosphere, and who were able to do so, left. The increased turnover of senior staff brought to administrative posts junior and inexperienced people who had no one competent to guide them. Instead of looking into the efficiency of matron's office, a psychoanalyst was called in who worked within a socio-therapeutic relationship – in itself a stressful situation for the staff.

The reviewer's solution was to bring in a competent matron, known and trusted by the nurses, who could restore self-confidence by re-establishing order in the nursing service.

According to another writer in the *Nursing Times*, Menzies's very limited study had immediate impact, causing 'much ruffling of professional plumage'.[29] This writer was also critical of the methods and conclusion of the study, the small place given to the patient, and the evidence presented that 'professional nursing' was somehow different to 'bedside nursing' in the eyes of the sociologist intent on analysing professional careers. As White has since pointed out, it is debatable whether Menzies's allegedly Freudian analysis derived from one large London hospital and untested, should have been so generalised. Yet, Menzies's critique of the *status quo* was widely disseminated and would become influential.[30]

The influence of Menzies's ideas was perceptible in a letter published in the *Nursing Times*, which described the traditional induction of nurses into the tradition of selfless dedication, the '*vocation theory*', as a 'pernicious manifestation' of a handed-on neurosis.[31] The 'recent work, done to show the psychodynamics of nursing', it stated, 'proves that far from being selfless, nurses are *selfish*': 'Dedication' was, in fact, the mark of a personality disorder. If older nurses thought that the younger generation lacked vocation, this is because the younger generation were less neurotic. The new generation of nurses were looking for different satisfactions: money, good hours, good conditions and lack of petty restrictions.

This letter provoked a reaction. An 'older nurse', argued that even though 'vocation' had become 'practically a rude word', it was no personal aberration to enjoy one's job.[32] Another respondent considered that in order to increase recruitment, nursing had two options: either to be judged as a profession with the main criterion for success being cash reward, or to stress the vocational aspect, not material reward but a reward of work done to the glory of God.[33] This letter was taken up by a suggestion that vocation be emphasised by teaching its meaning to the profession.[34]

However, there was weariness with this vocational argument. Letter writers suggested material security mattered more,[35] so did practical concerns, including incidents of low standards of care.[36] A *Nursing Times* editorial appeared to agree, suggesting that although research on administration and training were important, more important were practical matters: 'the prevention of pressure sores and incontinence; the bathing, dressing and feeding of helpless patients; the methods of rehabilitation and care and nursing treatment'.[37]

Abel-Smith, on the other hand, was keen to develop research-mindedness in the profession in order to investigate sociological aspects of nursing, administrative studies and studies of attitudes of doctors and patients towards nurses and vice versa.[38] He advocated the endowment of a nursing research institute that would be the bedrock of such research. Nursing needed to follow in the footsteps of North American nursing, discovering and analysing attitudes of patients, doctors and nurses. In his view the 'common sense' tradition of care could no longer be assumed as a basis for care. Indeed, he thought that attitude surveys would bring to light criticisms of the quality of patient care.

There were, however, more traditional approaches to nursing difficulties. R.W. Revans's study of *Standards of Morale* in hospitals thought that any problems of authoritarianism that junior nurses were experiencing could never be removed by externally imposed changes in syllabus, generous pay, or by any other administrative action.[39] Many nurses that Revans interviewed still thought of nursing as inherently a vocation.[40] One or two nurses said that 'nursing today was a "vocation only up to a point"', but, according to Revans, their view was exceptional. Revans concluded from his study that what was involved were cultural patterns, traditional beliefs and personal canons of conduct.

Although he suggested that psychotherapeutic techniques, then being developed, may have had a place, he saw the ultimate answer as lying in personal relations between individuals: 'True communication lies not so much in the physical passage of information ... as it lies in the will to communicate and in the desire to know whether the communication is serving the needs of those who seek it.' Problems would not be resolved by changing the entire culture but by altering the attitudes of senior staff in particular hospitals.[41]

Richard Titmuss's analysis of hospitals in the 1950s supported this view. He suggested that advances in applied scientific medicine, the growth of specialism, the fragmentation of services, alongside increasing organisational bureaucracy and, he thought, some failure in training, led to a lack of thought about the patient and his feelings. These attitudes, Titmuss believed, were neither deliberate nor conscious; they were 'done unthinkingly by people who are devoted to their calling, working unselfishly and for long hours in the interests of the sick'. In earlier times, when the hospital was a simpler institution, and when the natural, intuitive sympathies of doctors, nurses and others had not been overridden by long specialised courses of training, it was not perhaps necessary to emphasise elementary needs.[42]

Significantly, Titmuss commended Nightingale's *Notes on Nursing* and her insight into how the sick suffer mental pain – apprehension, uncertainty, waiting, expectation, fear of surprise – almost as much as bodily pain. Like Goddard, he appreciated her belief that the patient needed to be saved from worry by the nurse anticipating his needs. Because Nightingale never lost sight of the patient's fundamental needs, she sought factual tools to distinguish between the efficient and inefficient, an important part of her legacy to nursing.[43]

Challenging the *status quo*: professional division over the nursing 'revolution'

In June 1961 the practical part of the preliminary examination was abolished. There were further changes to part 1, to make it wider ranging, and part 2, to make it more comprehensive. In February 1962 the final examination also became more comprehensive. In 1962 a new syllabus was published.[44] This had three main sections: principles and practice of nursing including first aid; the study of the human individual; and concepts of the nature and cause of disease and principles of prevention and treatment.

The Guide to the newly revised syllabus explained that training schools had to submit a detailed scheme of both theoretical and practical training for approval by the GNC.[45] The preliminary examination was not included in the 1962 syllabus, because much of the content had been unrelated to practical nursing care and was quickly forgotten, and introductory schools were often separate from the overall teaching programme and the wards. The new syllabus sought to integrate all subjects throughout training. There was an increased emphasis on anatomy and physiology. The health service and social aspects of nursing were to be included under nursing history, and the ethics of nursing were to be introduced from the earliest stage of training.

Training was to start with an eight-week introductory course, and subsequent theoretical training in fourteen to sixteen weeks of study days or study blocks. Formal lectures were to be given by medical and specialist staff to introduce new material. Clinical teaching, group discussions and seminars should be increased. Teaching, observation and practice in nursing procedures, and testing of proficiency in them, was a major part of the syllabus which needed the closest cooperation between ward and classroom. All new work should be introduced by the fourth month of the third year. An intermediate examination should occur after fifteen months, assessing both ward and school work. Practical ward tests were to be observed from time to time by GNC inspectors.

The record of practical instruction was revised to allow for more individual entries by ward sisters and clinical instructors. By 1965 half the training schools of England and Wales were approved to use it. All needed to gain approval by 1968 because the last preliminary examination was held in October 1969.[46] The 1962 syllabus was a development of the apprenticeship system which built on previous syllabuses, and which relied on the central role of the ward sister. It affirmed that there should be no split between theory and practice. Classsroom learning should relate to practical ward experience and vice versa.

The previous unity within the nursing profession was, however, to break in 1964 with the Royal College of Nursing report, *A Reform of Nursing Education*, chaired by Sir Harry Platt.[47] Among the members of the committee were several forward-looking nurse tutors, keen to change the *status quo*. The remit of the committee was a complete reappraisal of the system of nursing education in Britain. Its proposals, in the words of the report itself, were 'revolutionary in character' and would require amending legislation because they were so 'drastic'. There was an urgency for the implementation of its recommendations to 'reform' of basic education. Further delay 'would endanger' the nursing service.[48]

The Platt Report argued that there was a need for more nurses as well as better-prepared nurses. As the largest professional group in the health service, nurses needed to be equipped to assume the responsibilities of leadership as well as be prepared to understand and perform increasingly complex techniques and procedures. Nurse education needed to prepare nurses with a background understanding and enable them adopt a critical approach to their work as well as adjust to changing conditions.

Society had changed over the last twenty years. Many more women were marrying and at a younger age, and so leaving the profession (which the committee predicted would continue). Many more professions were open to women. There were now increasing facilities for higher education. People entered nursing expecting a professional training that would stimulate and challenge them. If it did not students would become disillusioned and leave. It was vitally important that nursing provided courses that would attract and retain such students.

There was evidence of dissatisfaction and public concern about the state of the health service. Failure 'to provide a therapeutic environment' might be due to various factors, including a staff shortage and old buildings, but part of the dissatisfaction was due to 'traditional organisation, to the inflexibility of ward routine and the authoritarian approach'. The committee came to the 'inescapable' conclusion that the form of training failed to give the student an adequate understanding of human, social and psychological problems, and left her unprepared for certain technical procedures.[49] With regard to experimental degree courses, the committee suggested that a more concentrated educational programme would mean nurses could be registered in two years. The committee also thought that giving direct patient care was an essential element of professional education for the student, and that the principles of nursing could be taught as a university subject.

There was little factual evidence or relevant data to support the urgent desire of the committee for change.[50] Nevertheless, Platt's recommendations were 'revolutionary in character'. The committee proposed different grades of nurses: enrolled nurses prepared by a two-year apprenticeship, ward assistants (the old nursing auxiliary and ward orderly in one grade), and student nurses, who should undergo a two-year academic course with some supernumerary practical experience followed by a pre-registration year in full-time service under supervision. Schools of nursing should be managed and financed independently of hospitals under the auspices of regional councils. Student nurses would be 'students' in fact and not in name only. In the first two years student nurses should be financed by regional council grants, and in the third year they should receive two-thirds of the minimum staff nurse's salary. University degree courses were also to be established.

Platt was in line with the earlier RCN report *Observations and Objectives*.[51] The *Nursing Times* published a summary of the report and welcomed it.[52] Many of the opinions it sought, from a broad spectrum of professionals, were very positive, but there were some doubts raised about the accuracy of the report, as well as the implications.

Abel-Smith noted the similarity of Platt to Wood, although, and with irony, Wood's recommendations were regarded as 'pink peril' while the Platt Report in its blue covers was much more likely to be accepted.[53] Although he criticised Platt's report for its lack of statistical evidence, Abel-Smith agreed with the objective of improving recruitment by student status and was pleased with the principle of nursing degrees to prepare nurse leaders and administrators.

An educationalist, W.E.D. Stephens, was also critical of the lack of factual backing to the report.[54] A matron, B.B. Scott, was worried that the Platt recommendations would not produce a practical nurse and feared that if the recommendations were implemented, British nursing would become like North American nursing where the qualified nurse was deficient in practical skill. Practical skills were gradually and almost unconsciously acquired through practice and experience. Although technical skill was necessary for the modern nurse it was important that 'the milk of human kindness' should not be lost.[55]

A hospital management committee secretary, S.G. Hill, also found the report unconvincing. The assertion that the present system was responsible for the high wastage was unsubstantiated, and it was not clear that proposals would remedy this anyway. A retreat into academia would not provide practical nurses. And would the academic entrant still be called a 'nurse'? Hill wondered to what extent marriage, poor communication and human shortcomings were not more accurate causes of wastage. Hill was sceptical about the proposed educational hierarchy needed to implement Platt, and fearful about the philosophical change in nursing. The British nursing tradition needed to be preserved. No 'diehard reactionary', Hill argued for evolution rather than revolution. Nurses needed to be more practical, compassionate and understanding, rather than technical and theoretical: midway between junior doctors and practical nurses: 'We need nurses who *nurse*, and not nurses who are too over-educated to attend to a patient.'[56]

A meeting of the Student Nurses' Association highlighted anxiety that Platt's proposals would mean student nurses losing touch with patients, and that bedside care would be carried out by nurses of less academic attainment.[57] A student nurse who had left the profession welcomed the report, although the writer commented that many other student nurses were furious at the thought of the drudgery being taken out of nursing. This is what they had entered nursing to do. The *Nursing Mirror* also welcomed the Platt Report. [58]

But the Platt Report was not welcomed by the General Nursing Council for England and Wales who sent its considered comments to the Minister of Health in the Labour Government, Kenneth Robinson. On October 1, 1965, both the *Nursing Mirror* and the *Nursing Times* published the GNC response in full. As a news report in the *Nursing Times* stated, the GNC did not consider that there was a need for the drastic reform proposed by Platt. [59] The body responsible for nurse training said it was keeping nurse training under constant review and as a result a list of measures had been introduced. A 1962 syllabus of general training for student nurses had been introduced. Revised conditions for approval of training schools had been implemented from January 1964 which ensured a greater width of clinical experience. Tutor numbers were increased and compulsory refresher courses had been introduced. Clinical instructors were now employed, and it was hoped to increase the number, although this was dependent on resources. Standards of examination were being raised. Pupil nurse training was being encouraged with a revised syllabus from August 1964. Experimental schemes, under the jurisdiction of the GNC, were encouraged.

The GNC believed that the Platt Report was unrealistic in thinking that raising the educational requirements of student nurses would encourage entrants. This would reduce entrants, and if student nurses were given full student status there would be an inadequate number of pupil and enrolled nurses to take their place. It was essential to decide the desirable composition of the ward team regarding trained and ancillary staff, and there was no information available at that time. The GNC disagreed that there should be a higher proportion of less academic practical bedside nurses and a smaller proportion of nurses with higher academic qualifications who would become the leaders of the profession. Although there was a need for more girls who were practical bedside nurses, it was not true that fewer girls with higher educational qualifications would be needed to become State Registered Nurses. More attention should have been given to the training of pupil nurses.

In the view of the GNC, the 1962 syllabus and planned allocation had given hospitals a greater awareness of the needs of student nurses. Even so the success of this scheme, as with Platt's own proposals, depended on an adequate supply of staff to nurse patients. The GNC believed an adequate supply of tutorial staff and clinical instructors to supervise nurses would meet the Platt proposals, but this should be under the present system. The GNC also pointed out that a very great number of those who entered training as student nurses did so with a stronger desire to be a nurse than to be a student 'and that if too great an emphasis is placed on the student status of a nurse in training this may in fact act as a deterrent to recruitment'.[60]

The GNC's own proposals were for moderate experiments in higher education and student status. Entry to such courses would be by General Certificate of Education at 'A' Level rather than, as the Platt Committee had advocated, at 'O' Level. Apart from such experimental schemes, schools of nursing should not be financially independent. The GNC recommended immediate steps to explore the possibility of developing degree courses related to nursing to meet the needs of academic high-fliers, who would otherwise be lost to nursing, and who could not then obtain posts of international standing. The GNC wanted to retain responsibility of nurse training and did not believe this could be delegated to regional councils without the grave danger of introducing widely differing standards. But it called for greater powers and independence for Area Nurse Training Committees. The GNC was against the establishment of independent schools of nursing, except on an experimental basis, and saw the choice as one between a hospital-based apprenticeship training and a college-based education. The former was preferable. Whatever system of training was employed, the training and education of nurses must be in the hands of the ward sisters, who were themselves accountable to the matron.

The response from the GNC to the RCN committee, as Baly confirms,[61] argued for evolutionary rather than revolutionary change. Unlike previous reports, this had resulted in division in the profession about the nature of nursing. The RCN wanted to professionalise nursing by increasing its status and academic respectability, while the GNC wanted to preserve the service ethic. In the GNC's view, this was the real motive for choosing to become a nurse.

Correspondents to the nursing journals were broadly critical of the GNC memorandum. A group of student nurses from Bournemouth wrote to the *Nursing Times* calling for the implementation of the Platt Report and student status because the trainee role was 'abused'.[62] Further letters published in the *Nursing Times* expressed frustration and annoyance at the GNC rejection of the Platt Report.[63] An anonymous correspondent likened the GNC proposals to the cosmetic and symbolic changes of a totalitarian regime seeking self-protection against outside criticism.[64]

The *Nursing Mirror*, which had assumed an anti-traditional editorial policy under a new editor in 1963, criticised the GNC conservatism.[65] Its editorial suggested that six members of the newly elected and constituted GNC council had tabled a motion calling for the Platt Report to be reconsidered.[66] The editorial writer wondered how unanimous the original council members were in their criticisms of Platt, and how, given the *in camera* nature of meetings, their decisions were arrived at. Other editorials in the *Nursing Mirror* commended change, criticised older nurses, in that their reactionism hindered progress, and argued that progress in training and education could not be halted.[67] Yet, another view of the period, expressed in an award-winning essay, suggested that, despite having advanced with the times, nurses had retained the characteristics of the tradition. Nurses' professional values had remained unaltered, as had their faith in perpetuating the vocation of caring for the sick.[68]

The *Nursing Mirror* continued its criticisms of the GNC,[69] but was itself criticised by a correspondent who argued that the *Nursing Mirror* was too radical, and that bedside nursing must remain the essence of nursing.[70] An Open Forum debate in the *Nursing Mirror*, responding to Platt, showed the divisions within the profession. The defender of Platt argued, from personal experience, that intensive teaching and studying following post-basic training had led to personal fulfilment, and suggested there was a growing discontent with the second-rate 'ministering angel' nurse.[71] The opposer argued that problems in the profession were largely due to poor hospital administration and failure to implement GNC recommendations.[72]

The GNC during this period was itself divided, according to a history written by two of its members.[73] There were two distinct schools of thought in the council. The more conservative element worried about the disruption change would cause to training schools and nurse training, and therefore urged caution. On the other hand, more radical members were keen to show that there was neither consensus nor unanimity among the council members. The education department of the GNC was headed by Barbara Fawkes, and one of the authors of the history, Eve Bendall, served on the education committee,[74] and was also a member of the Platt Committee.[75] Both believed in radical change.

Feelings ran deep. One member of the Platt Committee was told by an opposing colleague 'that she might be forgiven in the next world but it was unlikely she would be forgiven in this one!'[76] Platt reflected the 1960s turmoil of a changing society with changing values, a period in which the concept of 'progress' involved a belief in radical change. As the *Nursing Mirror* editorial noted in 1965, the world was so rapidly changing that any attempt to preserve the *status quo* was 'doomed to failure and ridicule'.[77] And a nursing researcher, Doreen Norton, described the period as the 'rather crazy nursing world of the 1960s, during which time nursing was growing more professionalized, management was becoming more sophisticated and techniques and specialities were proliferating'. Norton, far from reactionary herself, as her seminal research on older people shows, was extremely worried that the character of nursing would be fundamentally altered, so that it would lose its crucial basic values.[78]

Reform of education involved a change of values. Monica Baly made this clear in her BMA award-winning essays in that year.[79] The apprenticeship involved cheap labour, suppressed critical questioning, and required a blind adherence to routine. 'It was unlikely that the profession would breed many revolutionaries.' Nurses were overworked and underpaid because their work was assumed to be 'Christian duty'. They were the subject of 'adulation and sentimental praise which was cloying to the art of self-criticism'.[80] There was a need for radical change. Baly suggested that there should be two types of training. The narrower preparation for State Registration should be via higher education, in which the student nurse's educational needs took precedence over service requirements. There should be fewer registered nurses but they would be better trained. The second type of training, the shorter, two-year training for the roll, would produce an understanding and safe practitioner. To prevent this group being exploited as cheap labour there would be non-nursing personnel to do non-nursing tasks. Student nurses would be replaced by enrolled nurses and orderlies.

This issue seems to have been worrying the profession even beyond Britain during that period. The Chief Nursing Officer of the World Health Organization, Lyle Creelman, quoted the editor of an American nursing journal who, about to undergo a surgical operation, observed that what she (or he) wanted were nurses who were kind and feeling and could respond as warm human beings. The editor did not want to feel alone.[81] While commending educational experiment and change, Creelman supported the idea of the qualified nurse continuing to remain close to the patient. She also alluded to the particular situation in Britain where the ward sister traditionally had an important teaching function. This needed to be retained. Despite a wide-ranging lecture commending nursing research and academic development, the bottom line of nursing should remain the practical, compassionate, bedside nurse.

In 1966 the Ministry of Health published the *Report of the Committee on Senior Nurse Structure*, chaired by Brian Salmon.[82] This committee was set up to advise on senior nursing staff structures in hospitals, their administrative functions, and methods for preparing staff to fulfil these functions.[83] A new management structure for nursing was proposed, with lines of top management, middle management and first-line management.

Organisational and managerial change was recommended. The professional function of the nurse (requiring a nursing qualification) was differentiated from both the administrative function of the nurse (coordinating jobs and the people who do them) and the personnel function of the nurse (relating to the welfare of subordinates).[84] The new role of chief nursing officer, envisaged by Salmon, did not specify the regular ward rounds for supervision of patient care and ward environment that had been the prime task of the former role of matron.[85]

The historical review of nursing administration, which provided the underlying premise, was explicitly drawn from Abel-Smith's nursing history: 'Much of the material in this chapter comes from this study.'[86] Although training and organisation in nursing history, particularly in the work of

Nightingale, featured in the report, and some religious influence was acknowledged, the importance of individual character was not: 'The discipline in the training came from the religious systems of the Continent and was perhaps influenced by the Army, but it had its justification in the conventions of the age: if educated women, that is, gentlewomen, were to be attracted to nursing, strict tutelage was necessary.'[87] The report treated the moral ethos of nursing as originating in a passing phase of history and culture, with little relevance to the present.

There were unresolved contradictions in the report. Nursing staff 'often expressed in evidence, a desire to remain "close to the patient" ' and it was noted that many nurses did not wish to exchange practical skills for managerial posts. Administrative nurses who longed to 'roll up their sleeves' were criticised for meeting their own needs rather than those of patients. Yet, the report did not address the significance of this desire among nurses, believing instead that the creation of managerial posts, by virtue of their perceived importance in serving a greater number of patients, would appeal to nurses with 'a developed sense of vocation'.[88]

One trenchant criticism of Salmon, by Dr J.W. Paulley, was that it undermined the 'real' nurse by the introduction of second-rate nurses as distant and detached administrators, divorced from direct patient care. It was also undemocratic:

> Distress is widespread at the consequences for British nursing of this folly foisted on a long suffering and greatly undervalued profession without ballot of its members and without the promised five-year pilot schemes. However, open protest by middle and senior nurses has been almost effectively silenced as if we live in a police state. Brave, indeed, the nurse who protests, knowing her promotion and prospects are firmly in the hands of the very people who regard Salmon as the new god and anything against him, blasphemy.[89]

The momentum for change: the Report of the Committee on Nursing (the Briggs Report) 1972

The Briggs Committee was set up in October 1970 by Richard Crossman, the Secretary of State for Health in the Labour Government, to relieve the government's embarrassment over the threat posed by nurses because of its prices and incomes policy. Arguably, this had indirectly led to the RCN 'Raise the Roof' campaign of 1969.[90] There was perceived to be a crisis in nursing. The remit of the committee was to review the role of the nurse and midwife in hospital and community, and look at the education and training needed to fulfil that role, to make best use of available manpower and so meet present needs as well as the needs of the integrated health service.[91]

Professor Asa Briggs, the historian, later to become Lord Briggs, was a surprising choice as chairman. In an overheard conversation at the House of Lords between Lady Summerskill and Lady Serota, formerly a minister under Richard Crossman, Lady Summerskill expressed surprise that Briggs would know anything about nurses and midwives. Lady Serota assured her that an independent chairman was the nurses' choice.[92]

In October 1972 the report was published. Its key recommendations were as follows. A single central body, the Central Nursing and Midwifery Council, was to be formed, responsible for professional standards, education and discipline for nursing, midwifery and health visiting in Great Britain. Colleges of nursing, midwifery and possibly health studies, were to be established. Education should be a continuous process. An eighteen-month introductory period followed by a modular course leading to registration was proposed. Nursing and midwifery education was to include knowledge of professions supplementary to medicine, including social work. The nursing and midwifery profession should become more research-based. More attention should be devoted to the recruitment of 'A' level, undergraduate and graduate entrants.[93]

The underlying assumption of the report was that the Nightingale tradition was outdated. Its historical perspective relied heavily on Abel-Smith's history of nursing,[94] although, like the Salmon Report, it referred to some writings of Nightingale. The view of the report was that inherited images of nursing were those of 'the lady with the lamp' or 'the ministering angel' – images from the late nineteenth century. This inherited image of the nurse, created by Nightingale among others, had the following features.

Nurses were subservient and ancillary to doctors and were considered their 'handmaidens'. Nurses had to fight 'sometimes ruthlessly' for their status. The essence of this fight was gender related because nurses were mostly women while doctors were mainly men. There was a class element in the traditional image: nineteenth-century women from higher social classes were those who chose to follow a 'vocation', providing a theme in itself, 'a theme, of course, with an older history leading back to the middle ages'. The nurse evolved 'her own distinctive code' which involved not money but service. She was usually described as 'dedicated'.[95] A direct quotation from Abel-Smith was used to underline the essence of the nursing code: 'the search for perfectionism and the attempt to achieve it by discipline'.[96]

Like Abel-Smith, the report had little sympathy with the Nightingale tradition of dedicated vocation, or its perpetuated moral ethos which still remained powerful. In the committee's view, the structure was hierarchical and authoritarian and the image of the matron remained the most powerful inherited image for the early 1970s.[97] While not all branches of nursing were seen in terms of such inherited images, the following section of the report intended to clarify the relationship between past and present. By listing the groups of people in 1970 who used the term 'nurse', the report concluded that 'Inherited images do not mirror this variety within nursing and midwifery. Yet not all images are inherited ones, and attitudes are changing all the time.'[98] Although, as Briggs argued, the traditional image of the nurse held by the public did not reflect reality, the report was not concerned to separate out image from fact, because it was inherited images which 'influence current attitudes and policies'.[99]

It has been argued since that the Briggs Report was a re-run of Bedford-Fenwick's professionalisation battle, now instigated by modern-day professionalisers.[100] There was a clear agenda to move nursing away from its apprenticeship tradition, and its underpinning values, as Briggs's speech to the Association of Hospital Matrons demonstrated.[101] Asa Briggs agreed with a *Nursing Times* editorial, that the role of the nurse needed to be clearly defined, but he was specific that this meant going beyond stereotypes.[102] In his view much more was required than merely to create a new image of Florence Nightingale: 'we are dealing in society with something more than images. The structures themselves require thorough review.'

Asa Briggs believed that the patient's viewpoint was important, but more important still was the motivation of nurses, not only then but in the future. This statement offers an important insight. Briggs was making the assumption that social relationships had changed in the previous ten years and would continue to do so. This, he believed, would affect the kind of people who would become nurses, their expectations and motivations. The 'thorough review' and complete revision intended by Briggs seemed to require not an updating of the Nightingale image, but its replacement. The report was intended to be prophetic, to presage the future rather more than reflecting on, and drawing lessons from, the past.

This was a contemporary view: it was fashionable to denigrate Nightingale at the time of the Briggs Report. This was made clear by Dr Wolstenholme, speaking in a lecture about Florence Nightingale given to the Royal Society of Medicine in 1970. The contemporary 'accusation' of Nightingale as a 'dreadful' woman, whose stress on nursing as a vocation hampered nursing, was unjustified.[103] According to Wolstenholme, she did not, as critics were claiming, suppress the economic and intellectual freedom of nurses. For Nightingale (as for many of the nurses who followed her) the idea of nursing as a calling did not rule out material rewards for nurses: 'I need scarcely add that nurses must be paid the market price for their labour, like any other workers; and that this is yearly rising.'[104] The idea that nurses needed to be obedient was not a demand for slavery. Rather, obedience was envisaged as the obedience of intelligence arising from a just and fair authority structure in the natural order.

It was against these rather negative assumptions about the Nightingale tradition, which historical evidence did not in fact support, that the Briggs proposals were published.

What evidence, then, from contemporary nursing was used to justify the proposals? The evidence selected by the committee seemed hardly to provide support for such radical changes. Concerns about recruitment were not founded in reality, the report admitted. Total numbers of nurses and midwives had increased through the 1960s and reached new heights each year. There was a greater proportion of nurses and midwives in the total working population than in the previous decade. Despite a fall in the number of eighteen-year-olds after 1965, the number of nurses in training had proportionately increased.[105] Indeed, as the general labour force was contracting, nursing recruitment was actually expanding.[106]

Briggs admitted that the prevalent concern over shortage and wastage rates in nursing was based on opinion and attitude rather than 'hard facts'. Worries were expressed about future needs as well as the education and training necessary to meet these hypothetical needs: 'In this connection we noted the sombre words at the beginning of the annual report of the Royal College of Nursing for 1971 that "all is not well with nursing".' It was this sense of urgency that precipitated the founding of the committee, and influenced its report.[107] The imperative to change was not, it seems, derived from factual evidence.

Neither were nurses as dissatisfied as many on the committee seemed to imagine they must be. The Briggs Committee was surprised that dissatisfaction with work, hours, shifts and promotion prospects were less prevalent than it expected.[108] Many nurses found enjoyment, satisfaction and a sense of doing something worthwhile in nursing. As one nurse wrote: 'I've never met a nurse who can't find something to moan about ... Yet whenever I am asked if I enjoy nursing ... I say, yes, it's a wonderful life. Compared with chasing after money, it is. Compared with the rat race of office life it is. Compared with living in luxury on a Pacific Island it probably isn't. But, then, who gets that chance?'[109]

These opinions, the report noted, were expressed in their questionnaire survey. But not all the evidence commissioned was actually published in the report. The Briggs Committee had commissioned its own research of nursing attitudes from an independent research organisation, Social and Community Planning Research (SCPR). The research data appears to be used selectively in the report. Other opinions expressed in the survey were not documented at all. The reason for the kind of enjoyment and satisfaction expressed by nurses, above, might have been found in answers to question 7a of their postal survey, which is included as an appendix, 'Can you say why you decided to take up nursing in the first place?'[110] Yet, no mention of the answers occurred in the report.

Why this should be so is not clear. In reply to a personal letter from the author asking where it would be possible to find the answers given by nurses in the survey to this question, Lord Briggs agreed that the answer to this question, which did not appear in the report, was not only interesting but important.[111] In fact, Social and Community Planning Research (SCPR) had prepared two reports for the Briggs Committee in 1971, according to the research director:[112] 'The first (our ref. 02.188)[113] was a report on a postal survey, on which the question "Can you say why you decided to take up nursing in the first place?" was asked. Unfortunately the results of this "open" question were not, it seems, written up in this report ... The second report (our ref.02.194) [114] was a report on depth interviews carried out with nurses.'

The postal survey showed general satisfaction with nursing as a career.[115] Despite the high level of satisfaction that people usually expressed with jobs they were currently doing, the researchers were surprised that only just over half of nurses said nursing was the only type of work that would satisfy them. Yet 45 per cent of respondents described themselves as 'very happy' in their work, and almost all the remainder described themselves as 'quite happy'.[116] In considering factors that affected nursing morale, the researchers found there was strong agreement that nurses' opinions were not adequately considered, and not enough care was taken of them, but there was less agreement with the statement that 'Routine tends to be more important than the welfare of the patient.'[117]

The introduction and first few pages of findings of the SCPR report dealt with nurses' motivations. The main reasons for women wanting to become nurses were expressed in the following statements: 'I always wanted to'; 'I wanted to help people'; 'I had been in hospital myself'; 'My mother/ sister was a nurse'. Most nurses were highly motivated, but for some, 'I drifted into it'; 'It was just a job'. Occasionally, the report found, for some nurses who wanted to help people, 'there was a sense of "mission"; more often it was simply a recognition that helping other people was a worthwhile field for a career.' This was the main source of personal satisfaction about the job once it had been entered into.[118]

The authors of the report, Jean Morton-Williams and Richard Berthoud, believed that:

> it is difficult to draw any firm conclusions about the sort of person who is most likely to take such a decision [to take up nursing], or what precisely it was that led to it. Many of the motives mentioned had the appearance of post-hoc rationalisation, or justification for the decision, and in many cases the event was too far in the past for the arguments to carry much weight.[119]

Whether this judgement interprets the nurses' testimony objectively seems questionable. In effect, as the authors admitted, the informal structure of the interviews together with the fact that it was a small, selected sample, meant that firm conclusions could not be drawn: 'We present what might be called an anthropological view of nurses' problems, as they appear to outsiders.'[120] They admitted to making their own interpretations of the opinions they were given: not as nurses saw nursing, but as the researchers did.

Clearly, potential nurses knew full well what being a nurse involved. The SCPR depth interview study noted that '*bedpans*', which they underlined, were the universal symbol of all that is worst in nursing, among both nurses and the laity: 'There was hardly a single interview which did not mention them. Perhaps it is their ordinariness which makes them so unpopular.'[121] Recruits were unlikely to be starry-eyed romantics.

Although the Briggs Report admitted that some of its own evidence had shown that 'most recruits learn about nursing not from literature (few admit to having been influenced by advertisements) but from personal contact, often with relatives',[122] it took no account of nurses' own opinions on motivation from its own survey, or the depth interviews carried out for the Briggs Committee by SCPR. Instead, it quoted the National Association of Head Teachers' statement that the public image of any trade or profession can influence considerably recruitment.[123]

The Briggs Committee perceived, independently of gathered evidence, a powerful public image and this proved basic to the report's analysis of nursing. The report stated that nursing recruitment was strongly influenced by media images in magazines, films and newspapers, and on television, of romantic, sentimental and glamorous portrayals of nurses. This anecdotal material was discussed in three lengthy paragraphs in the report.[124] According to the report, nurses portrayed in the media were always those working in acute general hospitals rather than those in other specialities, such as psychiatry, midwifery or the community.[125] In the view of the committee, 'Public images influence recruitment: they also predetermine attitudes at critical moments in the health history of individuals and families.'[126]

These fictional media images were not mentioned by SCPR, and one is led to question how much influence such portrayals actually had on recruitment, particularly as the report itself admitted that recruits in fact learned about nursing from personal contact, often from relatives. Potential recruits did not seem to have been influenced by media representations, or did not choose to admit to such influence. Why, then, did the committee give so much space in the report to details of impressionistic and fictional media images, yet ignore evidence of nurses' own opinions recorded by its own commissioned surveys?

The answer to this fundamental question may lie with the chairman's own presuppositions. Ten years later, at a major nursing conference, Briggs revealed his own preoccupation with nursing images.[127] He spoke not of the changing role of the nurse, but of the changing role of the image of the nurse. And he looked back to the Briggs Committee. In his mind, changing nursing involved changing public perception. This could only be achieved if the committee understood the image of the nurse held by the public. And this was not to be sought by collecting data from opinion surveys, rather it was to be found by immersing oneself in the kind of literature the public read about nurses: 'I encouraged members of my own Committee to read novels about nursing. I have about 40 or 50 of them, they are very strange, many of them, but they do appear to sell in quite large numbers. Articles appear on nursing. We have very well informed and interesting journals and I read those very regularly, and continue to read them myself now because I think it is of great importance'. By reading such material, fiction included, Briggs believed that it was possible to see the public face of nursing. It was this public face of nursing, its public image, that affected recruitment, patients and people in need of nursing care as well as people involved in political decision-making.

But, contrary to this belief that nurses were attracted by the media portrayal of a glamorous image, in fact the opposite was true. As the *Nursing Times* in 1972 pointed out, a then current publication entitled *Careers Advice for Teachers*, published by the National Union of Teachers, was quite negative about a nurse's life: 'Nursing is variously described as tiring, depressing, squalid and badly paid. The girl who has enough guts to get her SRN can then go on to make good money either in private nursing or in the higher posts and more especially abroad.'[128]

It seems that people in the 1970s, both lay and nursing, knew that the nurse's life was far from glamorous. The image of the bedpan was universally recognised. The life was known to be hard. Careers teachers would no doubt have pointed this out to potential nurses. Girls who chose to become nurses would have known they were entering a profession that demanded a dedicated commitment to a compassionate service. This may be described as 'a vocational attitude'. Ordinary people saw the nurse's life with a realism that belied the analysis given in the Briggs Report. It was this very realism, the endurance demanded of nurses, that made nurses so appreciated by the general public. As the report noted, current press coverage was highly favourable to British nursing. Unsolicited letters of criticism recognised that when nursing did fail the cause was directly related to issues of power which turned hospitals into institutions, and replaced 'ladies of the lamp' with 'dictatorial automatons'.[129]

The SCPR survey showed that the situation was more complex, and more positive, than the Briggs Report painted. Morton-Williams and Berthoud stated that: 'Nursing appeared to be a highly motivated career. The majority of nurses entered for positive reasons, and many did so to fulfil a long-standing ambition. Only a minority treated it as just a job. On the whole, nurses were happy with the theoretical instruction they received in training.'[130]

There were criticisms, of the amount of practical instruction received, staffing levels, and conditions of work, but most nurses did not seek higher promotion than that of sister 'since it would involve loss of contact with patients, and the abandonment of "real nursing"'. The one drawback that hindered this sense of satisfaction was the preoccupation with discipline and hierarchical status: 'To one or two respondents, it appeared that status and discipline were being used as a substitute for good leadership. Senior nurses were being put in charge of wards because of their qualifications in nursing as such; where these were not accompanied by the ability to lead a team, they were compelled to retreat behind a wall of stiffness and issue commands.' One respondent summed it up: 'Status seems so important in nursing, and it shouldn't – *nursing* should be the most important thing'.[131] Despite such criticisms, the researchers concluded:

> Almost all nurses were extremely satisfied with their choice of profession. The key to this was the satisfaction of caring for patients, either curing them or alleviating their suffering. The work was *interesting*, it was *rewarding* and it was *worthwhile*. Nurses were proud of their skill and enjoyed using it. They felt that their profession gave them status in society, or at least that it should do so.[132]

Although Morton-Williams and Berthoud used the word 'career' to describe nursing, this was their choice rather than nurses' own words. They admitted that, as social scientists, their own bias had some influence on their analysis. Nevertheless, the burden of evidence shows that nurses saw nursing differently from the way the Briggs Report portrayed it.

Surprisingly, despite commissioning this SCPR research, the Briggs Report stated that for evidence of nurses' motivations it was using the work of Jillian MacGuire,[133] one of its advisers, which it did not want to duplicate.[134] This collection of various studies on nurse recruitment and attrition was supervised by Brian Abel-Smith. But MacGuire's own previous work, which will be examined in the next chapter, found nursing to be still a vocation.[135] As she summarised her findings in 1961: 'Those who considered nursing to be a vocation had higher scores on the scale of commitment to nursing than did those who considered nursing to be a career.'[136] Briggs was selective in the use of this evidence also.

Broad statements were made by Briggs which do not appear to have been substantiated by data. Citing the evidence of nurses' opinions, Briggs stated that training 'tends to destroy initiative, common sense and dampens the enthusiasm which most nurses have to get to know and look after ill people'.[137]

But it is questionable whether evidence showed this to be a majority opinion. For example, nurses questioned by the SPCR attitude survey suggested that authoritarianism was the result of a failure in nursing leadership, rather than due to problems with training.

Briggs's radical review of nursing corresponded with the Royal College of Nursing's view, expressed in evidence to Briggs.[138] The RCN stated that the traditional image of the nurse as 'ministering angel' needed 'by adequate and forceful publicity' to be replaced by emphasising the wide range of opportunities open to the trained nurse. This premise may have partly originated from what the RCN understood to be an authoritarianism in nursing tradition which it saw as being 'alien to the liberal society of to-day'.[139] As the Royal College of Nursing hoped, the future of nursing was expected to lie in the social sciences and education, rather than biomedical science.

The Briggs Committee agreed that the future track of nursing was not the track of the paramedical nurse. Nursing care was separate from medical care, and indeed, referring to Nightingale, it was suggested that the nurse and not the doctor supplied the vital force of care. Scientific developments did not define the nursing role – the nurse 'is not one of the doctor's means of treating patients'.[140]

Indeed, the report seemed to reflect an anti-medical bias. Briggs detailed nine 'widespread complaints' against doctors that it had collected from nurses and midwives.[141] Doctors were possessive towards particular beds and admitted patients without consultation. There were too many separate medical rounds. There was poor communication between doctors and a lack of orientation of some overseas doctors. Doctors were reluctant to visit patients at night leaving decisions to nurses and midwives. Research that was planned and prepared by doctors involved nurses and midwives in considerable and unrecognised work. Equipment was installed without consultation but nurses and midwives were expected to monitor it. Doctors planned new developments without consultation on staffing implications.

But the following paragraph in the report appears to have contradicted this list of complaints.[142] Nurses had complained about only a minority of doctors, and indeed, 'a good deal of praise for doctors has also been forthcoming from nurses and midwives'. This praise, however was not detailed, and criticism was generalised: 'What we would hope to see in future would be a change of attitude among those doctors to whom one or more of the complaints listed above applies, so that ultimately all live up to the standards of the best.'

Having detailed complaints against doctors, however, the report did not discuss complaints against nurses. Instead it commented: 'Doctors could doubtless list large numbers of complaints about nurses and midwives. Cooperation is a two-way matter.'[143] But the report did not specify any such complaints. Instead, it pointed out that an opinion survey of nurses' experience of being valued by doctors varied widely in different settings. The rather tendentious conclusion drawn by the report was that 'such a range of variations [shows] there is obvious scope for improvement'.

The criticisms of medicine made by Briggs resonated with North American nursing in that period and its criticisms of the medical profession. This had led American nursing into a tension with medicine and a desire for professional autonomy. American nursing had rejected bedside care and subordination to physicians in favour of administrative responsibility and a career progression that would offer them at least equality with, and even superordination to, the medical hierarchy:

> We can therefore understand why it is that nurses who are preoccupied with attaining a fully independent status attempt to deprecate the Nightingale skills of bedside care – what was once called 'nursing' – pass them on to lesser workers, and specialize in administrative work. The practice of traditional nursing skills is ultimately contingent on the judgement of a superordinate profession and so cannot constitute the basis for autonomy. [144]

But Briggs was reticent about modelling the British nursing system on North America, because the efficacy of the United States nursing system was unproven: 'In the United States, where research is at a premium, the National Commission for the Study of Nursing and Nursing Education commented appositely that "we are dismayed that so little research has been done on the actual effects of nursing intervention and care; the profession has few definitive guides for the improvement of practice". '[145]

Changes in education were fundamental to the new professional status and this was clearly reflected in the Briggs Report.[146] The report recommended the setting up of colleges of health, free to employ specialists who were not nurses. The report envisaged the building of links between nursing, administration and management on the one hand, and psychology, sociology and pathology of ageing on the other hand, as well as with professions allied to medicine, in particular, social services. No explicit role for clinical doctors in nurse education was visualised. Nurses would instead be taught by academic physiologists and biologists, for example, who would probably not be clinical doctors.

Above all, the report proposed that nurse education, and the nursing curriculum, should no longer be standardised and universally applied. [147] Service and education were to be very definitely separate. This was the construction of a new kind of nurse. Nurse training in future should no longer be influenced by doctors and their medical teaching, neither would it be standardised. No longer a training at all, the focus was on the expansion of academic research and the need to recruit more 'A' level and graduate entrants.[148]

Progressive educational methods current in the 1960s were to underpin the new nursing education. As Lord Briggs later told the House of Lords: 'We also wanted some of the ideas which were at work in the educational world as a whole, about methods of learning, to be taken into the nursing profession.'[149]

The justification for these radical educational proposals was questionable, according to the report's own evidence. The report admitted that the majority of recently trained nurses and midwives rated both tutors' and doctors' teaching highly and only a minority were unhappy with the quality of instruction on the wards from staff nurses and sisters.[150] When asked whether they would like nursing theory to be taught in technical colleges and apart from the hospital, 75 per cent of nurses, both trainees and those recently trained, agreed with the statement: 'The only place to learn about nursing is in hospital.' Only 20 per cent agreed with the statement: 'It would be best if the theory was taught at a technical college.'[151]

These opinions from grass-roots nurses were consistent with other research findings from MacGuire,[152] which the next chapter will consider in more detail. She found that a more academic nurse education would negatively affect nurse recruitment. Despite this evidence, MacGuire's personal view was that liberal or further education for nurses could be advantageous,[153] and as nurses disliked 'the inclusive atmosphere of the school-within-the hospital', it might be possible in the future for schools of nursing to develop within local education authority structures.[154] Abel-Smith, too, was keen for nursing to move into higher education and was pleased to see nursing knocking on the doors of universities.[155] Briggs, similarly, seemed to take little account of the opinions of nurses who dissented from the view of the committee:

> Again it must be remembered that trainees have on the whole little experience of technical colleges; their views on the subject can be taken only as an indication of their possible attitudes to a particular change and not as conclusive evidence of its desirability or otherwise.[156]

The report's conclusion therefore discounted nurses' own opinions and recommended: 'Technical colleges, colleges of further education and sixth form colleges or their equivalent ... suitable centres.' It took no account of its own findings, that nurses wanted to care, they were not attracted by career development.[157] College-based education, which relegated and subordinated the place of bedside training, had no particular appeal for them.

The nursing establishment welcomed the Briggs Report.[158] The RCN response, now keen to improve the status of nursing, emphasised the crucial importance of 'selling' nursing by correcting the impression in the press, amongst teachers and elsewhere that academic qualifications were not a requirement for nursing. Young men and women needed to be recruited with 'O' and 'A' levels and university degrees.[159] Nurses should no longer be 'exploited as "pairs of hands" '.[160]

But there was some dissent. Dr J.W. Paulley, the fierce critic of Salmon,[161] argued that Briggs had failed to define the nurse's role, resorting instead to 'bureaucratic equivocation and windy managerial waffle'. He warned that the plans for education could result in colleges that were too big and impersonal, and the imposition of too much theory early on 'to break enthusiastic young hearts'. Moreover, the ward sister was: '"the key person" with the power to affect the morale of a whole ward (surprise, surprise!)'.[162]

The report had missed 'a golden opportunity of restoring job satisfaction and warmth in working relationships for those who actually nurse patients, as a *priority*'. It had rubber-stamped the managerialism of Salmon, and most of the references to Florence Nightingale were 'fashionably snide'. In Paulley's, view Briggs shared the same vision as Salmon. This was also suggested by a correspondent to *Nursing Times*, who argued that Salmon and Briggs were aiming to produce an academic profession rather than a practical nurse.[163]

Such dissenters were regarded as less than tolerable by those in favour of Briggs. An editorial in the *Nursing Times* suggested that any criticisms of the Briggs Report should be stifled for the sake of pushing the report through.[164] This was opposed and debate was called for.[165] But, this comment was itself vigorously questioned by a letter the following week from James P. Smith, then Principal Nursing Officer (Teaching) at Hammersmith Hospital.[166] Smith welcomed Briggs's emphasis on higher education: 'I have no reservations at all about Briggs', but he criticised dissenters, including the Principal Nursing Officer of St Mary's, who was also a recent chairman of the RCN's representative body, and others whom he called 'boat rockers':

> Of course I welcome constructive comments and debate. I just do not want professional people to rock the boat thoughtlessly for if we lose this wonderful opportunity for change presented by the Briggs Report we will not have another opportunity for decades to come ... I think it should also be remembered that the committee invited evidence from anyone, during its deliberations. I can only presume, since they submitted no individual evidence, that neither Mr. Holder nor Miss Illing personally felt very strongly about anything at the time. So what are they up to now?[167]

Brian Abel-Smith's history of nursing was used in a seminal way by both the Salmon and Briggs Committees, and therefore had an influence on policy changes affecting nursing in the 1970s. His historical study was part of a project into the demands and financing of medical care, and was carried out under Richard Titmuss.[168] But Abel-Smith was not merely a detached academic, he was a political adviser in the Department of Health and Social Security to Richard Crossman in the late 1960s and to Barbara Castle and David Ennals in the mid-1970s.[169]

He was, in fact, a close and influential friend of Richard Crossman: 'He has been my closest personal friend and without him I could have done very little in the past two years.'[170] As Barbara Castle, the minister charged with helping to pilot through the Briggs report recalled, Abel-Smith, Richard Titmuss and Peter Townsend were all enlisted as social reformers to plan changes in society, particularly regarding the role of women. The women's movement set the agenda to give women an independent voice. As most nurses were women, this agenda would obviously deeply affect nursing. Indeed, women were growing militant, and in Castle's view nurses were included in this militancy.[171]

Notwithstanding such challenges, traditional nursing values still held sway in that period: 'Nurses embodied to us the principle of service. We believed passionately that you must never exploit people who have such standards of service that they are not going to strike. They have a special claim on you.'[172] The RCN and the unions had set the agenda and called for a root-and-branch review of nursing pay in order to raise the status of the profession in the eyes of the public: 'They were not just nice girls with warm hearts looking after poor dears; they were a profession and a skilled and honourable profession. And I don't think they've ever lost this increased status.' The public esteemed the 'specialness' of the nurse. Professional leaders, on the other hand, wanted to raise their status. Status had become the key issue:

> We envisaged the nursing profession in terms of continuing education to develop the best opportunities for each individual nurse and to give the nurse within the profession choice of the various kinds of specialisation which the nurse in question could most effectively develop.[173]

But did Asa Briggs understand the real world of nursing, as opposed to some fictional and mythical image represented on television and by films, and in newspapers and novels? This is crucial to the validity of the report's analysis and hence to its recommendations. A decade later, in 1983, Lord Briggs admitted that he gained an authentic insight into nursing when his own daughter trained as a nurse in the years after his report was published:

> I heard a lot of things from her in the course of her training which did not have very much to do with the things I had written about in the Briggs Report! And she had a great deal of difficulty in disassociating herself with her father sometimes and wished that she had a totally different name, but she is a good nurse and from

> her, I learnt that the way in which the initiatory activities are carried out, the style of doing it, is almost as important as the content, to get it right in the feel and the style of it.[174]

She appeared to give him a genuine understanding of the significance of the traditional apprenticeship model, which he confessed he previously lacked. Through her, he realised how vital the ethos was to the training of the nurse. This acknowledgement had important implications for a way of nursing that was about to be ended.

Conclusion

The 1960s saw radical changes in the self-understanding of nursing, leading to the Briggs Committee. The report of this committee set in motion a new agenda for nursing and nurse education. It sought to develop a career progression away from the bedside into education, management and research. This involved a movement away from the apprenticeship method of learning: a massive shift away from the long-standing practical tradition of bedside care.[175] The impetus seemed now to be that of acquiring status for nursing, an attitude that would continue in the *Royal Commission on the National Health Service*.[176] Not only were Abel-Smith and MacGuire among those who assisted this commission, but as it stated, the commission drew heavily from the Briggs Committee Report in preparing the chapter on 'Nurses, Midwives and Health Visitors'.[177]

The movement of nursing was, therefore, not just at a professional level, it was at a government level too. In 1972 it was clear that a new track for nursing lay ahead. Was this new track in line with the wishes of ordinary nurses and patients during this period of radical change? This question will be examined in the next chapter.

Notes

1 Ministry of Health, Central Health Services Council, *The Pattern of the In-patient's Day*, HMSO, London, 1961; 'Pattern of the In-patient's Day', *Nursing Times*, 1961, p. 392, March 31; 'Ward Time-table: Revised Pattern, *Nursing Times*, 1961, p. 398–399, March 31; 'The Pattern of the In-patient's Day', *Nursing Times*, 1961, p. 440–442, April 7.

2 Ibid.

3 L.R.C. Haward, 'Selection of Nurses: A New Approach', *Nursing Times*, 1960, pp. 776–778, June 24.

4 'Teaching and Learning', editorial, *Nursing Times*, 1960, p. 771, June 24.

5 'Selection and Training of Nurses', A Nurse, *Nursing Times*, 1960, p. 857, July 8.

6 'Talking Point', Cyclops, *Nursing Times*, 1960, p. 810, July 1.

7 'Talking Point', Wrangler, *Nursing Times*, 1960, p. 600, May 13.

[8] 'What is Wrong with Apprenticeship?', *Nursing Mirror and Midwives Journal*, 110, 2881, 1960, p. 2185, September 16.

[9] J. Darwin, J. Markham, B. Whyte, *Bedside Nursing*, London, William Heinemann Medical Books, 1st edn 1964, 2nd edn 1967, 3rd edn 1971.

[10] S. Holder, 'Leader with a Common Touch', *Nursing Standard*, 8, 19, 1994, p. 46, February 2.

[11] B.B. Whyte, 'Home Thoughts from Abroad', *Nursing Times*, 1960, pp. 1351–1352, December 9.

[12] B.B. Whyte, 'Worm's Eye View', *Nursing Times*, 1961, pp. 332–333, March 17.

[13] M.L. Campbell, 'Home Thoughts from Abroad', letter, *Nursing Times*, 1961, p. 156, February 3.

[14] I.G. Duncan, 'Home Thoughts from Abroad', letter, *Nursing Times*, 1961, p. 252, February 24.

[15] J. Mackie, 'Home Thoughts from Abroad', letter, 1961, *Nursing Times*, pp. 315–316, March 10.

[16] 'The Student Nurse and the Bedpan Round', *Nursing Times*, 1963, p. 311, March 8.

[17] Nicusane (Northern Ireland, Canada, United States of America, Nurse-Teacher Exchange) 1960–1962, *Report of the Advisory Committee on a Pilot Scheme for the Exchange of Nurse Teachers*, Belfast, Northern Ireland Hospitals Authority, Royal Victoria Hospital; Boston, Massachusetts General Hospital; Toronto, Toronto Western Hospital, 1963.

[18] Ibid., p. 109.

[19] Ibid., p. 107.

[20] B. Abel-Smith, *A History of the Nursing Profession*, London, Heinemann, 1960.

[21] Ibid., p. 240.

[22] Ibid., p. 241.

[23] Ibid., p. 245.

[24] B.A. Bennett, 'A Sociologist Looks at Nursing (in England and Wales since 1800)', *Nursing Mirror*, 1960, pp. 2289–2290, September 23.

[25] W. Hector, *The Work of Mrs Bedford Fenwick and the Rise of Professional Nursing*, London, Royal College of Nursing, 1973, p. 35.

[26] I.E.P. Menzies, 'A Case Study in the Functioning of Social Systems as a Defence against Anxiety: A Report on a Study of the Nursing Service of a General Hospital', *Human Relations*, 1960, 13, pp. 95–121; I.E.P. Menzies, 'Nurses under Stress', *Nursing Times*, 1, pp. 141–142, February 3; *Nursing Times*, 2, pp. 173–174, February 10; *Nursing Times*, 3, pp. 206–208, 1961, February 17; I.E.P. Menzies, *A Case Study in the Functioning of Social Systems as a Defence Against Anxiety: A Report on a Study of the Nursing Service of a General Hospital*, Reprint of Tavistock Pamplet no. 3, London, Tavistock Institute of Human Relations, 1970.

[27] Ibid., p. 142.

[28] 'Defence Mechanisms in Nursing', review, R.M.N., *Nursing Times*, 1960, pp. 1078–1079, September 2.

[29] M.M. Edwards, 'Becoming a Nurse', *Nursing Times*, 1961, p. 1198, September 15.

[30] R. White, *The Effects of the National Health Service on the Nursing Profession, 1948–1961* London, King Edward's Hospital Fund for London, 1985, p. xv.

[31] 'Nursing – Neurosis or Vocation?', letter, Animus, *Nursing Times*, 1960, p. 1513, December 2.

[32] E.J. Ashe, 'Nursing – Neurosis or Vocation?', letter, *Nursing Times*, 1960, p. 1576, December 16.

[33] J.A.G. Lawrence, 'Vocation or Profession?', letter, *Nursing Times*, 1961, p. 97, January 20.

[34] 'Vocation *or* Profession', letter, W.C., *Nursing Times*, 1961, p. 157, February 3.

[35] E.S. Boyle, 'Vocation or Profession', letter, *Nursing Times*, 1961, p. 221, February 17.

[36] M. Sykes, 'Profession or Vocation?', letter, *Nursing Times*, 1961, p. 314, March 10.

[37] 'Research into Basic Nursing', editorial, *Nursing Times*, 1961, p. 327, March 17.

[38] B. Abel-Smith, 'Crisis in Nursing – 5: The Sociologist's View', *Nursing Times*, 1961, pp. 1262–1263, September 29.

[39] R.W. Revans, *Standards for Morale: Cause and Effect in Hospitals*, London, Oxford University Press, published for the Nuffield Provincial Hospitals Trust, 1964.

[40] Ibid., p. 43.

[41] Ibid., p. 83.

[42] R.M. Titmuss, *Essays on 'The Welfare State'*, London, George Allen & Unwin, 1963, p. 128.

[43] Ibid., p. 129.

[44] General Nursing Council for England and Wales, *Syllabus of Subjects for Examination for the Certificate of General Nursing*, London, General Nursing Council, 1962.

[45] General Nursing Council for England and Wales, *Guide to the Syllabus of Subjects for Examination for the Certificate of General Nursing*, London, General Nursing Council, 1962.

[46] E.R.D. Bendall, E. Raybould, *A History of the General Nursing Council for England and Wales 1919–1969*, London, H.K. Lewis & Co., 1969, pp. 183–186.

[47] The Royal College of Nursing and National Council of Nurses of the United Kingdom, *A Reform of Nursing Education: First Report of a Special Committee on Nurse Education*, Sir Harry Platt, Chairman, London, The Royal College of Nursing and National Council of Nurses of the United Kingdom, 1964.

[48] Ibid., p. 1.

[49] Ibid., p. 13.

[50] M.E. Baly, *Nursing and Social Change*, London, William Heinemann Medical Books Ltd., 1973.

[51] The Royal College of Nursing, *Observations and Objectives: A Statement on Nursing Policy*, London, Royal College of Nursing, 1956.

[52] 'The Platt Committee Report', editorial, *Nursing Times*, 1964, pp. 783–784, June 19; 'A Reform of Nursing Education', *Nursing Times*, 1964, pp. 813–814, June 19; 'A Reform of Nursing Education', *Nursing Times*, 1964, pp. 873–877, July 3; 'Preparation for Platt', editorial, *Nursing Times*, 1964, p. 1487, November 13.

[53] B. Abel-Smith, 'The Platt Report: Some Implications', *Nursing Times*, 1964, pp. 925–926, July 17.

[54] W.E.D. Stephens, 'An Educationist Looks at Platt', *Nursing Times*, 1964, pp. 1373–1374, October 16.

[55] B.B. Scott, 'The Platt Report', *Nursing Times*, 1964, pp. 1017–1018, August 7.

[56] S.G. Hill, 'A Reform of Nursing Education', *Nursing Times*, 1964, pp. 858–859, July 3.

[57] 'Platt and the Student Nurse', *Nursing Times*, 1964, p. 1550, November 20.

[58] 'A Reform of Nursing Education', *Nursing Mirror*, 1964, pp. 130, 147, November 6; 'Editorial', *Nursing Mirror*, 1964, p. 251, June 19. 'The Platt Report – A Vital Document', *Nursing Mirror*, 1964: pp. 271–273, June 19; pp. 287–289, June 26; pp. 307–309, July 3. 'Editorial', *Nursing Mirror*, 1964, p. 299, July 3; 'Nurses Discuss the Platt Report', *Nursing Mirror*, 1964, p. 313, July 3; 'Regional Action on Platt Report', *Nursing Mirror*, 1964, pp. 169–170, November 13; 'Student Nurses' Association Discusses Platt', *Nursing Mirror*, 1964, p. 174, November 20; 'News from Westminster: Next Move to Improve Nurses' Status', *Nursing Mirror*, 1964, p. 207, November 27.

[59] General Nursing Council for England and Wales, 'The G.N.C. Comments on the Platt Report', *Nursing Mirror*, 1965, pp. 17–19, October 1; General Nursing Council for England and Wales, 'Memorandum on the Platt Report', *Nursing Times*, 1965, pp. 1347–1349, October 1; 'No to Platt', *Nursing Times*, 1965, p. 1330, October 1; 'General Nursing Council for England and Wales', *Nursing Times*, 1965, pp. 1353–1354, October 1.

[60] General Nursing Council for England and Wales, 'The G.N.C. Comments on the Platt Report', *Nursing Mirror*, 1965, pp. 17–19, October 1; General Nursing Council for England

and Wales, 'Memorandum on the Platt Report', *Nursing Times*, 1965, pp. 1347–1349, October 1.

[61] M.E. Baly, *Nursing and Social Change*, London, William Heinemann Medical Books Ltd., 1973.

[62] 'Student Nurses Speak Out', *Nursing Times*, 1965, p. 1328, September 24.

[63] J.B. Price, 'The GNC and Platt', letter, *Nursing Times*, 1965, p. 1416, October 15; J.M. Martin, 'The GNC and Platt', letter, *Nursing Times*, 1965, p. 1417, October 15; A. McMillan, 'The GNC and Platt', letter, *Nursing Times*, 1965, p. 1417, October 15.

[64] 'The GNC and Platt', Iconoclast, letter, *Nursing Times*, 1965, pp. 1416–1417, October 15.

[65] Editorial, *Nursing Mirror*, 1963, p. 45, April 19.

[66] Editorial, *Nursing Mirror*, 1965, p. 323, December 3.

[67] Editorial, *Nursing Mirror*, 1965, p. 475, August 13; p. 275, November 19.

[68] E.M. Laws, 'What are Nurses for?' *Nursing Mirror*, 1964, pp. 178–180, November 20.

[69] Editorial, *Nursing Mirror*, 1965, p. 1, October 1.

[70] B. Ellicott, 'The G.N.C. and Platt', letter, *Nursing Mirror*, 1965, p. 219, October 29.

[71] E.M. Roberts, 'Open Forum: Views on the Platt Report: 1. The Defence', *Nursing Mirror*, 1965, p. 477, February 19.

[72] D.R. Barton, 'Open Forum: Views on the Platt Report: 2. The Attack', *Nursing Mirror*, 1965, pp. 477–478, February 19.

[73] E.R.D. Bendall, E. Raybould, *A History of the General Nursing Council for England and Wales 1919–1969*, London, H.K. Lewis & Co., 1969.

[74] 'General Nursing Council for England and Wales', *Nursing Times*, 1965, pp. 1353–1354, October 1.

[75] M.E. Baly, *Nursing and Social Change*, 2nd edn, London, William Heinemann Medical Books Ltd., 1980, p. 439.

[76] E.R.D. Bendall, E. Raybould, *A History of the General Nursing Council for England and Wales 1919–1969*, London, H.K. Lewis & Co., 1969, p. 202.

[77] Editorial, *Nursing Mirror*, 1965, p. 375, January 22.

[78] D. Norton, 'Research for Progress', *Nursing Mirror*, 1965, pp. 390–393, January 22.

[79] M. Baly, 'The Reform of Nursing Education', *Nursing Times*, 1965, pp. 867–868, June 25; pp. 955–956, July 9; pp. 977–978, July 16.

[80] Ibid., p. 868.

[81] L. Creelman, 'There is no Change without Challenge, *Nursing Mirror*, 1965, pp. 127–130, May 7; pp. 160–162, May 14.

[82] Ministry of Health Scottish Home and Health Department, *Report of the Committee on Senior Nursing Staff*, Brian Salmon, Chairman, London, HMSO, 1966.

[83] Ibid., p. 1.

[84] Ibid., p. 50, paras 5.37–5.39; p. 119, paras 23–25.

[85] W. Hector, *The Work of Mrs Bedford Fenwick and the Rise of Professional Nursing*, London, Royal College of Nursing, 1973, p. 67–70, Appendix A, sections i and ii.

[86] B. Abel-Smith, *A History of the Nursing Profession*, London, Heinemann, 1960.

[87] Ministry of Health Scottish Home and Health Department, *Report of the Committee on Senior Nursing Staff*, Brian Salmon, Chairman, London, HMSO, 1966, p. 11.

[88] Ibid., pp. 7–8, para. 1.13.

[89] J.W. Paulley, 'Is it Too Late to Scrap Salmon – A Charter for Incompetents?', *Nursing Times*, 1971, pp. 212–213, February 18.

[90] R. Dingwall, A.M. Rafferty, C. Webster, *An Introduction to the Social History of Nursing*, Routledge, London, 1988.

[91] *Report of the Committee on Nursing*, Professor Asa Briggs, Chairman, Cmnd.5115, London, HMSO, 1972, p. 1, para. 1.

[92] 'Why Briggs? asks Lady Summerskill', *Nursing Times*, 1970, p. 354, March 19.

[93] *Report of the Committee on Nursing*, Professor Asa Briggs, Chairman, Cmnd.5115, London, HMSO, 1972, pp. 212–217.

[94] Ibid., p. 24, para. 83d.

[95] Ibid., pp. 23–24, paras 81–83.

[96] B. Abel-Smith, *A History of the Nursing Profession*, London, Heinemann, 1960, p. 241; *Report of the Committee on Nursing*, Professor Asa Briggs, Chairman, Cmnd.5115, London, HMSO, 1972, p. 24, para. 83d.

[97] Ibid., pp. 23–24, para. 83.

[98] Ibid., p. 25, para. 87.

[99] Ibid., p. 26, para. 91.

[100] R. Dingwall, A.M. Rafferty, C. Webster, *An Introduction to the Social History of Nursing*, Routledge, London, 1988, p. 206.

[101] 'Briggs on Nursing', *Nursing Times*, 1970, pp. 1566–1567, December 3.

[102] 'I Use the Word Nursing for the Want of a Better', editorial, *Nursing Times*, 66, 40, 1970, p. 1249, October 1.

[103] G.E.W. Wolstenholme, 'Florence Nightingale: New Lamps for Old' in Shaw, R.M. , R.A. Bowen and G.E. Paget (eds), *All Heal*, pp. 201–215, London, William Heinemann Medical Books, for the Royal Society of Medicine, 1971.

[104] Ibid., p. 205.

[105] *Report of the Committee on Nursing*, Professor Asa Briggs, Chairman, Cmnd.5115, London, HMSO, 1972, p. 2, para. 5.

[106] Ibid., p. 2, paras 5–7; p. 123, para. 420; p. 125, para. 427.

[107] Ibid., p. 2, paras 6–8.

[108] *Report of the Committee on Nursing*, Professor Asa Briggs, Chairman, Cmnd.5115, London, HMSO, 1972, p. 33, para. 107.

[109] Ibid., p. 35, para. 108.

[110] Ibid., p. 245.

[111] Letter from Lord Briggs to Ann Bradshaw, 3 November 1994.

[112] Letter from Lindsay L. Brook, Research Director, SCPR, to Ann Bradshaw, 19 September 1995.

[113] J.R. Morton-Williams, R. Berthoud, *Nurses Attitude Survey: Report on Postal Survey*, ref. 02.188, London, Social and Community Planning Research, 1971, November.

[114] J.R. Morton-Williams, R. Berthoud, *Nurses Attitude Study: Report on Depth Interviews*, ref. 02.194, London, , Social and Community Planning Research, 1971, February.

[115] J.R. Morton-Williams, R. Berthoud, *Nurses Attitude Survey: Report on Postal Survey*, ref. 02.188, London, Social and Community Planning Research, 1971, November, p. 56.

[116] Ibid., p. 58.

[117] Ibid., p. 62.

[118] J.R. Morton-Williams, R. Berthoud, *Nurses Attitude Study: Report on Depth Interviews*, ref. 02.194, London, Social and Community Planning Research, 1971, February, pp. 1–7.

[119] Ibid., p. 4.

[120] Ibid., p. 3.

[121] Ibid., p. 5.

[122] *Report of the Committee on Nursing*, Professor Asa Briggs, Chairman, Cmnd.5115, London, HMSO, 1972, p. 31, para. 98.

[123] Ibid., p. 23, para. 81.

[124] Ibid., pp. 26–28, para. 91.

[125] Ibid., p. 28, para. 92.

[126] Ibid., p. 28, para. 93.

[127] A. Briggs, 'The Commitment of the Briggs Committee', in *A Time for Commitment*, Baroness Cox of Queensbury, Chairman, pp. 2–11, London, English National Board for Nursing, Midwifery and Health Visiting, 1983, November 15.

[128] 'The Image', editorial, *Nursing Times*, 1972, p. 1535, December 7.

[129] *Report of the Committee on Nursing*, Professor Asa Briggs, Chairman, Cmnd.5115, London, HMSO, 1972, p. 28, para. 91.

[130] J.R. Morton-Williams, R. Berthoud, *Nurses Attitude Suudy: Report on Depth Interviews*, ref. 02.194, London, , Social and Community Planning Research, 1971, February, p. 40.

[131] Ibid., p. 28.

[132] Ibid. p. 40.

[133] J. MacGuire, *Threshold to Nursing: A Review of the Literature on Recruitment To and Withdrawal from Nurse Training Programmes in the United Kingdom*, Occasional Papers on Social Administration No. 30, London, G. Bell & Sons, 1969.

[134] *Report of the Committee on Nursing*, Professor Asa Briggs, Chairman, Cmnd.5115, London, HMSO, 1972, pp. 28–29, para. 95.

[135] J. MacGuire, *From Student to Nurse – The Induction Period: A Study of Student Nurses in the First Six Months of Training in Five Schools of Nursing*, Oxford, Oxford Area Nurse Training Committee, 1961, September; J. MacGuire, *From Student to Nurse – Training and Qualification: A Study of Student Nurses in Training at Five Schools of Nursing*, Oxford, Oxford Area Nurse Training Committee, 1966, May.

[136] J.M. MacGuire, 'From Student to Nurse', *Nursing Times*, 1961, pp. 1297–1298, October 6.

[137] *Report of the Committee on Nursing*, Professor Asa Briggs, Chairman, Cmnd.5115, London, HMSO, 1972, p. 34, para. 107b.

[138] The Royal College of Nursing and National Council of Nurses of the United Kingdom, *Rcn Evidence to the Committee on Nursing*, London, The Royal College of Nursing and National Council of Nurses of the United Kingdom, 1971, pp. 10–11, para. 38.

[139] Ibid., p. 12, para. 46.

[140] *Report of the Committee on Nursing*, Professor Asa Briggs, Chairman, Cmnd.5115, London, HMSO, 1972, p. 47, paras 150–151.

[141] Ibid., p. 46, para. 145a–145i.

[142] Ibid., p. 46, para. 146.

[143] Ibid., p. 47, para. 147.

[144] E. Freidson, *Profession of Medicine*, New York, Harper & Row, 1970 p. 66.

[145] *Report of the Committee on Nursing*, Professor Asa Briggs, Chairman, Cmnd.5115, London, HMSO, 1972, pp. 38–39, para. 115.

[146] Ibid., pp. 103–114, paras 346–399.

[147] Ibid., p. 84, para. 262.

[148] Ibid., p. 108, paras 370–378.

[149] A. Briggs, 'The Essence of Briggs', *Nursing Times*, 1979, p. 345, March 1.

[150] *Report of the Committee on Nursing*, Professor Asa Briggs, Chairman, Cmnd.5115, London, HMSO, 1972, pp. 63–64, paras 209–210.

[151] Ibid., p. 69, para. 224.

[152] J. MacGuire, *From Student to Nurse – Training and Qualification: A Study of Student Nurses in Training at Five Schools of Nursing*, Oxford, Oxford Area Nurse Training Committee, 1966, May, p. 5d.

[153] Ibid., p. 5d.

[154] Ibid., p. 5f.

[155] B. Abel-Smith, 'The Platt Report: Some Implications', *Nursing Times*, pp. 925–926, July 17.

[156] *Report of the Committee on Nursing*, Professor Asa Briggs, Chairman, Cmnd.5115, London, HMSO, 1972, pp. 84, para. 262.

[157] Ibid., 159, paras 522–529.

[158] 'The Philosophy of Briggs', editorial, *Nursing Times*, 1972, p. 1305, October 19; 'By Briggs out of Nightingale', editorial, *Nursing Times*, 1972, p. 1401, November 9; 'Bendall on Briggs', *Nursing Times*, 1972, p. 1403, November 9.

[159] The Royal College of Nursing and National Council of Nurses of the United Kingdom (1973) *Rcn Comment on the Report of the Committee on Nursing*, London, The Royal College of Nursing and National Council of Nurses of the United Kingdom, 1973, February, p. 9 para. 38; p. 11, para. 43.

[160] Ibid., p. 15, para. 57.

[161] J.W. Paulley, 'Is it Too Late to Scrap Salmon – A Charter for Incompetents?', *Nursing Times*, 1971, pp. 212–213, February 18.

[162] J.W. Paulley, 'Masterly Report? Managerial Waffle?', *Nursing Times*, 1972, pp. 1374–5, November 2.

[163] T.L. Dann, 'The Briggs Debate', letter, *Nursing Times*, 1972, p. 1422, November 9.

[164] 'The Philosophy of Briggs', editorial, *Nursing Times*, 1972, p. 1305, October 19.

[165] M. Illing, 'Briggs Debate', letter, *Nursing Times*, 1972, p. 1388, November 2.

[166] J.P. Smith, 'The Briggs Debate', letter, *Nursing Times*, 1972, p. 1422, November 9.

[167] S. Holder, 'Masterly Report? Managerial Waffle?', *Nursing Times*, 1972, pp. 1374–5, November 2.

[168] B. Abel-Smith, *A History of the Nursing Profession*, London, Heinemann, 1960.

[169] C. Ham, *Health Policy in Britain*, Houndmills, Basingstoke, Macmillan, 1992, p. 109.

[170] R. Crossman, *The Diaries of a Cabinet Minister*, vol. 3, London, Hamish Hamilton and Jonathan Cape, 1977, p. 221.

[171] B. Castle, 'No Kitchen Cabinet', in Maitland, S. (ed.), *Very Heaven*, pp. 47–58, London, Virago Press, 1988, p. 55.

[172] A. Cole, 'Castles in the Air', *Nursing Times*, 89,29, 1993, pp. 16–17, July 21.

[173] A. Briggs, 'The Essence of Briggs', *Nursing Times*, 1979, p. 345, March 1.

[174] A . Briggs, 'The Commitment of the Briggs Committee', in *A Time for Commitment*, Baroness Cox of Queensbury, Chairman, pp. 2–11, London, English National Board for Nursing, Midwifery and Health Visiting, 1983, November 15.

[175] W. Hector, 'The Role and Preparation of the Teacher', *Nursing Times*, 1972, pp. 1460–1461, November 16.

[176] *Royal Commission on the National Health Service*, Sir Alec Merrison, Chairman, Cmnd. 7615, London, HMSO, 1979, p. 31, para. 4.11.

[177] Ibid., p. 184, para. 13.3.

Chapter 7

Behind the scenes: battle for the soul of nursing, 1960–1978

Correspondence, articles and editorials, published in nursing journals from 1960–1970 constitute a key body of evidence charting nursing opinion from all ranks of nurses. This material forms a testimony to the deep tension felt about the changes occurring to the ethos and practice of nursing. This evidence, together with important data from research studies into nurse and patient opinions recorded during this period, gives an important insight into the strong feelings, both positive and negative, about what was happening to nursing and its apprenticeship system of learning, and shows the mutual incomprehension these feelings aroused.

Modernising and redefining the vocational framework: voices from nursing journals 1960–1970

As the last chapter has shown, during the 1960s traditional nursing principles began to be thought of as outdated and unrealistically idealistic. Hence, for example, Evelyn Pearce's writing, thought of by some reviewers, past and present, as an invaluable resource for apprenticeship, the transmission of traditional values,[1] and whole patient care,[2] was criticised by others as outdated, even though the critics recognised her enormous influence on past generations of nurses.[3]

Here was a paradox at the heart of nursing: a desire for nursing to move away from past attitudes, but at the same time seeking not to lose what was acknowledged to be the tradition of quality care it had sustained. This dilemma is exemplified by the speeches, over a decade and a half, of Miss (later Dame) Muriel Powell, Matron of St George's Hospital. In 1955 she suggested that nurses were too keen to accept the *status quo* without questioning, and she was reluctant to use the word 'vocation': 'I hesitate to use the word "vocation" because many people think it merely implies working for a low salary ... I do not agree with that, and the nurse must believe in her work for otherwise she will not be able to lead others. Her conviction that her job is worthwhile must be bracketed with integrity in her work.'[4] In 1963 she spoke of the need for revolutionary changes in nurse education.[5] Four years later, she expressed her anxiety that nurses should not forget those qualities of mind and spirit, compassion, integrity and tolerance, which had sustained British nursing. The success of the nurse's care depended on her ability to see the patient as a whole.[6]

The issue was complex, as Powell acknowledged. The crucial question was whether the values would remain without the ethical framework to sustain them: 'In Britain the nursing profession has traditionally looked to the Christian religion for its concept of wholeness ... If this framework is removed, will the rules still be relevant? It is commonly assumed that they will; but it is a question to which we have paid little attention; and it requires an answer. Is the humanity and the humanism of our age enough?' The problem that leaders such as Powell were wrestling with was how to translate the nursing ideal to fit the present situation.[7]

Like many other eminent matrons of the period, including the matrons of St Bartholomew's Hospital, Guy's Hospital, University College Hospital, and the London Chest Hospital,[8] Muriel Powell was personally committed to the Christian faith and traditional moral principles of nursing.[9] But as a member of both the Salmon and Briggs committees, she was conscious of bringing nursing up to date in what she perceived to be a fast-changing world. More than once she pointed not only to the technological changes, but also to social changes. It appears that the lack of confidence in traditional values was accompanied by the fear that without traditional values altruism and service could not be sustained. The nursing journals from 1960 to 1970 charted these concerns and, particularly through their unsolicited correspondence, show the progressive change in nursing values.

The early period 1960–1962

From 1960 to 1962 writers appear to have been intent on defending nursing tradition against what were perceived to be criticisms of the established order, an undermining of the fundamental importance of vocation, and a questioning of the premises of religious faith. One correspondent suggested that nursing needed a 'moral re-armament' by a recommitment to God, 'the first point of change which prepared Florence Nightingale for the life of self-sacrifice resulting in her training as a nurse and all that followed'.[10] Another writer described her personal experience of becoming a nurse as a direct consequence of a distinct and unexpected calling, later in life.[11] This approach would become increasingly difficult to express as the decade proceeded.

In a series of articles for the *Nursing Mirror* in 1960, a sister tutor encapsulated this contemporary mood.[12] Nurses now had an easier life than ever before, and had become self-conscious rather than patient-conscious, no longer focused on the practical bedside care of the patient. The tradition of nursing as both a vocation and a profession was being lost as rules and structures had become ends in themselves: 'Every now and then an old argument sprouts again into the light – is nursing a profession or a vocation? Why "or"? Why can't it be both?'[13] These articles earned both praise and condemnation in letters from nurses.[14]

Although the majority of nurses still held nursing to be a vocational commitment, undertaken in a spirit of prayer and acceptance of the great responsibilities involved, the *Nursing Mirror* argued that this tradition was now subject to ridicule. According to the editorial, Virginia Henderson's definition of nursing, just published by the International Council of Nurses, captured this spirit: '[The nurse] temporarily is the consciousness of the unconscious, the love of life for the suicidal, the leg of the amputee, the eyes of the newly blind, a means of locomotion for the infant, knowledge and confidence for the young mother, a "mouthpiece" for those too weak or withdrawn to speak, and so on.' Nurses would recognise it as the expression of something which they as nurses, had always known, although they might not have been able to put it into words.[15]

A correspondent suggested that only the idea of nursing as a vocation was able to meet the demands of human suffering: 'Perhaps some effort will be made during 1961 to implicate nursing more as a vocation and less as a profession.'[16] Early-morning ward prayers were still timetabled into the regular general nursing day.[17] But the culture of the day and the mood of nursing were changing. In July 1961 the *Nursing Mirror* editorial suggested that increased promiscuity was the result of a breakdown in public morality, caused by the decline of religious belief and the sweeping away of codes of behaviour accepted by previous generations.[18] This argument was repeated the following December.[19] A gradual and almost imperceptible decline in morality had led to a decline in the general ideal of service. The editorial warned that although nursing had managed to maintain its ideals against the prevalent slide of society into a moral vacuum, these could only survive if they were sustained and nourished.

Changes preoccupied many nursing leaders. The Chief Nursing Officer, for example, Kathleen Raven, in a paper delivered to the Annual Conference of the Institute of Hospital Administrators, spoke on the changing structures of society, burgeoning building programmes, the advances of medical science, and demographic and social changes. Yet, even she took the tradition for granted: nursing was, for her, both a vocation and a profession.[20]

At a conference the editor of *Nursing Times* stated that there was felt to be an inability to translate vocation into the mid-twentieth-century idiom. Recruitment and retention problems were caused by nurses leaving the profession to marry, or else by faulty selection of applicants to nursing in the first place. Other speakers were equally preoccupied with this issue. Miss Spalding thought that a balance needed to be struck between the dedicated life and the idea of nursing as no less and no more than a profession: 'Neither will do'. Margaret Schurr argued that prospective nurses were not interested in pay and conditions, but in the atmosphere and the kind of life they would lead. On this issue, whether nursing was a calling or a job, rested the whole method of training. There was general agreement: 'By now the audience was largely as one with the speakers – particularly when Miss Nuttall said that to regard student nurses as students was the kiss of death, that they were apprentices to an honourable calling.'[21]

That the ethos of nursing was unambiguously rooted in a tradition was still assumed by many.[22] Buildings and equipment were not enough; personal and spiritual qualities were needed in a nurse, to carry the patient through the darkest days of his or her illness. Nurses were expected to absorb that loving care on which the tradition of the hospital was built, as they trained. The *Nursing Times* editorial in 1961 maintained that 'The western concept of nursing has its roots in Christianity.'[23] That this needed to be affirmed suggests a lack of confidence.

Perhaps a shortage of nurses was a reason for this defensiveness. In 1961 there was much in the nursing journals about the 'crisis' in nursing recruitment. The *Nursing Times* published a series of articles in September and October of that year under the title 'Crisis in Nursing', by authors from professions interested in nursing developments.[24] Contributors included a surgeon, a physician, an administrator, a medical economist, a nurse, a politician and a sociologist. All, in some way, called for a change in nursing, recruitment, preparation and organisation.

The politician, Kenneth Robinson, the Minister of Health, criticised the innate conservatism and traditionalism of nursing which made it reluctant to change. In his view, Isabel Menzies's work provided a 'rational explanation of the profession's resistance to change'. In this light, Robinson criticised working relationships between doctors and nurses as well as the hierarchical structure. His call for change, however, seems to be contradicted by his closing comments. He had visited hospitals in a dozen foreign countries, and been a patient in three: 'In none of them did I find a standard of nursing comparable with that of our own country.'[25]

An editorial in *Nursing Mirror* thought that this anxiety about recruitment was fuelled by the belief that women were no longer coming forward to be nurses because they did not have a sense of vocation. That nurses were not being recruited was, however, not supported by statistics. In 1949, the numbers of student nurses in training totalled 46,182. In March 1961, they numbered 53,088. The total nursing and midwifery force in hospitals had risen from 125,752 full-time and 23,060 part-time in 1949, to 162,611 full-time and

47,040 part-time in March 1961: 'These figures are sufficient evidence that more young people every year are taking up nursing, and indeed that more females and males, of any age, are serving in the various grades.'[26]

Although the rise in numbers was less spectacular for domiciliary midwifery and nursing services, there was an increase here too, except in midwifery where there was a decrease in the past eleven years of 200 to bring the number of domiciliary midwives to 8,000: 'So – let us shout this truth: in a world which every year offers women more chances of alternative employment more, not fewer, young women than ever before are taking up nursing.' Moreover, the editorial argued that 'there is just as much sense of vocation among the young people entering today as ever there was'. This was no sentimental image of nursing, but a clear-eyed dedicated approach to nursing, that 'is undertaken in the spirit of vocation'. This could not be made compulsory: 'Most nurses, we believe, regard their profession as a vocation – but that is an added bonus we have no right to demand, only be thankful for.'

During the early 1960s the *Nursing Mirror* regularly published articles on religious and biblical themes, often in series of half a dozen weekly articles by chaplains, eminent theologians and Christian writers, taken from radio broadcasts such as 'Lift up Your Hearts', and from sermons given at major services. In 1960, for example, were published series of articles on favourite hymns,[27] the life of St Paul,[28] Christian witness in the early centuries,[29] the service of God,[30] and the Bible.[31] In 1961 appeared series on religion, life and healing,[32] the gift of the spirit,[33] the ministry of the Christian nurse,[34] the parables of Jesus,[35] a sermon of the Bishop of Guildford,[36] and the Old Testament.[37] The following year, there were series on prayer,[38] the Bible,[39] the service of the five candles,[40] the resurrection appearances of Jesus,[41] the meaning of Christmas,[42] and the sermon to health-care workers by the Chairman of the Oxford Regional Hospital Board.[43]

The *Nursing Mirror* of this period was extremely supportive of nursing tradition. In an editorial in 1962 the editor referred to the crucial importance of the traditional values of service. The public appreciation of nurses, argued the writer, rested on the instinctive recognition that the nurse was primarily concerned with serving her patients. Nursing was still a vocation, a calling, to which people gave their hearts. It was not primarily for the expectation of a large pay packet. It was this freely-given service which made ordinary people concerned that nurses should be rewarded justly. But the editorial writer warned that if the emphasis ever shifted, so that salaries became more important than service, the special consideration, the heartwarming and ungrudging appreciation might well vanish. The writer did not anticipate that this would ever happen. Although it was now very fashionable to decry the idea of 'vocation', and talk instead about money in relation to nursing values, still there was no less 'vocation' than before.[44]

For twenty-five years the editor of the *Nursing Mirror* had been J. Elise Gordon. She retired at the end of 1962.[45] Usually, the editor's identity was kept secret 'in ghostly anonymity, behind their magnificent desks and function in isolated splendour as *The Editor*, unknown to all save a select few', as she wrote on her retirement.[46]

The winds of change 1963–1965

By 1963 the challenge to nursing tradition had grown stronger. The new editor of *Nursing Mirror*, Yvonne Cross, was undoubtedly a believer in change.[47] In one of her first editorials she decried the fact that 'Unquestioning obedience was once the chief attribute demanded of nurses ... life was made uncomfortable for those who held and expressed their own opinions.' Her call was for revolutionary thinkers, nonconformists, who would brave the difficulty of persuading society to accept their ideas. The policy encouraged under the new editorship was to challenge the traditional stand of the establishment.[48]

Nursing was affected by the changing ethos of society, in which even theology was being influenced by the radical ideas of the theologian John Robinson, a contributor to the *Nursing Mirror* in 1961.[49] It would not be surprising if such attitudes confused nursing leaders and nurses themselves. Old certainties were vanishing.[50] Devotional articles, which had been basic to the *Nursing Mirror* in 1961 and 1962, were gradually replaced by articles that sought to deal with readers' doubts. Hence, in 1963, although the *Nursing Mirror* published articles on biblical and religious themes,[51] it also published articles that considered religious doubt. [52]

The number of articles on a religious theme was noticeably less in 1963 than in the previous years, although they still continued. The *Nursing Times* included regular fortnightly features from the chaplain about the spiritual aspects of health and healing. But this too was questioned. The 'Chaplain's Diary' of May 1963, was a response to 'several letters' received by the editor 'asking why space should be taken up by "religious" rather than technical articles'. The chaplain defended the spiritual dimension of nursing care as a vital dimension of being that required a religious answer. And in a small paragraph inset into this article, the editor Peggy Nuttall also affirmed her belief in 'a trinitarian approach to healing ... we include regular articles on the spiritual aspects of man's welfare'.[53]

Letters in the *Nursing Mirror* in 1962 and 1963 argued over whether nursing was a job[54] or a vocation.[55] Writers were conscious of the changing world and the loosening moral structures of which contemporary nursing was part. The nurse's role in basic nursing care needed to be defended. This can be seen in an editorial in the *Nursing Times* in 1963 entitled 'The Bedpan Round'. The author described the importance of senior nurses meeting patients' most basic needs, and concluded: 'Many older nurses will recall being exhorted to "Carry that bedpan to the Glory of God"; if this is unacceptable to the humanists, then can we appeal to them to "Carry that bedpan to the dignity of Man"?'[56]

Humanistic ideas were becoming increasingly influential. In line with its new editorial policy, editorials in the *Nursing Mirror* in early 1963 stated that the modern nurse was no longer 'the submerged, "dedicated" creature that she was'[57] and should therefore no longer be expected to show 'Unquestioning obedience'.[58] To this end the *Nursing Mirror* was encouraging its readers to consider new ideas by introducing the 'Life and Living it' and 'Open Forum' series in the January edition. Readers were exhorted in the April editorial to 're-examine cherished ideas and practices and give fair consideration to new theories', particularly from younger colleagues. New ideas, theories and practices were introduced as replacements for devotional articles.

The *Nursing Times* was not so radical. In 1963, it reported the presidential address of Muriel Powell, who had argued that nursing was facing a difficult time; leaders felt the need to reaffirm moral and spiritual values in an increasingly technological society which was questioning all the old certainties in what Harold Macmillan called 'the winds of change'.[59] The *Nursing Times* editorial for that issue took Powell's speech as its focus, and quoted her: 'Perhaps we have laid too much emphasis on the technological advances of our time. Now we must get back to considering the moral and spiritual problems of the day'.[60] The editorial writer wondered if nursing of late has been too preoccupied with nurses 'being worthy of their hire', and reminded the profession that it 'expects more of its practitioners than mere skills and academic ability'.

The *Nursing Times* approach contrasted with that of the *Nursing Mirror*. An editorial in the *Nursing Mirror* later that year, suggested that prevailing concepts, such as 'winds of change', the 'need for progress', the 'need for human relationships', and statements about nurses 'as professional women', uttered by speakers from conference platforms and lecture rooms, were blindly accepted without questioning by most nurses. Without constructive criticism, the writer argued, the danger was that members of the 'captive, and perhaps somewhat somnambulant audience' not only accepted the practised phrases but repeated them in discussion as well as in their individual thinking. As the writer warned, such repetition meant that 'instead of minds we have a woolly mess of clichés, flowery phrases, and meaningless gestures'. Ordinary nurses seemed to be inclined to follow what they were told without questioning. In the light of earlier editorials that year, it may be deduced that the *Nursing Mirror* was not arguing for a critical approach to all ideas influencing nursing, but only to traditional ideas.[61]

Some fierce disagreement about the nature of radical change was seen in 1963. An article in May 1963 by Annie Unmack argued that nurses by virtue of their dedicated service rooted in Christian charity, were in a position to help orientate and reintegrate a world obsessed with its own selfish desires, and so restore the essential dignity of human beings.[62] This view was supported by the *Nursing Times* editorial the following week.[63] For five weeks correspondence ensued on this subject, strongly in support of the article, or strongly against it.[64] Amongst the letters attacking Unmack was one written by Claire Rayner, who supported the liberalising of morality.[65] In reply to her letter, Rosemary White argued that although ethics were constant a baseline needed to be maintained, and even if they were not practising Christians themselves, people needed to be aware that they were living in a Christian country.[66]

Following its two earlier editorials in 1963, the *Nursing Mirror* sought to re-articulate the idea of the vocation in an acceptable language for the contemporary world by seeking to play down any religious connotation.[67] Vocation was not a religious calling but a natural aptitude, even a desire, such as actors or comedians might have. Any connotation of dedication or sacrifice was also downplayed. Nursing had an equal right to reward as any other occupation.

There was now growing division within the profession about the moral requirement of the nurse. The editorial in the *Nursing Times* which appeared in December 1963, expressed this division.[68] Some matrons and tutors believed that nurses needed to conform to a higher moral standard than their contemporaries, whether shopgirls, secretaries or teachers. Others expected no difference. The General Nursing Council was itself unclear: 'Part of the difficulty here is to decide whether there is an ethic of nursing over and above ethics generally. And are ethical standards absolute or are they modified by the society in which we live?'

The central tenet of Nightingale's philosophy of nursing, that the nurse's moral character was fundamental to nursing, was being forcefully challenged. An article by a nurse tutor for student and pupil nurses reiterated the central tenet of the Nightingale tradition, that character was formed and tested through the apprenticeship training:

> Do not be perturbed if at first you feel no burning sense of vocation. If you ask any P.T.S. why its members became nurses the most conventional answers result. Ask them again three years later, and they will reply with greater frankness. One thing which emerges, especially if the school is a good one, is that some will have found a vocation during training ... The nurse's function, in addition to the part she may play in healing, is a spiritual one. It is a ministry of patience and cheerfulness and silent efficiency. These

> qualities are most likely to spring from a spirit which seeks something outside and above self.[69]

But the vocation was becoming less attractive to some nurses in leadership positions, and the American model, which had a different ethos, was of increasing interest. Such was the view of Sheila Collins, Principal Tutor of the London Hospital, later a member of the Briggs Committee.[70]

Meanwhile, nursing was becoming a subject of interest for social scientists. An editorial in the *Nursing Times* in April 1964 concerned the ever-increasing number of surveys, reports and investigations into morale in hospitals: 'The nursing profession seems to hold a remarkable fascination for research workers, sociologists and psychologists who continue to view the profession through the microscope.'[71] Few other occupations had been subjected to so many inquiries, and although interesting things were said about nurse wastage and the nursing hierarchy in hospitals, there were few concrete suggestions. Surprisingly little attention was paid to the medical profession and the effects of modern medicine on nursing staff.

Another editorial in the same journal in July 1964 noted the publication of 'yet another study of human relations in hospital'. It reflected that 'staff are weary, rather disheartened or even a little defiant at being hauled out in front of the class so often to be put to shame'.[72] This was not altogether negative, for some studies affirmed the strengths of the tradition. As the editorial noted, Revans's report of that year portrayed the efficient and competent nurse as also the nurse who had time to talk to patients.

An assistant matron, Anthony Carr, described the apprenticeship nature of nursing as hindering nursing from becoming a profession.[73] Yet, while he called for nursing to adopt student status and so fulfil the terms of a profession, he suggested that many people, particularly patients, saw nursing as an art, a vocation, or dedicated work, but rarely as a profession. In the same year, by contrast, another writer suggested that nurses were ordinary girls rather than the 'angels' which was the image they inherited. In fact the writer believed that the pressures in nursing turned nurses into 'fallen angels'.[74]

That year, an article on mental illness[75] provoked a correspondent to give a Christian religious viewpoint.[76] This letter was followed by strong disagreements.[77] So great seemed to have been the correspondence this issue raised, that two weeks later the *Nursing Mirror* devoted three-quarters of a page to replies, all of which asserted the importance of the Christian vocational tradition.[78]

Vocation was not restricted to a particular ethical or cultural group in nursing, as MacGuire's study had shown; nurses from all ethnic and cultural groups, and all classes held the same values.[79] This was clear in an article published in *Nursing Times*, which quoted Revans's research with West Indian

[sic] pupil nurses which showed them following in this same tradition. For example, one nurse was quoted: 'Personally I am so keen to do this course that I feel, with God's help, I will be able to surmount any difficulties.'[80]

Although articles on religious themes continued in the *Nursing Mirror* of 1964,[81] religious uncertainties increased. With increasing interest in the philosophy of humanism, an article entitled 'Christian humanism' tried to clarify the fundamental difference between humanism and Christianity, which was frequently being debated.[82] The focus was on the future, the question was to what extent this focus overturned the past.

In an editorial in May 1965, celebrating the golden jubilee of the *Nursing Times*, the writer affirmed that nursing must live in the present and look forward to the future. But she or he also affirmed nursing values to be immutable and unchanging: 'We are constantly reminded that we live in a time of change; but we also need to be reminded that it will only be to our detriment if the contemporary world rejects the values of the past: values that are immutable and unchanging in an unstable society.' The Hippocratic Oath was relevant: 'Strengthened by the Christian tradition in which nursing has its roots. The humanist will recognise the Christian ethic, the fruitful soil of so many welfare endeavours; the Christian will look beyond the ethic to the source.' This was the basis for providing nurses with 'pairs of willing, trained hands, educated minds and compassionate hearts'.[83]

For an increasing number of nurses change would mean the rejection of traditional values. In the *Nursing Mirror*, James P. Smith argued that the so-called problem of promiscuity was exaggerated by a prudish older generation. He even suggested that a conference on this subject may have been a safety-valve to allow this generation to release 'personal tension'.[84] Here was a new world of sexual liberation reflecting the culture of the 1960s.

It appears that the *Nursing Times*, edited by Peggy Nuttall, was more reticent about the changing ethos of nursing than the *Nursing Mirror*. The attitude of the *Nursing Mirror* to change, reflected in an editorial, was that in a rapidly changing world any attempt to preserve the *status quo* in nursing was doomed to failure and even ridicule: 'It will be discontent and criticism which will take us forward to greater things than we can yet dream of. Let us welcome both as two of the most productive human attitudes of all.'[85]

Similarly, an editorial concerned with recruitment was anxious to remove 'the mists of sentimentality and misunderstanding' of nursing's past reputation and image in order to project nursing as a profession like any other and thus with similar rewards.[86] As the *Nursing Mirror* argued, nursing needed to move with the times; change was being held back by older nurses who kept hold of a reactionary influence and would not retire gracefully.[87]

The theme of change as progress was often repeated. In a series of lectures entitled 'Politics in Nursing', delivered at the Royal Society of Health's

Congress, the Professor of Politics at Edinburgh University accepted Platt's premise that nursing should move into higher education. But in order to do so, he said, it needed to redefine its role and focus on administration. Nurses needed a change of emphasis in order to improve their bargaining position over salaries and conditions: 'Nearly all professions today suffer from a sense of malaise, induced by social change.'[88] If nursing was to improve its position, 'it, too, must set about acquiring a new dynamic, rather than sticking to old and tired ways'. Margaret Scott Wright, Matron of the Middlesex Hospital, and later a member of the Briggs Committee, agreed. As she described the increased demands on the nursing service, the effects on recruitment, education and administration, then she, too, pointed to the 'wind of change'.[89]

The *Nursing Mirror* was impatient with those who disagreed with change. Hence the General Nursing Council's Memorandum, which rejected the root-and-branch changes to nurse education proposed by the Platt Report was greeted negatively by the *Nursing Mirror* editorials.[90] Deprecating the tradition, the editorial writer of the *Nursing Mirror* called for nurses to exchange martyrdom for a proper reward. The past was 'cluttered with dust-covered, ancient momentoes': haloes made uneasy headwear with a comic look for modern times.[91]

Yet, during that year, nurses were writing to the *Nursing Mirror* because they were afraid that nursing was valuing technical skills rather than bedside care.[92] Some ordinary nurses did not seem to be striving for status. Indeed, there was considered to be 'appalling apathy among nurses regarding their conditions of employment or training, and their approach to active participation in professional organisations'.[93]

Changing times had brought a mood of insecurity, instability and apparent loss of confidence to the 'old school' of nursing leaders. This mood was reflected in a report on Christianity and nursing, which found that there was a lack of Christian witness to staff in hospitals.[94] Christian organisations were 'escapist and introspective', concerned with their own organisations.

Religious articles that appeared week by week in the *Nursing Mirror* in the early 1960s were less common. Several correspondents wrote to contradict what they felt to be an assumption expressed in a series of articles,[95] that evolutionary science and religion were mutually exclusive.[96] One of the writers stated that although the writer claimed to be value neutral, his articles were 'laced' with the 'New Morality' that was antagonistic to traditional Christian values.[97]

The atmosphere of change during this period brought uncertainty to nursing. After reading a report in the *Nursing Times* entitled 'When Waiting for Salmon and Platt', the correspondent wondered if members of the public and new recruits had a clear picture of what a 'proper' nurse was.[98] The following week a correspondent replied that while 'proper' nursing had always been difficult to define, it was 'Offering trust, acceptance and constructive assistance with humility, integrity and love.'[99]

Recruitment continued to preoccupy nursing leaders. A *Nursing Mirror* editorial in 1966 noted the Ministry of Health figures, recently released, which showed that in 1965 the number of full-time nursing staff had increased by nearly 6,000 and the number of part-time nursing staff had increased by 7,000.[100] The editorial itself was sceptical about the accuracy of these figures noting discrepancy between MoH and GNC statistics. Whatever the problems of recruiting nurses, the number of nursing staff increased by 3.7 per cent per annum up to 1969 and by 4.5 per cent per annum between 1969 and 1973. The number of nursing auxiliaries and nursing assistants rose from 20 to nearly 30 per cent from 1949 to 1973.[101]

The attack on tradition gathers force 1966–1967

As the decade progressed the ethos of nursing began to change more perceptibly. Following a report on a conference on nurse education,[102] a half-page letter from a ward sister expressed concern about the emphasis on education and the marginalisation of the patient as a person:

> I was unable to rid myself of the feeling of uneasiness which I and many of my colleagues have, concerning the degree of importance placed upon education. There seems to be a move afoot which aims at changing the face of nursing, from caring for the sick to reading for a degree, in order to attract new blood ... Many of us are far from convinced that higher education, Platt, extra duty payments, overtime payments, etc., etc., are the answers to finding, training, and keeping S.R.N.s.[103]

Her letter was strongly supported.[104] Even the *Nursing Mirror* seemed to see the dangers of losing the deeply implicit tradition. Despite its determination to move with the times, a passionate editorial was concerned with the preoccupation with research and 'stunned to note' that £3,000 was being spent by a university to find the causes of apathy among the elderly. The editorial not only questioned the financial costs and the ultimate value of research, but also the pressure that was placed on nursing by universities to research into such subjects as the authoritarian influence of Nightingale, or the charitable influence of the religious orders: 'Though research is a sophisticated and essential tool for progress, like any other tool it can be mis-used and mis-applied. There is evidence that we are growing to value it for its own sake, and failing to question the worth of the work resulting from its application.'[105]

Nurses were increasingly under pressure, it seems, to carry out research in order to prove themselves in their jobs. The editorial writer wondered if some nurses were drawn to research because they could not cope with the 'hurly-burly of a practical working situation', and because of the prestige of 'academic distinction'. Letters in following issues both supported and rejected the editorial.[106]

Vocational nurses did make an actual difference to patient care according to the writer of a column in the *Nursing Mirror*. Most nurses approached nursing as a vocation, although by the third year in training they had become split into two groups: the vocationalist and the careerist. The difference, the writer suggested, was one of attitude. The vocationalist was always with his or her patients, rarely got or sought recognition, and was kind and approachable to new staff. The careerist, on the other hand, was often 'hanging around the main office hoping to have a chat with the matron', and made sure that everyone knew what he or she was doing: 'Careerists naturally scoff and deride any notion that nursing can be vocational these days. It is just an occupation to them, where you can "skive" better than on any outside job.'[107]

In 1966, articles in the *Nursing Mirror* highlighted the effects on teenagers of promiscuity, drug addiction,[108] and an increase in venereal disease.[109] From inside the nursing profession, the roots of the vocational tradition were being widely attacked, as was observed in the Florence Nightingale Oration: 'The middle of the 20th century may well be called the day of the iconoclast. In so many ways attacks are being made on the traditions and the ethical and spiritual values of the past.'[110] Atheistic, agnostic and materialistic values, which now pervaded society, were attacking Nightingale and the tradition she stood for.

The consequence of this was that the spiritual was relegated to the purely personal. Spiritual values, which had formed a shared framework, were now reduced to interior piety. Hence, Phyllis Friend, Matron of the London Hospital, concluded her paper entitled 'Nursing in a Technological Age' with the comment that: 'Many young nurses have their own religious and spiritual values which will give them the support they need, but others do not and they will look to their seniors, to their medical colleagues and to their professional organisation for guidance, and this we must be prepared to give.'[111]

In the following year, 1967, the *Nursing Mirror* published an article which it thought to be controversial in its support for nursing as a vocation.[112] The author of the article argued that only the vocational basis for nursing could save it from becoming just a job like any other. Even in changing times, he argued, when the idea of the vocation was 'old hat' and the Christian ethic not so clearly defined, the imperative of love for one another should still be the basis for the nurse's attitude to care. In the past, even if nurses were not particularly 'religious', the 'inner compulsion' which motivated people to become nurses was rationalised by both nurses and the general public in Christian terms. Now, the materialistic mid-1960s, influenced by the growth of science, militated against the sacrificial and dedicated understanding of vocational nursing.

The author agreed that it was necessary for nurses to seek better conditions of work, and he admitted that the idea of nursing as a vocation was often misused by management to offset nurses' dissatisfactions. But he noted that when nurses moved into managerial roles they also tended to lose sight of the vocational part of their job: 'You have only to study some aspects of the Platt Report to see this materialistic attitude at work.' Only the idea of vocation could help nurses deal with the emotionally draining nature of their work and guard against the bureaucratisation that was increasingly occurring.

That this article was introduced as 'controversial' shows how far nursing had moved from an ethos that was taken for granted at the start of the decade. A letter from a nurse strongly agreed with the vocational aspiration expressed: 'He stated so clearly what every *real* nurse knows about dedication to her profession, even in this day and age.' Yet, she was from the older generation, and it was now very difficult to maintain this ideal.[113]

By 1966 the religious articles had dwindled. The publication of an article by a Congregationalist in a weekly column written by people from all walks of life, 'Life and Living it',[114] appears to have stimulated such interest from readers that it resulted in the author being commissioned to write a follow-up series of articles on religious themes.[115] By 1967, however, religious articles appear to have ceased apart from Christmas and Easter messages.[116]

Even in 1967 there were still hospitals where part of the student nurses' first teaching session was occupied by a prayer, or prayers of thanksgiving and dedication. The service was conducted by the nurse tutor. This tradition formed the subject of a *Nursing Mirror* editorial. The editorial writer understood that nurses with a religious conviction appreciated the opportunity to start their professional life in this way, but suggested that this posed a problem for nurses who were 'devout atheists (there is such a denomination), agnostics or convinced humanists'. Although they could opt out of these occasions, the editorial questioned the value of this approach, and indeed whether it was harmful. Was there a genuine choice for nurses who might be afraid of the consequences of not participating; did it encourage a 'dangerous precedent of enforced deceit'?[117]

Two weeks later the *Nursing Mirror* published a letter in support of its editorial which argued, citing evidence from Abel-Smith,[118] that religion and nursing were quite distinct entities.[119] In contrast, a letter commented on the lack of compassion of the editorial, and reminded readers that care of the sick grew out of Christian principles: 'Oh that more of us in the profession would publicise our Christian beliefs loudly.'[120]

The point of view of an agnostic nurse, published in the *Nursing Mirror*, which questioned the value of religious ritual generally, and hospitals employing chaplains particularly,[121] provoked a large response from readers. A page and a half of letters were published, expressing disagreement, and suggesting that nurses had a responsibility to meet patients' religious and spiritual needs without regard for their personal prejudices.[122] According to one of the correspondents, a sister tutor, agnostic nurses were in the minority: 'definitely you would be in the minority among the student nurses at this hospital, and for this I am thankful'.[123]

Two letters published in the *Nursing Mirror* became the subject of an editorial.[124] The first letter from an anonymous student nurse concerned the issue of a hospital service.[125] This had been conducted in the correspondent's introductory course by the hospital chaplain, was planned by the nurses themselves, and was much appreciated by the writer, an unnamed student nurse, and her set. No one had felt forced to participate, the writer argued, even though they each had different religious views. Calling for unity in the classroom, she suggested that nurses should not opt out of religious matters. The second letter concerned the use of nurses' Christian names by patients, which the writer felt to be inappropriate.[126]

The editorial writer was indignant at what was perceived to be a repressive attitude still in existence in nursing and exemplified by those two letters. Correspondents in the following weeks reflected their concerns at what they thought was the disparaging attitude of the *Nursing Mirror* to the tradition. Matrons were particularly critical: 'I have never read such a dictatorial Editorial as in *Nursing Mirror*, November 17. It was designed, it would appear, to distort deliberately the views set out in the two sincere letters'. [127] Another matron wrote:

> I have re-read the Editorial of November 17 over and over again and still find it difficult to believe that this was written by someone in a responsible position who has the opportunity of guiding and directing young minds. Her obviously un-Christian attitude is her own concern, provided she keeps it to herself, but she is not at liberty to use her professional position to foist her views on her readers, the majority of whom must, without doubt, find these very distasteful. [128]

A further letter, that same week, argued that the editorial had twisted the student nurse's letter, and disagreed with the editorial.[129] Student nurses wrote anonymously to say that most nurses enjoyed the opportunity of participating at a service and did not feel they would be 'blacklisted' if they did not attend.[130] But an article by a student nurse[131] and a letter by a charge nurse,[132] which suggested that Christian moral values helped them in their work of care, provoked an angry letter from a ward sister.[133] What seems significant is not that the ward sister disagreed with the views expressed by these nurses, but the hostile tone of her disagreement. As the decade progressed, the balance tilted away from vocational values. Some nurses were growing more militant.

Nursing militants 1968–1970

As was seen in the last chapter, the Briggs Committee was set up as a response to increased militancy in the nursing profession and, particularly, the RCN 'Raise the Roof' campaign. This campaign protested at the effect of the government's prices and incomes policy on money for nursing education and nursing salaries.[134] Patricia Veal, Administrative Sister at South Western Hospital, London, organised protest marches through the streets of London expressing nurses' unrest, fears for the future and consequently fears for the standard of patient care.[135] Nurses were marching for money. Interestingly, Monica Baly, the nursing historian, who had studied under Abel-Smith, and was influential in RCN politics, was also responsible for the campaign.[136] No longer was the vocational ideal to be a basis for nursing. This was expressed in an editorial in *Nursing Times* entitled 'The Summer of Our Discontent': 'Nursing is not a vocation, religious and therefore conveniently inexpensive. Nor is it a *pis aller* for the plain girl of the family. It is a profession which makes heavy demands on its members, but which in itself can be very attractive.'[137]

New nursing values were now openly expressed in the letters pages of the *Nursing Times*. Rosemary White wrote to express her solidarity with militant nurses, and her indignation at nurses' submissive attitudes to the medical profession.[138] The *Nursing Times* editions of August 23 and 30, and September 6, 13 and 20, all published letters about the march.[139] Many letters supported the march, but not all did. Some writers questioned the wisdom of the protest action. Anne Potter, a Nursing Recruitment Officer from the Royal National Orthopaedic Hospital in Stanmore suggested that the protest march would do more to damage nurse recruitment than low pay would.[140] She was supported in her view,[141] but her letter also provoked an angry response. Terence Wood, a Senior Nursing Officer at the Glenfrith Hospital in Leicester, described Anne Potter's attitude as archaic, and suggested attitudes like hers were the real damage to the nursing profession.[142] Referring to the editorial, 'The Summer of Our Discontent', he repudiated nursing's past adherence to vocation in any religious sense, and suggested that all people dedicated to society had a vocation. He wanted to remove any traditional religious understanding, and instead called for the need for nurses to open their eyes to changes in policies, attitudes and systems in the current age. This letter, and its rather angry tone, illustrates the profound changes that were now happening in nursing. The values inherent in the tradition were being increasingly marginalised as nurses became more politically aware.

Potter was moved to reply to Wood, 'in defence of my "archaic criticism"'.[143] She believed that grievances should have been negotiated in a dignified manner worthy of the profession: 'As nurses we do not want sympathy but definite realistic conditions befitting not only our traditions but the image of the modern well-educated nurse.' Potter saw nursing as an integration of the past tradition with the present. The *Nursing Times* published letters both in support of her and attacking her. A charge nurse from Bristol wrote to complain about the amount of coverage the *Nursing Times* devoted 'week after week to moans about pay, conditions on a "when are they going to do something for the workers" theme – some at great length'.[144]

No doubt there were real grievances at the way nursing was being treated by the government, particularly with regard to nurse education, as Dame Muriel Powell expressed in a letter to the *Nursing Times* in April 1968.[145] Earlier that month principal tutors of the London hospitals wrote to the Minister of Health to protest at the effect of government policy in devaluing nurse education.[146]

The question was whether change should be gradual reform, building on the past, or radical revolution, destroying it and starting afresh. Ordinary nurses in the late 1960s and early 1970s do not seem to have been in favour of radical change. As evidence has shown, the Briggs Committee was surprised to find so little dissatisfaction among nurses that they surveyed from 1970 to 1972, concerning work, hours, shifts and promotion prospects. This would seem to suggest that the nurses who took part in protest marches, or who wrote to journals such as the *Nursing Times*, were in a minority, albeit a vociferous one. But their influence had a powerful effect on the whole ethos of nursing, particularly as the Royal College of Nursing was spearheading the protest campaign, and the *Nursing Times* was their organ.

A letter from a nurse who described herself as having 'actively supported the RCN for many years' expressed extreme disappointment at the militant 'trades union' tactics used by the organisation.[147] Yet her letter was followed the next week by correspondents who rejected her criticism. One such letter suggested: 'If Miss Smith is motivated by a need to preserve her own image of altruistic dedication at the expense of an efficient nursing service, then it can only be regarded as an extremely selfish one.'[148] Several letters were in support of the new RCN policy, away from 'gentle and ladylike behaviour'.[149]

Perhaps the most telling comment on the situation comes from an article written in the *Nursing Times* by Margaret Lamb, the Chairman of the General Nursing Council for Scotland. She described the foundation of nursing as built on the ideal of service, and argued that service was of paramount importance.

The education of the nurse, her working environment, her own life and economic independence, came secondary:

> There are those who feel that the pendulum is swinging too much in the opposite direction and that something should be done to stop it. It is true, at this moment in time, that the aggrandisement of the nurse appears to be taking precedence over the ideal of service and that many senior nurses view this with misgiving but it is also true that there are many young people in the community with a very high ideal of service who never appear to have the case for nursing put before them.[150]

The tradition of nursing was waning. A *Nursing Times* editorial of 1970 suggested that the specifically Christian content of nursing had been diluted into secularism. The result of this was that the crucial concepts of 'Duty' and 'Obedience' had become dull uncompromising words no longer understood.[151]

By 1972 those who had sought to remove the concept of dedicated vocation from nursing seemed to have won the battle. A nurse, Dorothy Bishop, writing in the *Nursing Mirror* on the subject of why girls wanted to become nurses, described the idea of the 'dedicated' nurse as now unutterable: '*The Dedicated Nurse*: Ssh! Dirty word. This girl, in these materialistic days, would rather die than admit to having a vocation, so she pretends to be either giddy or hard-boiled.'[152]

It is perhaps not surprising then, that a district nurse should lament in the *Nursing Times* in January 1972 that the 'winds of change' sweeping through the nursing profession were causing some nurses to reject the giving of bedpans, changing soiled sheets and feeding patients as too menial. Were nurses filling their heads with so much technical information that they were forgetting 'the all-important objective of total patient care'?[153]

Nursing values 1961–1978: studies of nurses' motivations

Other evidence showed how integral and enduring traditional values were to the motivations of ordinary nurses during the period of the 1960s, and beyond. In 1961 Jillian MacGuire surveyed 300 student nurses in the first six months of training in five schools of nursing in the Oxfordshire area.[154] She was particularly interested to follow up the relationship of commitment to nursing by those who considered nursing a vocation and those who considered nursing a career. Students were followed up at intervals, and the second report was produced by MacGuire in 1966.[155]

Few student nurses admitted to being without religious affiliation. A total number of 292 nurses of different races were interviewed. Of these, 245 nurses

(84 per cent) were Protestant, 30 nurses (10 per cent) were Roman Catholic, 2 nurses (1 per cent) were of religions other than Christian, 7 nurses (2 per cent) were agnostic, and 8 nurses (3 per cent) did not state their religious affiliation. Over half the student nurses were Church of England, while 22 per cent belonged to other Protestant denominations.[156]

Over half of the student nurses interviewed by MacGuire in the Preliminary Training School (56 per cent), when asked whether nursing was a vocation or a career for them, replied that it was a vocation. 43 per cent thought nursing was a career and 1 per cent thought it both a vocation and a career. This was particularly true for girls from grammar schools: 'those who considered nursing to be a vocation were significantly more committed to nursing, according to their score on the commitment scale, than those who considered nursing to be a career'.[157]

Many of the student nurses could have gone into occupations which would have given them higher salaries after three years than nursing. MacGuire explained this by reference to the vocational ideal: 'It is surprising that so many of the entrants should have considered nursing to be a vocation for themselves. This explains, in part, why the hospitals can continue to attract student nurses despite the low remuneration and poor off-duty arrangements.' Among senior nursing staff, 'there are still traces of the attitude that a girl who enters nursing as a career is not so committed to nursing and does not make such a good nurse as one who considers nursing to be a vocation'.[158]

Nurses interviewed in the first study were broadly clear that a 'good' nurse was a nurse with personal qualities such as sympathy, kindness, patience, understanding and gentleness, as well as skill in nursing procedures, efficiency, ability to cope in emergency situations and carry out procedures correctly without unnecessary pain to the patient. The 'bad' nurse was characterised as lazy, untidy, unwilling, unkind, slovenly and ill-humoured. Over a third of nurses thought that a 'bad' nurse was one who was not interested in the patients she was dealing with.[159] 'The desire to help other people was the most important single motive for taking up nursing.'[160]

Five years later, MacGuire found sixty-nine out of 292 student nurses had withdrawn from training. She described this number as 'relatively small'.[161] In this latter study there was no mention of the vocational attitude. This is because MacGuire used a different terminology: she replaced the term 'vocation' with the term 'emotional identification'. Nevertheless, this ideal remained central and 'striking' among the nurses she surveyed: 'motivation' was one of the most striking and unchanging features.

MacGuire was struck by the great similarity in the motives of recruits for taking up nursing despite the wide diversity in their educational backgrounds. For a substantial majority, nursing was a positive choice rather than something decided on after other possible careers were eliminated. The decision was made early before a detailed knowledge of nursing could be known: 'An emotional identification with nursing as a practical humanitarian craft takes place and this is very difficult to shake.'[162]

MacGuire believed that the Platt recommendation for a higher educational standard and a more academic training was likely to alienate the majority of entrants who came from middle ability ranges. A consistently higher educational standard would probably not affect withdrawal 'though it would certainly affect the recruitment rate for state registration in an adverse direction'. This finding, MacGuire observed, was supported by another study, that of Marsh and Willcocks (considered below), who also thought that if nursing became too academic it would alienate potential recruits:

> What attracted students into nursing in the main was not the opportunity to study but the chance to do a practical, useful job of work with people ... The majority of entrants to nursing at present are, without a doubt, patient centred. Some of them could have gone to university or to colleges of education for teachers but they preferred to work directly with people and sick people at that.[163]

There was some frustration with the apprenticeship method, thought MacGuire, and there was a desire for rational explanations and understanding for reasons for procedures, rather than unquestioning obedience. Nevertheless, the majority of students enjoyed nursing, even if they became critical of some of the training programmes in some schools.[164]

MacGuire's work evidently provoked some upset within the profession she was studying; according to one commentator: 'We have not yet established a personality profile of the nurse, and when this was attempted by Dr J. MacGuire some years ago the profession was in uproar, because of possible intrusion into its privacy.'[165]

In 1965 Marsh and Willcocks's study in Nottingham found the same motivation amongst nurses as MacGuire had done: 'Those who became nurses were very much more likely to see it as a vocation, a view not shared by those few who *had been* nurses.'[166] Although the majority of school-leavers questioned thought nursing was a career rather than a vocation, a view held especially by the younger people, grammar school girls and girls from families at the upper end of the social scale were more likely to label nursing as a 'vocation'. A high proportion of nurses (45.8 per cent) and a majority of girls from grammar schools (52.8 per cent of twenty-year-olds and 72.5 per cent of sixteen- to nineteen-year-olds) described nursing as a vocation rather than a career or a job. Respondents who thought that nursing was a vocation spoke of the nurse needing to like her work despite its conditions and unpleasantness. They also thought nurses needed dedication and ability.

Marsh and Willcocks, social scientists at the University of Nottingham, judged this vocational ethos to be a negative finding for recruitment purposes. They thought that the emphasis on dedication in the vocational image of nursing would antagonise potential nurses interested in nursing as a career and would discourage recruitment.[167]

They devised a series of statements concerned with qualities people expected to find in a nurse, as well as perceived attitudes towards the nurse. Amongst the statements given to sixteen- to nineteen-year-olds, was the statement, 'Doctors do not respect nurses', to which 12.5 per cent agreed, but 80.6 per cent disagreed; 65 per cent of twenty-year-olds thought nurses were self-sacrificing (24.3 per cent disagreed); 71.2 per cent thought nurses were intelligent (22.1 per cent disagreed); 72 per cent thought nurses were very sympathetic and kind (15 per cent disagreed); 23.8 per cent thought nurses were full of self-importance (63.8 per cent disagreed); and 26.6 per cent thought nurses were more aware of their religion than other girls (56.4 per cent disagreed).[168] The evidence paints a picture of a respected profession held in high esteem by the young, and shows nursing values to be those of self-sacrifice, kindness, sympathy, intelligence, respect and lack of self-importance.

Marsh and Willcocks implied that such values bore no relationship to religious faith. They had developed a hypothesis, that religion was important to nursing, from their study of nursing journals.[169] But this hypothesis, they argued, was not supported by evidence from their data. Nurses were not more aware of their religion than most girls. Perhaps they drew their conclusion too readily, however. It may have been, as MacGuire found, that although nurses expressed a religious affiliation, its importance to the individual was unlikely to be articulated to researchers. Singh, as will be seen shortly, found religious beliefs to be important to nurses.[170]

That nursing still involved a commitment to the values of basic bedside caring was reflected in Ann Dutton's study on the factors affecting recruitment of nurse tutors, in 1968.[171] Dutton, a sociology lecturer, carried out the study for the RCN and the King's Fund. She found that ward sisters were reluctant to become sister tutors because they wanted to remain close to the patient's bedside. Ward sisters, who had originally become nurses through a humanitarian desire to help people, were reluctant to surrender their practical role for a more theoretical and detached position. This finding corresponded with MacGuire's research, that girls were attracted into nursing by humanitarian and altruistic motives. It also echoed the criticism made by the Salmon Report, that able nurses were reluctant to move into management and away from clinical practice. Dutton concluded that the reason why more ward sisters did not become tutors was because they were conscious of themselves as part of the Nightingale tradition:

> vividly conscious of their role as nurses in the Florence Nightingale tradition ... 'in touch with the deep issues of life.' As one of them said in an early interview, and as almost three-quarters of the respondents in the main survey agree, 'if you were a tutor you wouldn't have the same feeling of really helping humanity'. Many say it is difficult to think of tutors as really being nurses.[172]

Although the ward sisters in Dutton's study were committed to the Nightingale tradition, Dutton personally believed that the religious vocation was a cultural tool, employed at a period in history when hospitals were deplorable institutions. This was necessary, Dutton argued, to bring in the radical changes needed to dispel the drunken, promiscuous and dirty image of nursing. Only the heroic self-sacrifices of Nightingale's pupils would be enough to change the situation. Such discipline, Dutton believed, had continued in hospitals and nurses' lives although she thought it was now unnecessary:

> Often, still, as appears from a variety of personal stories and research reports, there exists an implicit assumption that because nurses are following a 'vocation' rather than a 'career' they should therefore be prepared unquestioningly to discount their own feelings and personal needs and be prepared to have them discounted by others.[173]

Dutton argued that tradition and ritual, associated with bureaucracy, uniformity, subordination of the individual, role differentiation and hierarchy, had no particular purpose, and were still characteristic of the Civil Service, the Army, and churches. Citing MacGuire, Revans and Menzies, this bureaucratic model, according to Dutton, led to emotional inhibition among nurses and hence caused ward sisters to conform to, and find emotional security in, the strict structured existence of hospital life.

Because Dutton believed the vocational ethos to be outmoded, she seemed to find it incomprehensible. Rather than seeking answers in moral reasons as to why nurses chose to stay at the bedside, she sought them in intellectual ones. Citing Abel-Smith, she suggested that the majority of girls became nurses because they were not academically gifted, and hence preferred to serve an apprenticeship for a 'practical vocation'. In her view, this was the cause of the conflict between those who wanted to 'up-grade' nursing by requiring higher educational standards, and those nurses who wanted nursing to retain the apprenticeship method of training. Most nurses just were not academically gifted, and did not want to increase the intellectual status of the profession. From Marsh and Willcocks's analysis she drew the conclusion that the generally accepted view of the 'intelligence' of nurses was not supported by school leaving results.[174] Lack of intelligence prevented nurses from seeking to become tutors.

Despite these criticisms, induction into the apprenticeship tradition and its values remained pivotal. This was demonstrated in a study published by Singh and MacGuire in 1971.[175] The majority of nurses ranked the opportunity to help people as their highest occupational value, and ranked social status, prestige and money as their lowest value. This finding was supported by Singh's earlier research, which compared student nurses on experimental courses to undergraduates (course entry autumn 1969) and found that student nurses prized human values and saw themselves as kind, sympathetic and unselfish:

> The average experimental student may, therefore, be defined as one who values other people for what they are themselves and not as a means of self gratification who regards love as itself the only suitable form of human relationship, and whose major motive for nursing is a humanitarian one.[176]

Such values ranked more importantly than economic ones. Hence, the nurse appeared to be a 'ministering angel'. And, in contradiction to Marsh and Willcocks, Singh argued: 'She also definitely values her religious beliefs and practices highly, and concern with religious matters seems to be one source of meaning and satisfaction (Religious value) to her.'[177]

The ideals of nursing remained strong amongst ordinary nurses, according to a psychiatrist writing in 1971. Motives underlying the decision to enter and stay in nursing evoked particularly strong feelings in a group discussion he organised. On one occasion, resentment was expressed towards a leader who was thought to be challenging the ideals and basic integrity of the nurse. Several members of the group regarded such attitudes as potentially dangerous and liable to undermine the confidence of vulnerable individuals.[178]

Indeed, in 1974, two years after Briggs was published, a study of 124 registered nurses by Lamond found that 92 respondents were quite content with their choice of worthwhile career, while 21 were not satisfied, 11 were disillusioned because it was not the 'image' they had imagined, and 16 were discontented with conditions of service. In addition, 6 nurses thought current criticisms were exaggerated; 26 found the job satisfying in terms of human relations, while 4 did not; 11 thought that nursing was a vocation or a calling which required dedication; 2 regretted the fading of the vocational ideals in their chosen career; 3 thought nursing had not attained professional status; 55 nurses talked of nursing as caring, either as 'assisting the patient to recovery' (29) or as 'helping the helpless' (26); and 29 nurses expressed their satisfaction with nursing at the patient's bedside, although 6 mentioned frustrations in not being able to do this properly. For 21 of the nurses the 'essence of nursing' was 'the individuality of the patient'.[179]

Lamond also found that the majority of respondents were very satisfied with the training in practical skills and procedures needed in clinical practice. These included oral hygiene for a critically ill patient, attending to the nutritional needs of patients, seeing that the patient came to no harm, drawing up, administering and recording intramuscular injections, and utilising up-to-date equipment. The majority of respondents thought each of these were part of the nurse's responsibility, and that training on the wards was adequate; 98 per cent thought oral hygiene training adequate; 96 per cent thought training in safety adequate; 97 per cent thought training in giving injections adequate; and 78 per cent thought training to use equipment was adequate. Only four nurses wanted to drop patient nutrition from nursing responsibility.[180]

Even in 1978, an attitude survey conducted by Wyatt found that the system of induction for student nurses was well organised towards the integration of the nurse into a normative team.[181] The survey found that the experiences of the student nurse and her total impressions of working on the ward produced a picture of 'what it takes to be a nurse'. There was no doubt about the practical orientation of the job. Theoretical knowledge was interpreted as a device to explain why something should be done. Student nurses saw themselves as communicators and a 'bridge' to frightened and vulnerable patients. With regard to their assessment, the students considered the report from the ward sister to be more important than the level of achievements documented.

Wyatt identified key nursing qualities as 'common sense', 'punctuality' and 'attitude to patient and visitors'. According to Wyatt: 'Nursing as a profession can be seen to be defined by the character and behaviour of the nurse rather than by her intellectual quality.' The ward sister undoubtedly chose not only to show students how to perform an activity, but also to tell them why it was done. The system was well adapted to encouraging and reinforcing certain character traits. One particular wry comment to the researcher from a student nurse showed the current perception: 'You don't need 'A' levels to give out bed-pans.' There was a general anti-intellectualism amongst the group of students Wyatt interviewed.

The system was not change-orientated, rather it perpetuated a tradition. Other social scientists found this reactionary and inhibiting, but Wyatt argued for its value. Although the educational process could be re-examined and the remoteness of nurse tutors reduced, the tradition should be sustained: 'the student nurses have one great advantage over many other students in further and higher education, their commitment to their calling. Any changes should not in my opinion damage this most valuable asset.'

The views of patients: the public opinion of nurses and nursing care

If nurses and student nurses in the 1960s were broadly satisfied with the ethos of nursing and nurse training, so were patients. In 1961, an experimental survey of the patient's view of the Crumpsall Hospital, Manchester, by Haywood et al., found that only 11 per cent of patients surveyed were critical of their nursing care:

> By and large it was remarkable that so many patients had so much praise for the standard of nursing care in a hospital which suffers from a shortage of nursing staff. Almost two-thirds of them were genuinely enthusiastic, and critics were in a small minority here. [182]

In 1961 McGhee also found that patients were, on the whole, satisfied with their physical care.[183] From her responses she found it impossible to differentiate between the two functions of nursing – physical care and emotional support: 'The two are interdependent; and the patient's judgement of the standard of physical care appeared to be strongly influenced by the way in which it was given.'[184] Many patients emphasised instances of exceptional nursing given to them or to some seriously ill patient: 'There was no reservation in the patient's mind about the high quality of technical skill, although sympathy in applying these skills seemed to be lacking on occasions.'[185] Yet such criticisms were often felt to be related to nurses' working conditions and training programme, directed largely at inadequate staffing levels and the inflexibility of the ward organisation.

McGhee found that patients were unhappy with nurses who were not kind and compassionate, no matter how skilful they were. What counted for patients above all else appeared to be the kindness and compassion of the nurse:

> A nurse might be inexpert at using a hypodermic syringe, but if her approach to the patient relaxed him, her lack of skill was forgotten. Conversely, the good technician lost much of the credit for her ability when with a 'matter of fact "roll-over" she threw in the dart'. [186]

If a nurse 'became hard' it was felt she became insensitive as a result of her experience.[187] It was not the personal character of the nurse that was criticised, but the effect on her of methods of training and conditions of work and leisure. McGhee concluded that a good quality of nurse at all grades was potentially available to patients in any hospital:

> In the present study, the quality, kindness, courtesy, cheerfulness and willingness of the young student nurse was never in question.

> The question, unanswered, but put in many forms to the interviewer, was 'what happens to them on the way up?'

When asked to describe the way nurses looked after them, a study by Cartwright, in 1964, found that 53 per cent of patients were unreservedly enthusiastic, using phrases such as 'like angels' and 'real champion'.[188] Only 3 per cent were mainly critical; although when asked for an occasion when nurses could have done more for them, 23 per cent made some critical comment and 15 per cent made some further qualification, although not a criticism.

Patients told frequent stories about nurses' sympathy and understanding. For example, a female patient described the kindness of a nurse who put her arms around her and comforted her when she was lonely.[189] Only a minority of patients criticised the nurses and described occasions when nurses were unkind, impatient, inconsiderate and unsympathetic. Cartwright concluded that:

> Most patients were grateful for the way the nurses had looked after them. Dissatisfaction among the minority may have stemmed from three sources: unreasonably critical or demanding patients; individual nurses who were unsympathetic or otherwise inadequate; and unsatisfactory working conditions for the nurses. It is not possible to distinguish between these possible reasons for discontent.

Over half the patients in Cartwright's study described the way nurses looked after them enthusiastically: 'This is a tribute to the devotion of most nurses.'[190]

In 1965 Winifred Raphael found that patients were broadly very satisfied with their care.[191] What mattered most to them was the kind of relationship they had with the nurse, and her competence. They valued kindness, gentleness, sensitivity and serenity. Nursing tasks that were considered most important were bringing the bedpan quickly and care given to old people: helping them eat and drink, cutting toenails, and so on. As Raphael wrote: 'It was these unglamorous activities that were mentioned by the patients rather than technical skill.'[192]

A patient satisfaction study carried out by Raphael four years later, in 1969, and repeated with revised questionnaires in 1973 and 1977, supported these conclusions.[193] Raphael found that patients were broadly very satisfied with their nursing care. Patients recorded comments such as 'superb nursing', 'gentle and kind, gay and amusing'[194] and 'I cannot speak too highly of the way I was cared for by all', 'doctors, sisters and nurses are tops', 'the team spirit was marvellous' and 'I will remember the staff in my prayers'.[195] Raphael regarded these as typical. Human factors were most important to patients. As she wrote in the next edition of the survey, which had the same statistical conclusions:

> Perhaps the most striking finding of the whole survey is that 93 per cent of matters liked best [by patients] depend on human factors (including organisations) and only 7 per cent on physical factors such as food or the ward. The happiness of patients seems to depend on the skill, ability and kindness of other people far more than on physical factors or finance.[196]

Both nurses and patients seemed to have had a similar and very clear idea of what made a good nurse. A study by Anderson in the early 1970s found that both nurses and patients thought that the main things a patient expected of a nurse were: 'kindness', 'understanding', 'availability', 'gentleness', 'tenderness', 'patience', 'sympathy' and 'consolation'. Patients also frequently mentioned 'civility', 'courtesy' and 'politeness'. Values were constantly reiterated.[197]

To what extent patients' opinions were taken into consideration in shaping nursing policy is debateable. As one author suggested, 'patients' views, although they may contribute useful insights, are but one facet of the many ingredients which, together, constitute high quality care'.[198]

It may be that patients did not like to express negative opinions about nurses, but during the period of the 1960s, serious abuses of care also came to light. In 1964 Gerda Cohen wrote *What's Wrong with the Hospitals?*,[199] and in 1967 Barbara Robb wrote *Sans Everything*.[200] Cohen argued that patients had no rights, no dignity and no status. Cohen's work was a personal and anecdotal view of a hierarchical hospital system and the power of the tradition of nursing rooted in what she called 'the Nightingale myth'.[201] Robb's criticisms were so serious that committees of enquiry were set up, even though the accuracy of her criticisms was questioned.[202]

In 1966 the Ministry of Health asked the RCN to undertake empirical studies to develop measures for the quality of nursing care, an enormously complex task.[203] But according to a psychologist, writing in Robb's book, answers lay elsewhere: 'Our concern and relationship with our fellow-men must surely be a moral and religious problem. ("For as much as ye have done it unto the least of these, ye have done it unto me.")'[204] Recommitment to the traditional moral principles of the profession was the only solution when deficiencies occurred.

Conclusion

The body of evidence examined in this chapter gives a window into the feelings of nurses and patients. The desire for radical change to the status of the profession that developed during the 1960s, and led ultimately to the publication of the Briggs Report, was not uniform. During this period, which encompassed the major cultural movement towards secularisation, there was a remarkable tenacity by those who sought to maintain the vocational spirit of nursing. This continued into the next decade.

Editorials in nursing journals shifted their position as the decade advanced, but a large volume of letters disagreed with this shift. Research studies found that nurses and patients thought that the principles underpinning the practical apprenticeship tradition were fundamental to the quality of nursing care. Many nurses and their patients were in the main, if not always, contented with nursing and nurse training. Shortcomings should be remedied by reform and a recommitment to those principles. Evidence has shown that there was undoubtedly perceived to be a 'battle for the soul of nursing'. But the tide had turned. Those in power were now wedded to fundamental change. The next chapter will show the direction nursing would take.

Notes

1 J.P. Brown, 'Faith and Nursing', *Nursing Times*, 1965, p. 1428, October 15.

2 'Nurse and Patient: A Study in Human Relationships. Evelyn C. Pearce', *Lancet*, 1953, p. 380, August 22; K.L.B., 'Nurse and Patient by Evelyn Pearce, Second Edition', *Nursing Mirror*, 1963, p. vii, November 8.

3 M. Clarke, 'Nurse and Patient, Human Relations in Nursing, Second Edition. Evelyn Pearce', *Nursing Times*, 1963, pp. 1422–1423, November 8; T.A.K., 'Nurse and Patient by E. Pearce, Third Edition', *Nursing Mirror*, 1969, pp. 44–45, September 26.

4 'The Changing Scene', *Nursing Times*, 1955, pp. 1225–1228, October 28.

5 M.B. Powell, 'Nursing Training and Standards of Care', *Nursing Times*, 1963, pp. 1081–1082, August 30.

6 M. Powell, 'The Challenge of Nursing Education', *Nursing Mirror*, 1967, pp. 551–554, March 17; pp. 581–584, March 24.

7 T. Crawford, 'Foreword', in Powell, M., *Patients are People*, pp. 9–11, Reading, Educational Explorers, 1975.

M.B. Powell, 'Nursing – its Contribution to Society', *Nursing Times*, Part 1, 1969, pp. 113–116, July 17; Part 2, pp. 117–118, July 24.

8 O.V. Buxton, 'A Day Off in the Life of a Matron', *Nursing Mirror*, 1960, p. 641, November 18; 'Miss Loveridge of Bart's: A Profile', *Nursing Times*, 1967, p. 1032, August 4; 'Helen Downton', *The Daily Telegraph*, 1994, p. 29, November 23; H. Downton, 'Divine Healing: The Nurse and Spiritual Healing', *Nursing Times*, 1959, p. 851, September 11; E. MacManus, *Matron of Guy's*, London, Andrew Melrose, 1956.

9 M. Powell, *Patients are People*, Reading, Educational Explorers, 1975.

10 A. Davis, 'Moral Re-armament', letter, *Nursing Times*, 1960, p. 479, April 15.

[11] E. Dainty, 'Back to School at Thirty-Seven', *Nursing Mirror*, 1960, pp. 59,64, October 7; pp. 167–168, October 14.

[12] 'You Hear it Said, Platitude 1, Nurses are Different!' *Nursing Mirror*, 1960, p. 1915, August 26; 'Platitude 2. Nurses are Practical People', *Nursing Mirror*, 1960, p. 2005, September 2; 'Platitude 3. Nurses Have to be Tough!', *Nursing Mirror*, 1960, p. 2105, September 9; 'Platitude 4. Nurses Find it Hard to Express Themselves!', *Nursing Mirror*, 1960, p. 2197, September 16; 'Platitude 5. Nurses are Not What They Used to Be', *Nursing Mirror*, 1960, p. 2287, September 23; 'Platitude 6. Nurses Need Discipline', *Nursing Mirror*, 1960, p. 2370, September 30; 'Platitude 7. Nurses are not Professionally Minded', 1960, *Nursing Mirror*, p. 64, October 7.

[13] Ibid., p. 2287.

[14] 'Selection of Letters from Readers on our Controversial Series of "Platitudes", *Nursing Mirror*, 1960, p. 65, October 7; p. 352, October 28.

[15] 'The Vigil and the Vow', editorial, *Nursing Mirror*, 1960, p. 1141, December 30.

[16] J.A.G. Lawrence, 'Vocation or Profession?', letter, *Nursing Times*, 1961, p. 97, January 20.

[17] 'Ward Time-table: Revised Pattern', *Nursing Times*, 1961, pp. 398–399, March 31; Ministry of Health, Central Health Services Council, *The Pattern of the In-patient's Day*, London, HMSO, 1961.

[18] 'A Shocking Situation', editorial, *Nursing Mirror*, 1961, p. 1399, July 28.

[19] 'Pointers for 1962', editorial, *Nursing Mirror*, 1961, pp. 233, 250, December 29.

[20] K.A. Raven, 'The Future of the Nursing Profession', *Nursing Mirror*, 1961, pp. 739–740, May 26; pp. 843–845, June 2.

[21] 'Who will Nurse the Patients of Tomorrow?', *Nursing Times*, 1961, pp. 946–947, July 21.

[22] 'Wolfson School of Nursing', *Nursing Times*, 1961, p. 392, March 31.

[23] 'Professional Roots', editorial, *Nursing Times*, 1961, p. 1557, December 1.

[24] B. Abel-Smith, 'Crisis in Nursing – 5: The Sociologist's View', *Nursing Times*, 1961, pp. 1262–1263, September 29; H. Gainsborough, 'Crisis in Nursing – 4: The Physician's View', *Nursing Times*, 1961, pp. 1228–1229, September 22; F. Hart, 'Crisis in Nursing – 1: The Administrator's View', *Nursing Times*, 1961, pp. 1119–1120, September 1; S.A.S. Malkin, 'Crisis in Nursing – 2: The Surgeon's View', *Nursing Times*, 1961, pp. 1150–1151, September 8; K. Robinson, 'Crisis in Nursing – 3: The Politician's View', *Nursing Times*, 1961, pp. 1195–1196, September 15; J. Seale, 'Crisis in Nursing – 6: The Medical Economists's View', *Nursing Times*, 1961, pp. 1286–1288, October 6; Anonymous, 'Crisis in Nursing – 7: A Nurse's View', *Nursing Times*, 1961, pp. 1324–1325, October 13; Anonymous, 'Crisis in Nursing – 8: A Nurse's View 2. Long-term Policy', *Nursing Times*, 1961, pp. 1358–1359, October 20.

[25] K. Robinson, 'Crisis in Nursing – 3: The Politician's View', *Nursing Times*, 1961, pp. 1195–1196, September 15.

[26] 'No Sense of Vocation Today?', editorial, *Nursing Mirror*, 1961, pp. 99,120, November 10.

[27] J.H. Bodgener, 'Some Familiar Hymns', *Nursing Mirror*, 1960, p. 426, April 29; p. 605, May 13; p. 691, May 20; p. 774, May 27; p. 869, June 3.

[28] S. Perowne, 'Paul – An Apostle of Jesus Christ', *Nursing Mirror*, 1960, p. 2194, September 16; p. 2292 , September 23; p. 2372, September 30; p. 56, October 7; p. 180, October 14; p. 269, October 21.

[29] J. Foster, 'Christian Witness in the Early Centuries', *Nursing Mirror*, 1960, p. 1230, January 8; p. 1316, January 15; p. 1406, January 22; p. 1496, January 29; p. 1590, February 15.

[30] R. Pitter, 'In the Service of God', *Nursing Mirror*, 1960, p. 2070, March 11; p. 2162, March 18; p. 2250, March 25; p. 55, April 1; p. 166, April 8.

[31] M. Stocks, 'The Unread Best-seller', *Nursing Mirror*, 1960, p. 1488, July 22; p. 1568, July 29; p. 1654, August 5; p. 1752, August 12; p. 1832, August 19; p. 1918, August 26.

[32] M. Wilson, 'Religion, Life and Healing', *Nursing Mirror*, 1960, p. 1156, December 30; 1961, p. 1251, January 6; p. 1348, January 13; p. 1444, January 20; p. 1538, January 27; p. 1632, February 3.

[33] J. Robinson, 'The Gift of the Spirit', *Nursing Mirror*, 1961, p. 1544, September 8; p. 1566, September 15; p. 1580, September 22; p. 1594, September 29; p. 15, October 6; p. 6, October 20.

[34] G. Abell, 'The Ministry of the Christian Nurse', *Nursing Mirror*, 1961, p. 156, April 14; p. 254, April 21; p. 338, April 28; p. 432, May 5; p. 542, May 12; p. 554, May 19.

[35] D. Stewart, 'The Parables of Jesus', *Nursing Mirror*, 1961, p. 1823, February 17; p. 1906, February 24; p. 2004, March 3; p. 2118, March 10; p. 2216, March 17; p. 2308, March 24.

[36] G. Reindorp, 'Hold Fast That Which Thou Hast', *Nursing Mirror*, 1961, pp. 137–138, November 17.

[37] M. Stocks, 'Favourite Tales from the Old Testament', *Nursing Mirror*, 1961, p. 1036, June 16; p. 1144, June 23; p. 1232, June 30; p. 1324, July 7; p. 1378, July 14; p. 1396, July 21.

[38] M. Wilson, 'The Purpose and Practice of Prayer', *Nursing Mirror*, 1962, p. 13, October 5; p. 38, October 12; p. 63, October 19; p. 88, October 26; p. 110, November 2; p. 136, November 9.

[39] M. Stocks, 'Living World of the Bible', *Nursing Mirror*, 1962, p. 394, August 17; p. 415, August 24; p. 436, August 31; p. 456, September 7; p. 480, September 15.

[40] H.M. Lloyd, 'The Service of the Five Candles', *Nursing Mirror*, 1962, p. 480, March 16; p. xvi, March 23; p. x, March 30; p. 13, April 6; p. 35, April 13; p. 54, April 20.

[41] N. Earle, 'The Resurrection Appearances of Jesus', *Nursing Mirror*, 1962, p. x, April 27; p. 88, May 4; p. xvi, May 11; p. 136, May 18; p. xvi, May 25.

[42] Bishop of Lichfield, 'The Festival of Love and Worship. Series of three articles on the meaning of Christmas', *Nursing Mirror*, 1962, p. 244, December 14; p. 264, December 21; p. 280, December 28.

[43] G. Schuster, 'Service of Dedication to Workers in Oxford', *Nursing Mirror*, 1962, p. 184, November 23; p. 203, November 30.

[44] 'For Whom the Train Stopped,' editorial, *Nursing Mirror*, 1962, p. 481, September 21.

[45] J.E. Gordon, 'The Nurse's Contribution to the Community', *Nursing Mirror*, 1963, pp. 92–94, May 3; pp. 113–115, May 10; pp. 139–141, May 17; pp. 161–162, May 24.

[46] 'Vale Atque Ave', editorial, *Nursing Mirror*, 1962, p. 267, December 28.

[47] 'Miss Virginia Henderson in London', *Nursing Mirror*, 1963, p. 243–244, June 14.

[48] 'Editorial', *Nursing Mirror*, 1963, p. 45, April 19.

[49] J. Robinson, 'The Gift of the Spirit', *Nursing Mirror*, 1961, p. 1544, September 8; p. 1566, September 15; p. 1580, September 22; p. 1594, September 29; p. 15, October 6; p. 6, October 20.

[50] A.J.P. Taylor, 'Seventy Years On', in Barker, L.M. (ed.), *Pears Cyclopaedia 1967–68*, p. vii–x, London, Pelham Books Limited, 1967.

[51] G. Reindorp, 'How do you Read your Bible?', *Nursing Mirror*, 1963, p. 538, March 22; 'Tiresome Types', p. 560, March 29; 'No Work Today', p. 32, April 12; 'The Waters of Comfort', p. 75, April 26; 'Remember Lot's Wife' p. 134, May 17.

[52] E. Patey, 'Has Science made Religion out of Date?', *Nursing Mirror*, 1963, p. 476, March 1; 'Can We Prove the Existence of God?', p. 514, March 15; 'The Search for Truth, pp. 385–386, August 2.

[53] H. Booth, 'A Chaplain's Diary', *Nursing Times*, 1963, p. 658, May 24.

[54] E. Messer, 'Nursing is a Job', letter, *Nursing Mirror*, 1962, p. 34, April 13; E. Lockyer, 'Taking a Vocation Too Far', letter, *Nursing Mirror*, 1963, p. 59, April 19.

[55] E.A. Mole, 'A Vocation and Profession', letter, *Nursing Mirror*, 1962, p. 89, May 4; D.A. Buckley, 'A Question of Vocation', letter, *Nursing Mirror*, 1963, p. 102, May 3.

[56] 'The Bedpan Round', editorial, *Nursing Times*, 1963, p. 281, March 8.

[57] 'Editorial', *Nursing Mirror*, 1963, p. 311, January 11.
[58] 'Editorial', *Nursing Mirror*, 1963, p. 45, April 19.
[59] 'An Outward Look', *Nursing Times*, 1963, p. 689, May 31.
[60] 'Giving a Lead', editorial, *Nursing Times*, 1963, p. 665, May 31.
[61] 'Editorial', *Nursing Mirror*, 1963, p. 313, July 12.
[62] A. Unmack, 'Chastity and Charity', *Nursing Times*, 1963, p. 651–652, May 24.
[63] 'Giving a Lead', editorial, *Nursing Times*, 1963, p. 665, May 31.
[64] Letters, *Nursing Times*, 1963, p. 687, May 31, pp. 715–716, June 7, p. 756, June 14, pp. 786–787, June 21, p. 816, June 28, p. 849, July 5.
[65] C. Rayner, 'Chastity and Charity', letter, *Nursing Times*, 1963, pp. 715–716, June 7.
[66] R. White, 'Chastity and Charity', letter, *Nursing Times*, 1963, pp. 786–787, June 21.
[67] 'Editorial', *Nursing Mirror*, 1963, p. 87, May 3.
[68] 'A Fit and Proper Person', editorial, *Nursing Times*, 1963, p. 1623, December 27.
[69] A. Stevens, 'So You're Going to be a Nurse', *Nursing Mirror*, 1963, pp. 280–281, June 28.
[70] S.M. Collins, 'Exchange of Nurse Teachers', *Nursing Times*, 1964, pp. 370–372, March 6.
[71] 'Morale in the Ward', editorial, *Nursing Times*, 1964, p. 421, April 3.
[72] 'For Immediate Action', editorial, *Nursing Times*, 1964, p. 849, July 7.
[73] A. Carr, 'It is not Professional', *Nursing Mirror*, 1964, p. 258, June 19.
[74] S.M. Johnson, 'Fallen Angels', *Nursing Mirror*, 1964, p. xvi, August 7.
[75] M. Davie, 'Mental Illness', *Nursing Mirror*, 1964, p. 464, August 21.
[76] D. Repton, 'Spiritual Help', *Nursing Mirror*, 1964, p. 538, September 11.
[77] 'A Question of Faith', letters, *Nursing Mirror*, 1964, p. 584, September 25.
[78] 'A Question of Faith', letters, *Nursing Mirror*, 1964, p. 46, October 9.
[79] J. MacGuire, *From Student to Nurse*, Oxford, Oxford Area Nurse Training Committee, September, 1961.
[80] J.L. Martin, 'West Indian Pupil Nurses and their Problems in Training', *Nursing Times*, 1965, pp. 1079–1082, August 6.
[81] G. Macleod, 'Confession is Good for the Soul', *Nursing Mirror*, 1964, p. 376, January 24; 'Intercession', p. 417, February 7; 'Interior Prayer', p. 500, February 28; 'What Happens when you Shut your Eyes?', p. 3569, January 17.
[82] T. Corbishley, 'Christian Humanism', *Nursing Mirror*, 1964, p. 237, June 12.
[83] 'Pairs of Hands', editorial, *Nursing Times*, 1965, p. 11, May 7.
[84] J.P. Smith, 'Promiscuity, Morality and all That', *Nursing Mirror*, 1965, p. iv, January 1.
[85] 'Editorial', *Nursing Mirror*, 1965, p. 375, January 22.
[86] 'Editorial', *Nursing Mirror*, 1965, p. 471, February 19.
[87] 'Editorial', *Nursing Mirror*, 1965, p. 475, August 13; p. 275, November 19.
[88] H.J. Hanham, 'Politics in Nursing', *Nursing Mirror*, 1965, pp. 553–555, September 3.
[89] M. Scott Wright, 'Politics in Nursing', *Nursing Mirror*, 1965, pp. 163–170, October 15.
[90] 'Editorial', *Nursing Mirror*, 1965, p. 1, October 1; p. 323, December 3.
[91] 'Editorial', *Nursing Mirror*, 1965, p. 365, July 16.
[92] 'Bedside Nursing', letters, *Nursing Mirror*, 1965, p. 533, August 27; p. 151, October 15.
[93] 'Conference Discusses Supply and Demand', *Nursing Mirror*, 1965, pp. 387–389, July 16.
[94] 'Christianity and Nursing Today', *Nursing Mirror*, 1965, p. 346, January 8.
[95] P. Rhodes, 'Society, Culture and Reproduction,' *Nursing Mirror*, 1965, pp. iv–vi,xvi, May 28; pp. vii–ix, June 4; pp. i–iii, June 11.
[96] 'Evolution and Christianity', letters, *Nursing Mirror*, 1965, p. 593, March 19; p. 594, March 19; 'Anthropology of Man', letters, *Nursing Mirror*, 1965, p. 269, June 11; p. 310, June 25.
[97] Ibid., p. 310.
[98] M.W. Peake, 'A Proper Nurse?', letter, *Nursing Times*, 1965, p. 1087, August 6.

[99] W.J. Kirkpatrick, 'A Proper Nurse', letter, *Nursing Times*, 1965, p. 1114, August 13.
[100] 'Editorial', *Nursing Mirror*, 1965, p. 217, December 9.
[101] B. Watkin, *The National Health Service: The First Phase*, London: George Allen & Unwin, 1978, p. 50.
[102] 'Educating for Nursing – Aims and Objectives', *Nursing Mirror*, 1966, pp. 528, 549–550, February 4.
[103] A. Fothergill, 'Why Education for Nurses?', *Nursing Mirror*, 1966, p. 695, March 18.
[104] C.M. Robertson, 'Education for Nurses', letter, *Nursing Mirror*, 1966, p. 43, April 8.
[105] 'Editorial', *Nursing Mirror*, 1966, p. 57, April 22.
[106] M. Dibb, 'Research Waste', letter, *Nursing Mirror*, 1966, p. 163, May 20; A. Altschul, 'Value of Research', letter, *Nursing Mirror*, 1966, p. 234, June 10.
[107] A. Jones, 'Careerist or Vocationalist', *Nursing Mirror*, 1966, p. 576, September 16.
[108] A. Benton, 'Drug Addiction in a 19-year-old Youth', *Nursing Mirror*, 1966, p. 562, February 11.
[109] J. Fluker, 'Venereal Disease and the Young Woman', *Nursing Mirror*, 1966, pp. 633–636, March 4; pp. 663–666, March 11.
[110] J.E. Headberry, 'Florence Nightingale and Modern Nursing', *Nursing Mirror*, 1966, p. xiii, September 2.
[111] P. Friend, 'Nursing in a Technological Age', *Nursing Mirror*, 1966, p. 145, November 11.
[112] N. Goodland, 'Is Nursing a "Vocation"?', *Nursing Mirror*, 1967, pp. 372–373, January 20.
[113] M. Harrison-Thomas, 'Vocation', letter, *Nursing Mirror*, 1967, p. 467, February 17.
[114] F.W. Bell, 'Life and Living it', *Nursing Mirror*, 1966, pp. 309–310, July 1.
[115] 'All the World's a Stage', *Nursing Mirror*, 1966, p. 561, September 9; 'No Standing on the Top Deck', p. 586, September 16; 'It all Adds up to Something', p. 602, September 23; 'This Side of Innocence', p. 622, September 30; 'All the World's a Stage and all the Men and Women Merely ...', p. 16, October 7.
[116] E. Patey, 'All in it Together', *Nursing Mirror*, 1967, p. 573, March 24; 'A Time for Revaluation', p. 282, December 22.
[117] 'Editorial', *Nursing Mirror*, 1967, p. 83, October 27.
[118] B. Abel-Smith, *A History of the Nursing Profession*, London, Heinemann, 1960.
[119] R. Sangar, 'Nurses and Religion', letter, *Nursing Mirror*, 1967, pp. 150–151, November 10.
[120] 'Vespers', 'Religion for Nurses', letter, *Nursing Mirror*, 1967, p. 174, November 17.
[121] 'View of an Agnostic Nurse', *Nursing Mirror*, 1967, p. 149, November 10.
[122] 'In Reply to Agnostic Nurse', letters, *Nursing Mirror*, 1967, pp. 200–201, November 24; '... and Criticism', letter, *Nursing Mirror*, 1967, p. 252, December 8.
[123] Ibid., p. 201.
[124] 'Editorial', *Nursing Mirror*, 1967, p. 155, November 17.
[125] 'Religion for Nurses', letter, *Nursing Mirror*, 1967, pp. 174–175. November 17.
[126] I.W. Thornton, 'No Christian Names', letter, *Nursing Mirror*, 1967, p. 175, November 17.
[127] M. Hulme, 'Dictatorial Leader', letter, *Nursing Mirror*, 1967, p. 225, December 1.
[128] M.M. Pearce, 'Un-Christian Attitude', letters, *Nursing Mirror*, 1967, p. 252, December 8.
[129] B. Hovenier, 'Un-Christian Attitude', letters, *Nursing Mirror*, 1967, p. 252, December 8.
[130] 'Religion for Nurses', letter, *Nursing Mirror*, 1967, p. 199, November 24.
[131] V. Dolan, 'How can I Nurse without Knowing my Lord?', *Nursing Times*, 1967, p. 398, March 24
[132] D. Smith, 'How can I nurse ...', letter, *Nursing Times*, 1967, p. 496, April 14.
[133] C. Belsey, 'How can I nurse ...', *Nursing Times*, 1967, p. 573, April 28.
[134] 'Raise the Roof!', editorial, *Nursing Times*, 1968, p. 753, June 7.
[135] 'News of the Week. 1,000 March on Whitehall', *Nursing Times*, 1968, p. 1126, August 23.
[136] C. Hancock, 'The Lady of the Lamp', *Guardian*, 1998, p. 22, November 20.

[137] 'The Summer of our Discontent', editorial, *Nursing Times*, 1968, p. 1125, August 23.

[138] R. White, 'Protest March', letter, *Nursing Times*, 1968, p. 1180, August 30.

[139] Letters, *Nursing Times*, 1968, p. 1150, August 23; p. 1180, August 30; p. 1211, September 6; p. 1250, September 13, pp. 1279–1280, September 20.

[140] A. Potter, 'Protest March', letter, *Nursing Times*, 1968, p. 1150, August 23.

[141] C. Mullen, 'Protest March', letter, *Nursing Times*, 1968, p. 1211, September 6.

[142] T. Wood, 'Protest March', letter, *Nursing Times*, 1968, p. 1211, September 6.

[143] A. Potter, 'Protest March', letter, *Nursing Times*, 1968, p. 1250, September 13.

[144] H. Wilkey, 'Two Types of Letters', letter, *Nursing Times*, 1968, p. 1249, September 13.

[145] M. Powell, 'Nursing Education', letter, *Nursing Times*, 1968, p. 574, April 26.

[146] 'To the Rt Hon Kenneth Robinson MP Minister of Health', *Nursing Times*, 1968, p. 512, April 12.

[147] S. M. Smith, 'Raising the Roof', letter, *Nursing Times*, 1969, p. 1499, November 20.

[148] R. Holt, 'Raising the Roof', letter, *Nursing Times*, 1969, p. 1559, December 4.

[149] R. Fisher, 'Raising the Roof', letter, *Nursing Times*, 1969, pp. 1559–1560, December 4.

[150] M. Lamb, 'The Image of British Nursing', *Nursing Times*, 1969, pp. 1523–1524, November 27.

[151] 'A New Beginning', editorial, *Nursing Times*, 1970, p. 385, March 26.

[152] D. Bishop, 'Why Do You Wish to be a Nurse?', *Nursing Mirror*, 1972, p. 44, August 25.

[153] S. Daniels, 'What *are* Nursing Duties?', *Nursing Times*, 1972, p. 121, January 27.

[154] J. MacGuire, *From Student to Nurse – The Induction Period: A Study of Student Nurses in the First Six Months of Training in Five Schools of Nursing*, 43 Banbury Road Oxford, A report published by the Oxford Area Nurse Training Committee, September, 1961.

[155] J. MacGuire, *From Student to Nurse – Training and Qualification: A Study of Student Nurses in Training at Five Schools of Nursing*, Old Road, Headington, Oxford, A report published by the Oxford Area Nurse Training Committee, May, 1966.

[156] J. MacGuire, *From Student to Nurse – The Induction Period: A Study of Student Nurses in the First Six Months of Training in Five Schools of Nursing*, 43 Banbury Road, Oxford, a report published by the Oxford Area Nurse Training Committee, September, 1961, p. 30.

[157] Ibid., p. 38.

[158] Ibid., pp. 40–41.

[159] Ibid., p. 70.

[160] Ibid., p. 81.

[161] J. MacGuire, *From Student to Nurse – Training and Qualification: A Study of Student Nurses in Training at Five Schools of Nursing*, Old Road, Headington, Oxford, a report published by the Oxford Area Nurse Training Committee, May, 1966, p. 21.

[162] Ibid., p. 56.

[163] Ibid., p. 57.

[164] Ibid., pp. 57–58.

[165] M.P. Bowman, 'Nursing by Lamplight', *The Health Services*, 1983, pp. 10–11.

[166] D.C. Marsh, A.J. Willcocks, *Focus on Nurse Recruitment: A Snapshot from the Provinces*, London, Oxford University Press, published for the Nuffield Provincial Hospitals Trust, 1965, p. 28.

[167] Ibid., pp. 28–29.

[168] Ibid., p. 38–39.

[169] Ibid., p. 40.

[170] A. Singh, 'The Student Nurse on Experimental Courses – III: Basic Values', *International Journal of Nursing Studies*, 8, 1971, pp. 207–218.

[171] A. Dutton, *Factors Affecting Recruitment of Nurse Tutors*, London, King Edward's Hospital Fund for London, 1968.

[172] Ibid., p. 58.

[173] Ibid., p. 67.

[174] Ibid., p. 72.

[175] A. Singh, J. MacGuire, 'Occupational Values and Stereotypes in a Group of Trained Nurses', *Nursing Times*, 1971, pp. 165–168, October 21.

[176] A. Singh, 'The Student Nurse on Experimental Courses – I: Attitudes Towards Nursing as a Career', *International Journal of Nursing Studies*, 7, 1970, pp. 201–224; 'The Student Nurse on Experimental Courses – II: Personality Patterns', *International Journal of Nursing Studies*, 8, 1971, pp. 189–205; 'The Student Nurse on Experimental Courses – III: Basic Values', *International Journal of Nursing Studies*, 8, 1971, pp. 207–218.

[177] A. Singh, 'The Student Nurse on Experimental Courses – III: Basic Values', *International Journal of Nursing Studies*, 8, 1971, pp. 207–218.

[178] W.Ll. Parry-Jones, 'Human Relations Training in the General Hospital', *International Journal of Nursing Studies*, 1971, 8, pp. 153–162.

[179] N. Lamond, *Becoming a Nurse: The Registered Nurse's View of General Student Nurse Education*, London, Royal College of Nursing, 1974, pp. 16–17.

[180] Ibid., pp. 12–35.

[181] J.F. Wyatt, 'Sociological Perspectives on Socialization into a Profession: A Study of Student Nurses and their Definition of Learning', *British Journal of Educational Studies*, 3, 1978, pp. 263–276, October 3.

[182] S.C. Haywood, R.E. Jefford, R.B.K. MacGregor, K. Stevenson, G.D.E. Wooding Jones, 'The Patient's View of the Hospital: An Experimental Survey,' *Hospital*, 57, 1961, pp. 644–650, October.

[183] A. McGhee, *The Patient's Attitude to Nursing Care*, Edinburgh, E. & S. Livingstone, 1961.

[184] Ibid., p. 44.

[185] Ibid., p. 46.

[186] Ibid., p. 47

[187] Ibid., p. 48.

[188] A. Cartwright, *Human Relations and Hospital Care*, London, Routledge & Kegan Paul, 1964.

[189] Ibid., p. 35.

[190] Ibid., p. 45.

[191] W. Raphael, 'Patient Care', *Nursing Times*, 1965, pp. 1606–1608, November 26; pp. 1654–1656, December 3; pp. 1686–1687, December 10; pp. 1725–1727, December 17; pp. 1759–1761, December 24.

[192] Ibid., pp. 1686–1687.

[193] W. Raphael, *Patients and their Hospitals*, 1st edn, London, King Edward's Hospital Fund for London, 1969; 2nd edn, 1973; 3rd edn, 1977.

[194] Ibid., 1969, p. 35.

[195] Ibid., p. 33.

[196] Ibid., 1973, p. 41.

[197] E.R. Anderson, *The Role of the Nurse*, London, Royal College of Nursing, 1973, p. 40.

[198] J.C. Hayward, 'Nursing Research', In Allan, P. and M. Jolley (eds), *Nursing, Midwifery and Health Visiting Since 1900*, pp. 196–214, London, Faber & Faber, 1982, p. 204.

[199] G. Cohen, *What's Wrong with Hospitals?*, Harmondsworth, Penguin, 1964.

[200] B. Robb, *Sans Everything*, London, Thomas Nelson & Sons, 1967.

[201] G. Cohen, *What's Wrong with Hospitals?*, Harmondsworth, Penguin, 1964, p. 31.

[202] Minister of Health, National Health Service, *Findings and Recommendations following Enquiries into Allegations Concerning the Care of Elderly Patients in Certain Hospitals*, London, HMSO, July, 1968. 'Ministry of Health Allegations about Care of Elderly Patients in Seven Hospitals', *Nursing Times*, 1968, p. 943, July 12.

[203] J.K. McFarlane, *The Proper Study of the Nurse*, London, Royal College of Nursing and National Council of Nurses of the United Kingdom, 1970, pp. 12–13.

[204] M.D. Enoch, 'Afterword, Ready for the Scrapheap', in Robb, B., *Sans Everything*, pp. 136–140, London, Thomas Nelson & Sons, 1967.

Chapter 8

The end of the nurse apprentice, 1969–1979

This chapter reaches the end point for the apprentice nurse system. The reasons behind the break with the tradition are explored as are the philosophical ideas that influenced nursing leaders at the General Nursing Council. An Act of Parliament put in place a formal mechanism for restructuring nursing as a self-regulating profession. This initiated a new educational approach and new values to replace the apprenticeship training and the ethic of vocational service. The significance of this radical redirection of nursing and nurse preparation will have important implications for the role and purpose of the nurse and so for the care of patients.

Continuity and change

According to Celia Davies, a sociologist involved in later educational change in nursing, the mid-1960s brought striking disagreement about the nature of nurse education amongst the professional bodies.[1] She believed this was politically motivated, with bodies such as the General Nursing Council issuing its angry and defensive response to the Royal College of Nursing's Platt Report because it felt its sphere of influence was under threat.

Like Davies, White thought that political issues rather than altruism determined policy in health care and nursing.[2] With that in mind, she has suggested that matrons lost the ethic of dedication and service as early as 1948, and became politicised in order to resist a loss of control and status. Matrons dominated the policy-making bodies of the GNC and RCN, imposing their concepts of 'reality', which differed from nurses who were still socialised into the service ethic.[3]

Minutes of matrons' meetings from the GNC, quoted by White, seem to show no such dichotomy, however. The matrons appeared to express genuine concerns about the selection of suitable candidates, the needs of the patient, the need to maintain standards, the importance of nursing being practical, and the need to maintain a balance between practical skills and theory.[4] All this was consistent with perpetuating the service ethic. Indeed, evidence from earlier chapters seems to point to a genuine concern by the GNC to sustain rather than abolish the Nightingale tradition, particularly through the ethos of apprenticeship training, and to reform it as necessary for the good of patient care.

The service ethic was sustained in the revisions of the national nursing syllabus necessary to address changing patient needs. In 1969 the syllabus for state registration was revised slightly. The syllabus of subjects for examination no longer appeared as a separate booklet, but was integrated with the record of practical instruction and experience. Minimum teaching time was increased, and psychiatric or geriatric, and community care or obstetric experience was included. Nursing procedures now included care of the dying and care of paralysed patients; first aid and treatment in emergencies added cardiac arrest; and the syllabus was no longer separate, being appended to the nurse's record of practical instruction and experience.[5] The principles of the apprenticeship method of training, and the importance of total patient care, preventative health care, and the patient as part of the community, all consistent with nursing tradition, were affirmed in the revised 1969 syllabus, as the preface to the syllabus explained.

The 1969 syllabus, compulsory from 1971, was reprinted in 1973, 1974 and 1976, and was still used in 1977.[6] From 1973 onwards the final page of the syllabus was printed with a section detailing the 'Final State Practical Examinations'. Four ward-based practical assessments, examined by the training school, replaced the practical state examination which had been conducted by GNC examiners. These four sections were: 'Aseptic Technique', 'Drug Administration', 'Nursing Care' and 'Communication and Organisations'. The examiner was instructed to enter and sign the date of the assessment and the result (pass, referred or fail). The page was counter-signed and dated by the training school.

The 'Guide to the Teaching of the Syllabus of Subjects for Examination for the Certificate of General Nursing', included at the end of the syllabus, reaffirmed the need for adaptation to meet changing methods of treatment and care. The underlying principle remained the concept of 'total patient care', and the guide emphasised that this should be stressed throughout the training period.[7]

The philosophical shift in nurse education had reached the General Nursing Council by the late 1960s. In 1968 a joint working party of the King's Fund and the GNC criticised current methods of student nurse assessment. Alleged confusion and concern over standards of assessment of student nurses were blamed on resistance to change. One recommendation was to bring in a team approach to assessment,[8] which would inevitably undermine the ward sister's position as the main supervisor of practice. It appears to have been this report which led to the change in practical assessment in the revised syllabus of the GNC the following year.

The philosophy underpinning changes in nurse training

Two highly influential nursing educationalists, Barbara Fawkes and Eve Bendall, were instrumental in such changes. Barbara Fawkes was Chief Education Officer of the General Nursing Council from 1959, when she had replaced the previous Officer, Marjorie Houghton, the textbook author. Fawkes had been a night sister in the early 1940s at Stoke Mandeville Hospital, where she was amazed at the understanding and encouragement given by even inexperienced student nurses to young paraplegic men. She believed that the importance of the development of cheerful, kindly and sympathetic attitudes in student nurses could not be too strongly emphasised. Notwithstanding her personal experience of caring nurses from decades earlier, she thought that modern educational methods were the key to developing these attitudes.[9]

Students came into nursing with basic humane attitudes, wrote Fawkes, but they needed to learn more professional approaches; and this they were reluctant to do. According to Fawkes it was difficult to persuade students of the need to do this. She cited the views of a North American educationalist, who argued that teachers in schools and communities in the last third of the twentieth century needed skills and attitudes 'vastly different' from their traditional predecessors. Modern education was more complex because factors were more diverse.

Fawkes had studied in North America, and seemed persuaded such that modern educational techniques needed to be implemented in nurse education. She called for less formal lectures and more seminars, group discussion and student project work supplemented by videos, tape-recordings and films. Nurse teachers needed to be prepared in educational psychology, teaching methods and the practice of education as well as in the study of basic sciences. Multidisciplinary courses were helpful, so that nurse teachers would be prepared alongside teachers of crafts, industrial skills, sciences and the humanities. But she held to some fundamental traditional principles: teaching had to be 'patient-centred', and attitudes of cheerfulness, kindness and sympathy were vital attributes of the nurse, and should form part of the selection process.

Eve Bendall, Chairman of the Examination and Education Committee of the GNC in 1969, was Registrar at the General Nursing Council from 1973. In 1981 she was appointed Chief Executive Officer of the newly formed English National Board for Nursing, Midwifery and Health Visiting.[10] In 1969 she gave her opinion to *Nursing Times* on what she hoped the next fifty years would bring nursing.[11]

Bendall believed that the two grades of nurses, registered and enrolled, needed to be maintained, and that a smaller number of Registered Nurses should be educated to lead. The role of the nurse needed to be defined by research, and consideration needed to be given to whether student status was appropriate, and whether student nurse preparation should be part of further education. In this case the rethinking of hospital ward staffing was crucial.

Bendall was keen to see a 'radical change in the syllabus'. Individual training schools should assess their own students, and she hoped for a swing away from the current emphasis on the patient's requirement for physical care, towards much more of a focus on psychological and social needs. She thought student nurses should be encouraged towards individual thought, discussion and professional accountability, rather than as at present being mainly trained to respond to given situations.

That same article contained other views. A hospital matron, Monica Pearce, who was Chairman of the Registration Committee of the GNC, hoped the following century would bring an end to the 'folly of the 'permissive society'; a respect for the family and sanctity of marriage and human life, born and unborn, and nursing as a vocation. She hoped for a return to respect

> for the Almighty Creator, who, for long enough, has been patient with a world that is rejecting Him. Only so will the 'modern civilization' survive. Through all this, the nurse must remain true to her vocation (for such it is), seeing the sick person, in whatever area she meets him, as a human being, possessed of human rights, entitled to live a dignified life while it lasts, and entitled to die a dignified death, when it comes. Wherever she may be, whatever she may do, one thing remains certain, she must continue to 'comfort always'.[12]

This traditionalist view from a hospital matron shows the polarity that now existed in the GNC. The opinions of Bendall and Pearce mark the sharp contrast in attitudes towards nursing, its ethos and function, that occurred in that seminal period of change. This would take place despite the belief, echoed in the same article by the Chairman of the Finance Committee of the GNC, that the British nurse was regarded as the 'best trained and most efficient in the world'.[13]

Bendall would seem to have dissented. She subsequently undertook a research study, supervised by educationalists from the Institute of Education, London University, published in 1975.[14] This study explored the assumptions on which written examinations were based. Her presupposition, stated in her introduction, was that 'caring', both for the needs of patients and the needs of learners, 'is not an outstanding characteristic of many of our hospitals today'.[15] One symptom of what she called this 'dis-ease' was her belief that the way nurses in training described nursing care on paper was quite different from what they did in practice. With echoes of Nightingale, but with a very different perspective and solution, Bendall suggested: 'A "good" test paper is no guarantee that a learner would give "good" care, nor vice versa.'

From research in organisational sociology, Bendall developed her hypothesis that the 'ideal', which nurses were taught in the introductory courses, conflicted with the 'reality' of the ward. The more idealised the school ideology, the greater the conflict with reality. A dichotomy resulted 'in the individual's perception, theoretical nursing being seen as useful only for exams and real nursing for work'. This led to theory being adapted or disregarded by the student nurse and led to 'the conflicting value system'. Bendall's research sought to analyse 'the distance between the ideal and the real'.[16]

From her data, Bendall found that nursing itself satisfied the large majority of subjects although it fell below expectation for over one quarter. She also found general satisfaction with training. Nurses gained most satisfaction from helping patients. Their main aim was being a good nurse rather than passing exams or completing their training. Over a third of nurses thought the ward sister spent a lot of time with patients, while just over a third did not know how the ward sister spent her time. Bendall recorded that 40 per cent of nurses said: 'Nursing is everything I hoped it would be'; 34 per cent said: 'Nursing is better than I expected'; 23 per cent said: 'Nursing is not as good as I expected'; and 3 per cent said: 'Frankly I am disappointed in nursing'.[17]

Bendall argued that the more conservative and traditional the student the more satisfied the student was. The conservative student respected established ideas and was tolerant of traditional difficulties. It was the radical, analytical trainee, 'labelled' early in training, in whom differences in satisfaction were most obvious. Disenchantment over the training period was likely to be experienced more by those who were radical, less trusting and conciliatory, and who had passed more formal examinations. This was linked to the perception of decreasing relevance of theory to practice, and to the increasing perception that relationships between school and wards were poor. She believed that this was probably linked with the trainee's perception of progress, since it was the training context and training process that disenchanted rather than nursing *per se*.[18]

In Bendall's view, the nurse's role had developed solely to 'serve the doctor and supply patient care'.[19] The supreme status figure was the sister, while the training school provided status for the student nurse. The national syllabus of training, devised by the GNC from the one in use in a leading training school in the early 1920s, was largely based on medical science (anatomy, physiology, hygiene, pharmacology and so on, as well as signs, symptoms and treatment of disease), because nursing had no body of knowledge. The role of the nurse tutor was developed to teach this, but became out of touch with the reality of clinical practice, as were the GNC members who drew up the syllabus. Faced with providing a national training programme, and with little common ground on the actual practice of nursing:

> They fell back on medical and scientific knowledge and an ideal concept of 'total patient care', which they themselves had never practised and which was not carried out in the wards of their hospitals, but with which all would agree since it typified the reification of the reason for the existence of nursing.

Bendall argued that this was a comfortable solution: 'superficially it provided a body of nursing knowledge; most nurses subscribed to its idealism; since the practice had little basis in reality, its implementation could be accepted without difficulty'. Inspectors' reports on training schools rarely spoke of actual nursing practice, but focused instead on such factors as numbers of beds, ratio of trained staff to trainees, attrition, examination pass rates and physical ward amenities.

Tutors liked this idealised approach because it meant they could teach 'comprehensively' and describe situations of care which trainees rarely experienced but which sounded reasonable and which increased knowledge. Bendall concluded that a dichotomy persisted between what happened in the wards and what was prescribed in the syllabus, taught in the schools, and questioned in the final examination.

Although Bendall admitted that nurses were happy with the traditional system, she herself was extremely critical of it. In their efforts to aspire to professional status, nurses had 'reified' the thing called nursing. Statements such as 'good nursing care', 'a good nurse', and 'nursing standards', were merely emotional weapons that had no basis in reality. They had a strong emotional appeal to nurses as well as large sections of the public: 'The "overworked, underpaid angel of mercy" does not really exist in 1973 but the public like to think that she does, and nurses do little to shatter the concept'. Training schools inculcated a subjective idealism which conflicted with their high disillusionment and 'objective and factual criticisms'. Although this statement was not supported by the findings of her study, Bendall argued that within the training school all were 'socialized into a common way of thought and a common expressed purpose "to maintain the standard of nursing"'.[20]

Trained staff and trainees shared similar backgrounds, culture, social class and school type. The organisation had a strong unchanging tradition which had altered little. There was a unanimity of purpose among nursing administrators, tutors and senior ward staff. Outwardly, at least, all worked to the same end. This resulted in a highly cohesive organisation which produced 'missionaries to carry the precious symbols to others less fortunate'.

Bendall rejected as a myth the traditional conception of a person as 'suitable' to be a nurse. There was no ideal type of nurse. In her view the only measurable criterion was educational background. She noted that one lobby of opinion, supported by the Royal College of Nursing, called for a raising of this minimum standard, while the General Nursing Council sought to encourage special courses for graduates or combined nursing and degree courses. By this, it was hoped to influence head teachers to send their brighter pupils into nursing. However, another lobby of opinion, 'equally strong or stronger', was anti-intellectual, and held that nursing could only be learned by experience. They argued that there was an inverse relationship between academic and practical ability.

Organisations were confused about the qualities required of potential recruits. So were tutors, who were torn between the view that experience and practical ability were crucial, and the need to raise educational standards. There was a further problem in that, according to Bendall, raised educational standards did not always lead to success in the final examination. Bendall interpreted the measure of this confusion as the fact that no tutors in her survey believed their job entailed helping students pass exams.[21]

Bendall proposed a rethinking of the examination system. It was no longer sustainable to accept that a trainee's nursing ability could be assumed from her written papers and her recall of information. She saw two alternative strategies; to accept the conflict between the ideal and the real and alter the examination, or to seek ways of resolving the conflict. With the first strategy the conflict would continue, and a formula would be needed to lessen its effects by restricting the knowledge to be examined to factual knowledge (physiology, drugs, signs and symptoms of disease).

Such objectivity, Bendall believed, would be more difficult to obtain in assessing performance in the real situation. Responsibility for this had already begun to be transferred to training schools in the four ward-based assessments. But, according to Bendall, these were not free of the ideal–real conflict. Assessment criteria were laid down in many cases by school staff, and were often not present in the everyday situation so that the assessment became a 'performance' laid on for the occasion. This differed from the actual care patients received even the day before or the day after.

Bendall thought that the second strategy offered most promise. To resolve the conflict between the ideal and the real, a redefinition of the whole process of training in terms of the work required of trainees in and after training, was imperative. Much that was in the current syllabus, in terms of knowledge, was probably unnecessary while what was not in the syllabus, in terms of skills, was required.

Bendall recommended a reappraisal of the syllabus based on objective research findings and not on current opinion, and possibly based on skills (manual, observational, technical, organisational, relational and teaching). 'Patient-centred care' should be tried, but if this was not possible it should be rejected in favour of a job-centred approach. Teaching of nurse tutors needed to focus on facilitating teaching in the real situation rather than the classroom, and the skills they required were to be defined. Trainers needed to recognise their needs as learners, more money required to be spent on training, and individual nurses should be given the skills to assume individual responsibility for patient care. This strategy would have to be adopted if the Briggs Report were to be implemented successfully.[22]

Research into the kind and content of syllabus in relation to the ward situation should be conducted. Parameters needed to be developed for measuring differences between organisations and how staff, trainees and patients were affected. The nature of these situations as 'highly emotive and laden with value judgements' meant that a sympathetic approach to change was needed to lessen the trauma for individuals. No 'patch-up' of the existing system, would do, rather root and branch change was needed.

Bendall had argued that the vocational tradition was an ideology whose effect was to make a virtue out of dedication and mechanical obedience, and which needed to be challenged and changed. She had also disregarded the significance of the nurse's record of practical instruction as a method of teaching skills and procedures. Moreover, she appeared to take no account of research studies of the period, that showed nurses were satisfied with their training as a preparation for practical competence.[23] The key principles of the apprenticeship tradition were disputed. Although Bendall later admitted to her fear that British nurse education might supplant its moral base in 'effective caring' with 'education, 'research', and 'management',[24] she saw no link with her own work, and its proposal to put in place a radical departure from nursing tradition, its values and ideals.

Other critics were also important persuaders for change. The sociologist Celia Davies, although not a nurse, became Project Officer to the United Kingdom Central Council for Nurses, Midwives and Health Visitors which replaced the GNC. In 1986 she helped draw up the report *Project 2000*, which formed the future direction of nurse preparation.[25]

Davies believed that the deliberate occupational strategy of nursing was to be a dependent occupation rather than an independent profession. She attributed this to historical legacy, female values, and the pragmatic problem-solving approach to the everyday work and organisational situation. Davies admitted that this strategy had not lost any of its functional validity over 150 years, but she speculated whether it would continue in the 'contemporary climate of introspection and change'.[26]

A year later Davies built on this theme. Humility and vocation in nursing history precluded change in nursing. Even modern developments such as Salmon and Briggs, she argued, were not radical enough. She looked towards the United States, and the different model of clinical nurse specialists. The creation of nurse practitioners, she argued, would give nursing occupational control. The continuity of British nursing, which had perpetuated a routinised work system and hierarchical control, should be ended.[27]

Davies influenced the work of Joan Fretwell on ward teaching which occurred at the end of the 1970s. Fretwell argued that the ideal of nurse training through apprenticeship did not work in reality. Ward sisters, the 'key to nursing', on whom nursing training relied, did not have time to supervise and instruct nurses in practical skills. Traditional patterns of ward organisation concentrated on delegating repetitive nursing work, essentially basic nursing, to learner nurses which militated against learning. Educationalists argued that a precondition to learning was the belief that there was something to find out; routine basic nursing dulled this precondition. Traditional hierarchical task allocation practised in the wards was inconsistent with learning. Routinisation stifled the spirit of enquiry. Nurses found the basic nursing work easy to do, felt fully competent to do it, did not feel it was important for their education, but did recognise that it was important for the patient.[28]

According to Fretwell, frequent repetition led nurses to do work automatically, without thinking, and routine relieved anxiety, often leading to the objectification of the patient. Nurses were socialised into valuing 'cure' over 'care', preferring the technical, difficult, but 'clean' tasks over the 'basic' and easy work. And they were constantly searching for learning experiences. She concluded that the ward environment was inconsistent with learning and needed to change from a traditional to a new order.

The effect of this critique was cumulative. Bendall's criticism of nursing tradition as an imposed ideology which prevented progress was supported by Davies and later Fretwell. Davies was keen for nurses to gain political control over their profession. Fretwell argued that the apprenticeship method with its repetition and routinisation was stifling learning, even though nurses themselves appreciated its significance for patients. The century-long principles of the apprenticeship tradition, the high ethical ideals, the correct balance of theory and practice, and the thorough mastery of nursing techniques, formerly regarded as essential to train nurses into both the art and science of care,[29] were now under threat and, indeed, about to be dismantled.

The end of the nurse apprentice

In 1977, five years after the Briggs Report, the final syllabus of the General Nursing Council was published.[30] The preface stated that the syllabus set out in broad terms the subjects to be studied during training for the general part of the register maintained by the General Nursing Council for England and Wales. The concept underlying the syllabus was 'that of total patient care', but for convenience the syllabus was divided into three main sections: nursing, the study of the individual, and the nature and cause of disease together with its prevention and treatment. These three aspects of patient care should be learned concurrently through training.

Bendall was able to put her own educational theory into practice in the new syllabus. What changed, and was made clear by the GNC in 1977, was that the syllabus document would be printed without the pages for the record of practical instruction and experience.[31] Training schools were required to draw up statements of learning objectives and opportunities for each clinical experience area. The GNC considered that these were more effective tools for learning and assessing achievement than the previous practical record. This apparently small change, the removal of the record of practical instruction and experience, which had developed from the Nightingale School nurse's record, was of immense significance. The systematic and mandatory process of individualised assessment of proficiency was ended.

The document contained a statement of educational policy designed by a working party set up in December 1975. No major decisions had been made about the Briggs Report, but there were now nursing directives from the European Economic Community, which constrained the GNC from making major changes to nurse education. Nevertheless, the working party sought to make modifications to educational policy. The reasons given were: the increasing conflict arising from the condition of learners as employees; poor morale within the Health Service following reorganisation and economic crisis; continued inadequacy of sufficient numbers of trained staff able to give supervision during clinical experience; and deteriorating numbers of nurse teachers.

The 1977 syllabus introduced fundamental changes to nurse training, as Bendall had intended. The nursing process was imported from North America and integrated into the syllabus.[32] The balance between health and disease was shifted. There was more attention to psychology and emotions, particularly the nurse's emotions, and to sociology. References to diseases and sickness were minimal. There was explicit reference to nursing research. Nursing ethics was omitted. The student was termed the 'learner', and the training was termed 'the experience'. These ideas reflected Bendall's influence, as a later speech of hers would confirm.[33] Although the apprenticeship method of learning continued with this 1977 syllabus, the GNC no longer prescribed the assessment process. Individual institutions were allowed flexibility to decide how practical skills were to be assessed and, indeed, which practical skills would be assessed.

During this period the modular system replaced the arbitrary block system.[34] Bendall stated that the block system was still used by 17 per cent of training schools in 1983. The desire for 'better' methods, including views expressed in the Briggs Report, led to the development of the modular system. In this system a set period of twelve to fourteen weeks was devoted to a particular speciality. The first week was spent in theoretical discussion, the following weeks were spent on experience in the clinical area and the final week was again theoretical, pulling together all the problems that had arisen.

The module was self-contained, focused on one discrete area, correlating theory and practice. In some schools this was linked with the development of continuous or progressive assessment, assessing the nurses as they passed through the training period during each module. By 1983, 15 per cent of training schools had reached the modular system. Some had continuous assessment which, according to Bendall, was a long, difficult and trying process involving everybody in the training school. The remaining 67 per cent of training schools at that time were somewhere between the block system and the modular, with certain parts of the programme on one system, and others still left on the other.[35]

Examiners from one central organisation, the General Nursing Council, were no longer responsible for overseeing that the registered nurse had reached a uniform national standard of theoretical knowledge and practical skill. Neither were they responsible for ensuring that the nurse's qualities or virtues of character were attested to, although there would continue to be character references prior to registration. Despite such changes, however, the 1977 syllabus was broadly a continuation of the traditional model of nurse education with its synthesis of practical skill and biomedical theory. It remained, fundamentally, an apprenticeship pattern of training.

The supernumerary nursing student

The break with the past was finally accomplished in 1979, with the passing of the Nurses, Midwives and Health Visitors' Act 1979, which provided the legal mechanism for change. The Queen's Speech in November 1978 announced the government's intention to introduce a Bill on the regulation and training of nurses, midwives and health visitors, based on the recommendations of the Briggs Report, nearly seven years earlier.[36] Introducing the Bill, David Ennals, Secretary of State for Social Services, stated that the Bill did not itself make any change in the substance of professional education, rather, it paved the way for the professions themselves to initiate a new system of integrated training on the lines recommended by the Briggs Report.[37]

The debate took place against the background of a fall in nurse training recruitment during the previous two years, which was now being arrested and even reversed. This fall in recruitment was partly caused by the reduction of courses in training schools, not part of government policy, according to Ennals. It had been undertaken in a number of areas, and worried the government, which thought it a dangerous policy.[38] Shortages appeared to be due primarily to cuts in training places, rather than a failure of recruits coming forward. It was difficult to know how many of those who even entered training would actually come into the service. Ministerial experience a decade earlier showed that as soon as people qualified they married and left the National Health Service.[39]

Members of Parliament expressed doubts as to whether the legislation would improve patient care; indeed they were concerned that the patient was not mentioned.[40] It was questioned how the setting up of a central council would improve care of patients: 'Its intention is not for members of the nursing profession to impress one another with what they can do in their internal organisation.' There was general satisfaction with nursing standards. It was considered that empire-building by nurses' professional bodies might cause unhelpful competition with other health professions and was not in patients' best interests.[41] The public was not dissatisfied with nursing.[42]

Despite these fears, Members of Parliament admitted that they had little knowledge of the profession and were happy to devolve its regulation and training requirements to the profession itself.[43] There was also concern expressed as to whether there was any real demand from nurses at the grass roots for the new monolithic structure. The best nurses, it was felt, did not necessarily want to become administrators but would rather stay at the bedside practising clinical nursing skills. Proposed changes to nursing were reflective of the climate in the 1960s and 1970s, when the country lived under the 'white heat of the technological revolution' in which all kinds of reorganisations took place with centralisation and an extension of bureaucracy.[44]

Members of Parliament assumed that people who entered nursing were dedicated to the care of patients.[45] The devotion and skill of nurses in 1978 were recognised, their standard of care was second to none throughout the world. The urgent need was to restore to the nursing profession their morale, their taste for the job, their sense of vocation. They needed to be reassured by those who ran the public affairs that 'their sense of vocation is not being taken for granted'.[46]

One of the most heated issues, not yet resolved, was whether nurses should be pure trainees or whether their training should have a service input.[47] It was feared that proposed educational changes would mean that student nurses would be less liable to duties on the ward. They would concentrate more on their training which would be contrary to the interests of patients: 'The first concern in any hospital should be the patients, not the training of nurses. I appreciate that in some ways there are clashes between those two views, but I think that patients must have absolute priority.' There was a psychological element to this matter. A student saw learning as exclusive and adopted a more lighthearted attitude towards her duties and to life than a fully trained, qualified person. Nurses should be employees and realise their duties and responsibilities. The role of the student nurse was different from that of the medical student. Medical responsibility was taken by the house physicians and surgeons and so medical students could be dispensed with. This was not so with nurses who were responsible for the patient.[48]

The issue of student status was problematic. The Briggs Committee had not been clear what student status meant. Some trainees thought it would mean having a students' union, others that it meant receiving a government grant instead of a salary, which 'put a dampener on enthusiasm for change'. Student status would seem to suggest that students and pupils should learn theory in a college, and work on the wards only as a source of practice rather than to staff them. The government had set up the Briggs Coordinating Committee to look into these matters, but 'it was not able to define what it really meant by "student status". From that point of view it ran into a number of problems.' There were tensions between those who wanted to use students or learners in a service capacity, which they needed in order to learn, and those who wanted to use them for entirely educational purposes. The matter was to be left to the profession to decide.[49]

Lord Briggs made his maiden speech in the debate when the Bill reached the House of Lords. Looking back over the years he denoted six aspects of his report. These included the attempt to set out clear principles about recruitment into the nursing profession. Recruitment conditions varied and obstacles were placed in the way. The committee had also noted that there was no system of training and education in relation to nursing, forms of education varied. Urgent action was needed to increase the supply of nurse tutors. Continuing education was considered important, and the idea of a generic nurse was rejected. Rather, a basic nurse education was envisaged so that specialised forms of nursing education could be developed. The committee wanted to bring into nursing modern educational ideas and methods of learning. It also emphasised the need for continuing research to identify nursing needs. Conditions of work and community nursing were also considered.[50]

Other members of the House of Lords expressed criticisms. The medical profession was being marginalised.[51] During this two-year struggle for medical representation on the Briggs Coordinating Committee, a letter was received which caused anxiety. It stated that the committee recognised the part the medical profession 'could play' in nurse education and training. And it was these two words, 'could play' that seemed to spell out a rather off-hand dismissal of the traditional cooperation which the medical profession had given and still sought to give nursing.

Briggs responded that, although doctors, or scientists, were important to the new body, the future improvement of nursing rested specifically and uniquely in nurse teaching. The role of the nurse tutor needed to change, not only because of changes in medicine, but to take account of the 'changes in the nature of the educational system and the way in which this approaches the learning process'.[52]

The GNC was replaced during the years 1980–1983, following the passing of the 1979 Nurses, Midwives and Health Visitors' Act. The United Kingdom Central Council for Nursing, Midwifery and Health Visiting was established in 1982. From 1980 to 1983 the shadow English National Board for Nursing, Midwifery and Health Visiting set out its new philosophy of nurse education in England.[53] The ENB proposed a collegiate approach to the setting of standards for education and practice, rather than prescriptive, hierarchical attitudes to the supervision and provision of education.

This philosophical change was not, however, without criticism from within the profession. From 1981 to 1982, it was noted, there were profound concerns from nurse tutors and midwives as well as health authorities and professional education outside the NHS about the proposals which: 'generated a degree of concern / suspicion / insecurity which has its roots in deeper issues than those actually outlined in the document'.[54]

On the surface, the ENB suggested, this could be seen as a power and status conflict, but there was a deeper issue: the dichotomy between the end point of the 'educated' nurse and the end point of the delivery of patient care. In neither group did the one appear to be seen as the means to the other. Specific comments from the RCN and the National Association for Health Authorities were supreme examples of this dichotomy. The goal of producing an educated nurse, as against the goal of delivery of patient care, were acknowledged as mutually exclusive by those on both sides of opinion. Because of this polarisation, decisions on change were shelved.

That same year, at the shadow English National Board conference, Lord Briggs also argued that tradition was inimical to innovation and progress.[55] Nursing members of the ENB, one of whom was Bendall, expressed the urgent need for a change in nurse education. In particular, they sought a change in educational methods, from the didactic and prescriptive to the experiential and flexible.[56] The English National Board was being attacked because its members were not democratically elected.[57] The early work of the board was 'hammering out the beliefs and values and ideals which should guide it in its work'. The 'relationship of equals' which was fundamental to the new nursing philosophy, deliberately rejected the 'strong sense of hierarchy which the profession had developed'. Competency had been redefined by the Briggs Coordinating Committee. In line with the nursing process approach adopted by the GNC in 1977, competency centred around general concepts: the nurse needed the capability to observe, interpret, plan and evaluate care. If she was able to do this she would be deemed competent. Unlike the old system, the new system did not specify how standards of competence were to be set, measured or tested.

Nursing was not just concerned with the physical needs of the patient, but with the psychological, social and spiritual needs also; an implication that this was new, rather than the essence of the tradition. The new educational system would be based on principles of autonomy and individualism, which required a

> self actualising learner, a learner who goes out and searches, learns by discovery, sets their own objectives and becomes responsible for their own learning experience and I do not think that that can be accomplished in the old systems of authoritative and didactic teaching and I think that hierarchies tend to perpetuate those authoritarian regimes, not inevitably so but possibly so ...[58]

Although Bendall had been instrumental in altering nurse training, in 1983 she admitted to problems of recent origin. Newly qualified staff were not as effective on qualification as they used to be. They wanted further and continuing training, which, she argued, showed they lacked confidence and the feeling for responsibility that had been theirs in the past. Staff involved in post-basic clinical specialities were having to fill in the gaps of students' knowledge and skill that had been left after basic training. They even had to remedy some basic wrong learning.[59]

British nursing had begun to adopt the North American model of nursing and nurse education. Simultaneously, North American nursing was asking questions of its own efficacy. As earlier chapters have shown, many nurses as well as other commentators had argued in earlier decades that British nursing should not take this path and lose its practical unity. North American writers lent support to these warnings. The ethical tradition of nursing was replaced by the learning of techniques, a 'doctrinal conversion', and North American nurses, schooled in the social sciences, were no longer trained in the art of basic practical care.[60] As the Briggs Report had noted, the efficacy of the North American system was not then proven.[61]

The greatest change ushered in by the new Act was the change of purpose. As Members of Parliament had noticed, the primary purpose of nursing, the patient, was now scarcely mentioned in debates on the future of the profession. The newly formed shadow ENB was preoccupied with achieving professional autonomy.

The decisions that were shelved by the ENB in 1982 were now gradually taken. There was a fundamental reorientation of nursing over the next decade during which the apprentice nurse would finally be replaced by the supernumerary nurse. This would take several years to accomplish, but was set in motion in 1986 when nurses 'persuaded government to put in place *Project 2000*, and adopted new but untested philosophies, at a time when the demands on their profession were altering radically'.[62]

Conclusion

In 1979 the nursing profession became self-regulating. The Nurses, Midwives and Health Visitors Act 1979 replaced the General Nursing Council with a new council and boards. The apprenticeship model of nurse training was gradually replaced by an educational system with newly defined values and in which professional status was central. Formal hierarchies, the uniform national examination, biomedicine, traditional structures, methods and procedures were exchanged for individual responsibility, flexibility and the dynamic creativity of social science. Theory would take precedence over practice in the preparation of students. Both the art and science of nursing would be affected. The mutually cooperative community in which apprenticeship operated would be replaced by a system of learning based on autonomy and individualism.

This radicalisation occurred even though many doubts were expressed about whether these changes were in the best interests of the patient. The consequence was that the single-minded purpose of nursing, the altruistic calling of service to the practical needs of the patient, which had defined the profession for a century, was now clouded. Improving the status of the nurse, ostensibly to improve recruitment, was to become the primary motivation. This involved a major departure from the underlying value system of nursing, the implications of which would be far-reaching in redefining the nursing profession itself.

Notes

1 C. Davies, 'Past and Present in Nursing Education', *Nursing Times*, 1980, pp. 1703–1707, September 25.

2 R. White, 'Political Regulators in British Nursing', in White, R. (ed.), *Political Issues in Nursing*, vol 1, pp. 19–43, Chichester, John Wiley , 1985.

3 R. White, *The Effects of the National Health Service on the Nursing Profession, 1948–1961* London, King Edward's Hospital Fund for London, 1985; R. White, 'From Matron to Manager: The Political Construct of Reality', in White, R. (ed.), *Political Issues in Nursing*, vol. 2, pp. 45–68, Chichester, John Wiley, 1986.

4 R. White, *The Effects of the National Health Service on the Nursing Profession, 1948–1961* London, King Edward's Hospital Fund for London, 1985, p. 39.

5 General Nursing Council for England and Wales, *Syllabus of Subjects for Examination and Record of Practical Instruction and Experience for the Certificate of General Nursing*, London, General Nursing Council, 1969.

6 General Nursing Council for England and Wales, *Syllabus of Subjects for Examination and Record of Practical Instruction and Experience for the Certificate of General Nursing*, London, General Nursing Council, 1969, reprinted 1973, 1974, 1976.

7 Ibid., p. 67.

8 'Student Nurse Assessment', *Nursing Times*, 1969, pp. 119–120, July 24; King's Fund Hospital Centre, *A Study of Student Nurses' Progress*, King's Fund, London, November, 1968.

9 B.N. Fawkes, 'Needs of Education and Training in Nursing', *Nursing Times*, 1972, pp. 69–71, May 4.

[10] 'Bendall on Briggs', 1972, *Nursing Times*, p. 1403, November 9; English National Board for Nursing, Midwifery and Health Visiting, *The End of the Beginning*, London, ENB, 1983.

[11] E.R.D. Bendall, 'The Next Fifty Years', *Nursing Times*, 1969, p. 152, January 30.

[12] M.M. Pearce, 'The Next Fifty Years', *Nursing Times*, 1969, p. 153, January 30.

[13] C. Montacute, 'The Next Fifty Years', *Nursing Times*, 1969, pp. 153–154, January 30.

[14] E.R.D. Bendall, *So You Passed, Nurse*, London, Royal College of Nursing and National Council of Nurses of the United Kingdom, 1975.

[15] Ibid., p. 8.

[16] Ibid., pp. 11–12.

[17] Ibid., p. 44.

[18] Ibid., p. 51.

[19] Ibid., pp. 61–64.

[20] Ibid., pp. 64–65.

[21] Ibid., pp. 65–66.

[22] Ibid., pp. 67–68.

[23] N. Lamond, *Becoming a Nurse: The Registered Nurse's View of General Student Nurse Education*, London, Royal College of Nursing, 1974, pp. 16–17.

[24] E.R.D. Bendall, 'The Future of British Nurse Education', *Journal of Advanced Nursing*, 2, 1977, pp. 171–181.

[25] United Kingdom Central Council for Nursing, Midwifery and Health Visiting, *Project 2000: A New Preparation for Practice*, London, UKCC, 1986.

[26] C. Davies, 'Experience of Dependency and Control in Work: The Case of Nurses', *Journal of Advanced Nursing*, 1, 1976, pp. 273–282.

[27] C. Davies, 'Continuities in the Development of Hospital Nursing in Britain', *Journal of Advanced Nursing*, 2, 1977, pp. 479–493.

[28] J.E. Fretwell, 'Hospital Ward Routine – Friend or Foe?', *Journal of Advanced Nursing*, 5, 1980, pp. 625–636; J.E. Fretwell, *Ward Teaching and Learning: Sister and the Learning Environment*, London, The Royal College of Nursing, 1982.

[29] L.R. Seymer, 'Florence Nightingale's Writing on Nursing', *Nursing Mirror*, 1948, pp. 81–82, May 8.

[30] General Nursing Council for England and Wales, *Training Syllabus Register of Nurses: General Nursing*, London, General Nursing Council, Amended 1977.

[31] General Nursing Council for England and Wales, *Educational Policy: Syllabus and Practical Experiences Required for Admission to the General Part of the Register, Revising Council's Circular 69/4/3, 77/19/B*, London, General Nursing Council, 1977.

[32] C. de la Cuesta, 'The Nursing Process: From Development to Implementation', *Journal of Advanced Nursing*, 8, 1983, pp. 365–371.

[33] E.R.D. Bendall, 'Commitment to What?', in *A Time for Commitment*, Baroness Cox of Queensbury, Chairman, pp. 35–42, London, ENB, November 15, 1983.

[34] Ibid.

[35] Ibid.

[36] House of Lords Parliamentary Debates (Hansard), *Queen's Speech*, London, HMSO, 1978, November 1.

[37] House of Commons Parliamentary Debates (Hansard), *Nurses, Midwives and Health Visitors Bill*, London, HMSO, 1978, November 2, 13.

[38] Ibid., c.37–40, November 13.

[39] House of Commons Parliamentary Debates (Hansard), *Nurses, Midwives and Health Visitors Bill*, London, HMSO, 1979, February 7, c.474.

[40] House of Commons Parliamentary Debates (Hansard), *Nurses, Midwives and Health Visitors Bill*, London, HMSO, 1978, November 13, c.41, 53–56, 66–67.

[41] House of Commons Parliamentary Debates Standing Committee (Hansard), *Nurses, Midwives and Health Visitors Bill*, London, HMSO, 1978, November 28, c13, 87–88.

[42] House of Commons Parliamentary Debates (Hansard), *Nurses, Midwives and Health Visitors Bill*, London, HMSO, 1978, November 13, c.88–89.

[43] Ibid., c.56–57.

[44] Ibid., c.71, 73–76, 78.

[45] Ibid., c.93.

[46] Ibid., c.111, 113–114.

[47] House of Commons Parliamentary Debates Standing Committee (Hansard), *Nurses, Midwives and Health Visitors Bill*, London, HMSO, 1978, November 30, c.81–83.

[48] House of Commons Parliamentary Debates (Hansard), *Nurses, Midwives and Health Visitors Bill*, London, HMSO, 1979, February 7, c.477–478.

[49] Ibid., c.479–480.

[50] House of Lords Parliamentary Debates (Hansard), *Nurses, Midwives and Health Visitors Bill*, London, HMSO, 1979, February 19, c.1660–1664.

[51] House of Lords Parliamentary Debates (Hansard), *Nurses, Midwives and Health Visitors Bill*, London, HMSO, 1979, March 13, c.504–508, 513, 516–517.

[52] Ibid., c.513–514.

[53] English National Board for Nursing, Midwifery and Health Visiting, *The End of the Beginning*, September 1980–September 1981, London, ENB, 1983.

[54] English National Board for Nursing, Midwifery and Health Visiting, *The End of the Beginning*, September 1981–September 1982, London, ENB, 1983.

[55] A. Briggs, 'The Commitment of the Briggs Committee', in *A Time for Commitment*, Baroness Cox of Queensbury, Chairman, pp. 2–9, London, ENB, 1983, November 15.

[56] E.R.D. Bendall, 'Commitment to What?', in *A Time for Commitment*, Baroness Cox of Queensbury, Chairman, pp. 35–42, London, ENB, November 15, 1983; J.K. McFarlane, 'The Commitment of the First English National Board for Nursing, Midwifery and Health Visiting', in *A Time for Commitment*, Baroness Cox of Queensbury, Chairman, pp. 13–19, 45, London, ENB, November 15, 1983.

[57] J.K. McFarlane, 'The Commitment of the First English National Board for Nursing, Midwifery and Health Visiting', in *A Time for Commitment*, Baroness Cox of Queensbury, Chairman, pp. 13–19, 45, London, ENB, November 15, 1983.

[58] Ibid., p. 45.

[59] E.R.D. Bendall, 'Commitment to What?', in *A Time for Commitment*, Baroness Cox of Queensbury, Chairman, pp. 35–42, London, ENB, November 15, 1983, p. 36.

[60] J.P. Smith, *Virginia Henderson: The First Ninety Years*, London, Scutari Press, 1989, pp. 38, 49, 68, 72. F. Davis, 'Professional Socialization as Subjective Experience: The Process of Doctrinal Conversion among Student Nurses', in Cox, C. and A. Mead (eds) , *A Sociology of Medical Practice*, p. 116–131, London, Collier-Macmillan, 1975.

[61] *Report of the Committee on Nursing*, Professor Asa Briggs, Chairman, Cmnd.5115, London, HMSO, 1972, pp. 38–39, para. 115.

[62] G. Rivett, *From Cradle to Grave: Fifty Years of the NHS*, London, King's Fund, 1998, p. 481.

Conclusion: lessons from history and the significance of the nurse apprentice

The first major system of nurse training, which began at St Thomas's Hospital in 1860 and spread worldwide, developed from what were perceived as Nightingale's principles. It was understood and accepted that nursing was a vocation, a moral activity, dependent on the character of the nurse and her high ideals. The system embraced technical, practical and scientific knowledge, and relied on the thorough mastery of techniques. Equally essential was intelligence. No task could be considered menial, or less important than any other, because all were necessary to provide the unity of patient care.

A model of leadership, the ward sister was the key person in training nurses how to nurse, and to induct them into the values and ideals to which all nurses should aspire. She was the trustee of the tradition which was organic rather than individualistic. Right relationships to colleagues and seniors, to matrons and doctors, based on authority and respect, were vital, because the one objective that united all was responsibility towards the patient. The patient's welfare was the sole purpose which nurses and doctors were expected to serve. The apprenticeship system of training nurses grew from this avowed purpose.

By the end of the nineteenth century there were divisions around the further development of the profession in Britain, although there was no such division on the principles which should underpin it. Consensus was reached, and following the Nurses Registration Act of 1919, the apprenticeship training became the basis for the national system of examination adopted for state registration by the General Nursing Council for England and Wales, and set out in its successive syllabuses.

Until the 1970s, potential nurses were selected for training according to their moral qualities as well as their intellectual capability, determined through references and on interview by matrons and heads of training schools. The ward sister oversaw not only each individual's practical performance but also the manner and attitude of the nurse, and this was attested to before training could be completed. Lectures on subjects relevant to the patient's condition and treatment were given by medical staff. This knowledge was synthesised in the teachings of ward sisters, nurse tutors and later clinical instructors, and integrated with practical knowledge, skills and techniques. Supervised clinical experience ensured that relevance to patient care was maintained.

Learning was graduated and incremental. First, the student nurse learned basic knowledge, for example elementary hygiene, anatomy and physiology. At the same time she learned basic skills, such as bed-making, bedbathing and mouth care. As she grew in experience, the complexity of her knowledge, both intellectually and practically, increased. She was taught more complex theory, diseases and their treatments, and concurrently learned more complex procedures such as catheterisation and passing naso-gastric tubes. As the student nurse gained knowledge and skill, and experience in practice, so she would be able to take on increasing responsibility. At each stage she worked with more senior nurses, and even as a staff nurse was supervised by the ward sister. The manner of performance was as important as the content of her knowledge.

Knowledge and skill were tested, prior to a nurse becoming registered, by oral and written examination as well as by continuous assessment. Training was individualised according to the training needs of each student. Clinical experience of tasks, techniques and procedures was entered and signed in the student nurse's personal record book, which recorded performance and levels of achievement. The practical examination tested competence of the student's performance. The State Registered Nurse was trained to be competent and proficient in both basic and technical care, which were considered to be inseparable aspects of patient requirements.

Structures gave the nurse a pattern in which she could be confident. If she followed the routines and procedures as she was taught, and as they were ingrained into her, they should become second nature. The argument was that such repetition was neither oppressive nor mechanical. Rather, it was liberating, freeing the nurse to use her intelligence and intellect to reflect critically on the individual needs and circumstances of the patient. Structures gave the patient the security of knowing that detailed attention to his needs would be automatic and not haphazard.

This form of training came under scrutiny and criticism as being authoritarian, routinised and restrictive. It was argued that the vocational tradition was adversely affecting recruitment. But many leaders in the profession vigorously defended the tradition. The reason for the shortages of nurses was that the need for the nursing service was growing. The numbers of registered nurses and student nurses in training was, in fact, increasing year by year. By the middle of the twentieth century, however, supporters of the apprenticeship tradition were becoming increasingly defensive in a social climate which questioned traditions generally. To some nurses, North American models of nursing and nurse education, with their emphasis on autonomy, appeared attractive by contrast.

Shortcomings in North American nursing concerned many British nursing leaders and commentators. British nursing, they argued, should remain united, and not follow the divided American model, in which graduate nurses, practical nurses and nursing aides all specialised in different aspects of patient care. In America graduate nurses, educated in the liberal arts and status driven, preferred to move away from the bedside. Basic and technical aspects of care were disconnected. Patient care was fragmented. And bedside caring *de facto* if not *de iure* had become devalued as menial work of the lowlier ranks. Against this, the British trained nurse, to whom the soul of nursing was still bedside care, was regarded globally as second to none. Critics feared that specialisation and rationalisation would destroy this soul, as had happened in the United States, making nurses, to use Max Weber's words, into 'specialists without spirit'.

Within the British nursing profession the consensus was to sustain the apprenticeship tradition until the 1960s. By then there was a loss of confidence in its vocational values, even though total nursing numbers had reached new heights during that period, and the number of nurses in training, as a proportion of their age group, had increased substantially. Divisions grew: those who wanted to sustain the tradition, both inside and outside the profession, advocated reform. Others, perhaps influenced by social scientists, argued that the tradition was oppressive, and nursing needed an entirely new direction urgently.

Many senior, as well as grass-roots, nurses were not in favour of a radical redirection of the profession; recruits were still largely motivated by vocational values, ward sisters were generally keen to remain at the bedside, eschewing career advancement, and patients were on the whole satisfied with their care. Against this evidence, the Briggs Report in 1972 set out an agenda for a revaluation of nursing's status and career orientation with proposals for a different educational system. The final syllabus under the apprenticeship system was published in 1977. The Briggs Report was put into practice by an Act of Parliament in 1979 which set out a new mechanism for professional self-regulation. Thereafter, a gradual movement occurred, away from practice-based training, towards a college-based system of education; from the nurse apprentice to the supernumerary nurse. The objective of nursing, once clearly understood as a service to the practical needs of patients, would become less clear, and vocation would no longer be relevant as a social driver for becoming and being trained as a nurse.

The apprenticeship training was significant for both the patient and the nurse. For the patient, the system brought a clarity of purpose to care which was practical, efficient and medically orientated. The public esteemed nurses because nursing was not just a job. It was perceived as being based on values higher than the merely pragmatic. Nurses were regarded in a special way, which might be described as quasi-religious. As regards the nursing profession itself, this caused a tension. The aura of transcendence fell out of favour as a value system and professionalisation clashed with vocation. It was this that led to the call for change by some sections of the profession, a call that was far from unanimous. Those who disagreed doubted that altruism could be professionalised. Here lay the paradox: increasing the professional status of the nurse meant decreasing the vocational ethic and attracting a differently motivated recruit. Such doubts have become increasingly significant, and 140 years after Nightingale's model of nursing began in Britain, the implications of withdrawing it, for quality in patient care, nurse education and the future direction of the nursing profession, have yet to be fully realised. History will judge whether revolution rather than reformation was the right way forward.

Bibliography

Primary sources

Books and pamphlets

Anderson, E.R. (1973), *The Role of the Nurse*, London: Royal College of Nursing.

Barclay, J. (1946), *Why No Nurses?*, London: Faber & Faber.

Bendall, E.R.D. (1975), *So You Passed, Nurse*, London: Royal College of Nursing and National Council of Nurses of the United Kingdom.

Box, K. Croft-White, E. (1943), *Recruitment to Nursing: an Inquiry into the Attitudes of Student Nurses to their Profession with Special Reference to the Present Recruiting Campaign*, Regional S.7 London: Wartime Social Survey for Campaigns Division of the Ministry of Information, October.

Carter, G.B. (1939), *A New Deal for Nurses*, London: Victor Gollancz.

Cartwright, A. (1964), *Human Relations and Hospital Care*, London: Routledge & Kegan Paul, 1964.

Cohen, G. (1964), *What's Wrong with Hospitals?*, Harmondsworth: Penguin.

Crossman, R. (1977), *The Diaries of a Cabinet Minister*, vol. 3, London: Hamish Hamilton and Jonathan Cape.

Dutton, A. (1968), *Factors Affecting Recruitment of Nurse Tutors*, London: King Edward's Hospital Fund for London.

Farnworth, M. (1952), *A Study of the Social Prestige of Nursing*, London: report submitted to the Medical Research Council.

Lamond, N. (1974), *Becoming a Nurse: The Registered Nurse's View of General Student Nurse Education*, London: Royal College of Nursing.

McFarlane, J. K. (1970), *The Proper Study of the Nurse*, London: Royal College of Nursing and National Council of Nurses of the United Kingdom.

McGhee, A. (1961), *The Patient's Attitude to Nursing Care*, Edinburgh: E. & S. Livingstone.

MacGuire, J. (1969), *Threshold to Nursing: A Review of the Literature on Recruitment To and Withdrawal from Nurse Training Programmes in the United Kingdom*, Occasional Papers on Social Administration No. 30, London, G. Bell & Sons.

MacGuire, J. (1961), *From Student to Nurse – The Induction Period: A Study of Student Nurses in the First Six Months of Training in Five Schools of Nursing*, Oxford: Oxford Area Nurse Training Committee, September.

MacGuire, J. (1966), *From Student to Nurse – Training and Qualification: A Study of Student Nurses in Training at Five Schools of Nursing*, Oxford: Oxford Area Nurse Training Committee, May.

MacManus, E. (1956), *Matron of Guy's*, London: Andrew Melrose.

Manchèe, D. (1946), *Whatever Does the Almoner Do?* London: Baillière, Tindall & Cox.

Marsh, D.C. and A.J. Willcocks (1965), *Focus on Nurse Recruitment: A Snapshot from the Provinces*, London: Oxford University Press, published for the Nuffield Provincial Hospitals Trust.

Menzies, I.E.P. (1970), *A Case Study in the Functioning of Social Systems as a Defence Against Anxiety: A Report on a Study of the Nursing Service of a General Hospital*, Reprint of Tavistock Pamplet no. 3, London: Tavistock Institute of Human Relations.

Morton-Williams, J.R. and R. Berthoud (1971), *Nurses Attitude Study: Report on Depth Interviews*, ref. 02.194, London: Social and Community Planning Research, February.

Morton-Williams, J.R. and R. Berthoud (1971), *Nurses Attitude Survey: Report on Postal Survey*, ref. 02.188, London: Social and Community Planning Research, November.

Nightingale, F. (1851), *The Institution of Kaiserswerth on the Rhine, for the Practical Training of Deaconesses, under the Direction of the Rev. Pastor Fliedner, Embracing the Support and Care of a Hospital, Infant and Industrial Schools, and a Female Penitentiary*, London: London Ragged Colonial Training School.

Nightingale, F. (1860), *Suggestions for Thought to the Searchers after Truth among the Artizans of England*, in 3 vols, London: Eyre & Spottiswode, privately printed.

Nurses Christian Movement Working Party (1963/1964), *Christianity and Nursing Today*, London: Epworth Press.

Nutting, M.A. and L.L. Dock (1907), *A History of Nursing in Two Volumes*, New York and London: The Knickerbocker Press, G.P. Putnam's Sons.

Oxford, M.N. (1900), *A Handbook of Nursing*, 1st edn, London: Methuen & Co. Ltd., 8 edns 1900–1923 (8th edn revised Sheldon, F.A.).

Osler, W. (1904), *Aequanimitas*, London: H.K. Lewis.

Osler, W. (1905), *Counsels and Ideals*, 1st edn, London: Humphrey Milford, Oxford University Press, 2nd edn.

Osler, W. (1910), *Man's Redemption of Man*, London: Constable & Co., 1910.

Osler, W. (1919), *Medicine and Nursing*, London: Humphrey Milford, Oxford University Press.

Powell, M. (1975), *Patients are People*, Reading: Educational Explorers.

Raphael, W. (1969), *Patients and their Hospitals*, 1st edn, London: King Edward's Hospital Fund for London, 3 edns 1969–1977.

Revans, R.W. (1964), *Standards for Morale: Cause and Effect in Hospitals*, London: Oxford University Press published for the Nuffield Provincial Hospitals Trust.

Robb, B. (1967), *Sans Everything*, London: Thomas Nelson & Sons.

Worcester, A. (1927), *Nurses and Nursing*, Cambridge: Harvard University Press.

Nursing textbooks

Ashdown, A.M. (1917), *A Complete System of Nursing*, 1st edn, London: J.M. Dent & Sons Ltd., 4 edns 1917–1943.

Bailey, H. (1933), *Surgery for Nurses*, 1st edn, London: H.K. Lewis, 8 edns 1933–1954.

Clarke, M. (1971), *Practical Nursing*, 11th edn, London: Baillière Tindall.

Cochrane, M. (1930), *Nursing*, London: Geoffrey Bles.

Croft, J. (1873), *Notes of Lectures at St Thomas's Hospital*, London: St Thomas's Hospital, Blades East & Blades.

Dannatt, A. (1893), *How to Become a Hospital Nurse*, London: The Record Press, Limited.

Darnell, L.M. (1959), *Nursing*, 1st edn, London: Robert Hale Limited, 2nd edn, 1961.

Darwin, J., J. Markham and B. Whyte (1964), *Bedside Nursing*, 1st edn, London: William Heinemann Medical Books, 3 edns 1964–1971.

Domville, E.J. (1885), *A Manual for Hospital Nurses*, 5th edn, London: J. & A. Churchill; 7th edn, 1891; 9th edn, 1907.

Fisher, E. (1937), *The Nurse's Textbook*, London: Faber & Faber.

Fox, E.M. (1914), *First Lines in Nursing*, 1st edn, London: Scientific Press, 2nd edn, 1924.

Fretwell, J.E. (1982), *Ward Teaching and Learning: Sister and the Learning Environment*, London: Royal College of Nursing.

Gration, H.M. (1944), *The Practice of Nursing*, 1st edn, London: Faber & Faber, 6 edns 1944–1959 (3rd edn with D.L. Holland).

Gullan, M.A. (1920), *Theory and Practice of Nursing*, 1st edn, London: H.K. Lewis & Co., 8 edns 1920–1961 (8th edn revised by Gould, M.E.).

Hadley, W.J. (1902), *Nursing: General, Medical and Surgical*, 1st edn, London: J. & A. Churchill, 1902, 2nd edn, 1907.

Hector, W. (1960), *Modern Nursing*, 1st edn, London: William Heinemann Medical Books, 7 edns 1960–1982.

Heather-Bigg, M. (1918), *Home Nursing*, London: St John's Gate.

Houghton, M. (1938), *Aids to Practical Nursing*, 1st edn, London: Baillière, Tindall & Cox, 10 edns 1938–1065 (10th edn with M. Whittow).

Humphry, L. (1889), *A Manual of Nursing: Medical and Surgical*, London: Charles Griffin & Co.

Kropotkin, P. (1902), *Mutual Aid a Factor of Evolution*, London: William Heinemann.

Landale, E.J.R. (1893), *Points for Probationers*, London: Record Press.

Lees, F.S. (1874), *Handbook for Hospital Sisters*, Acland, H.W. (ed.), London: W.S. Isbister & Co.

Lewis, P.G. (1890), *Nursing: its Theory and Practice*, 1st edn, London: Scientific Press, 11 edns 1890–1899.

Lückes, E.C.E. (1886), *Hospital Sisters and their Duties*, 1st edn, London: J. & A. Churchill, 4th edn, 1912, London: Scientific Press.

Lückes, E.C.E. (1889), *What will Trained Nurses Gain by Joining the British Nurses' Association?*, London: J. & A. Churchill.

Lückes, E.C.E. (1892), *Lectures on General Nursing*, London: Kegan Paul, Trench, Trübner & Co.

Lückes, E.C.E. (1898), *General Nursing*, 4th edn, London: Kegan Paul, Trench, Trübner & Co.

Moroney, J. (1950), *Surgery for Nurses*, 1st edn, Edinburgh: E. & S. Livingstone, 15 edns 1950–1982.

Morten, H. (1888), *Sketches of Hospital Life*, London: Sampson Low, Marston, Searle & Rivington.

Morten, H. (1893), *How to Become a Nurse and How to Succeed*, London: Scientific Press.

Morten, H. ((1913), *The Nurse's Pronouncing Dictionary*, revised Burdett, M.L., London: Scientific Press.

Nightingale, F. (1860), *Notes on Nursing*, 1st edn, London, Harrison.

Pearce, E.C. (1937), *A General Textbook of Nursing*, 1st edn, London: Faber & Faber, 18 edns 1937–1971.

Pearce, E.C. (1953), *Nurse and Patient*, 1st edn, London: Faber & Faber, 3 edns 1953–1969.

Pringle, A.L. (1905), *A Study in Nursing*, London: Macmillan and Co.

Riddell, M.S. (1914), *Lectures to Nurses*, 1st edn, London: Scientific Press, 6 edns 1914–1936.

Riddell, M.S. (1931), *A First Year Nursing Manual*, 1st edn, London: Scientific Press, 5 edns 1931–1939.

Scales, M. (1952), *Handbook for Ward Sisters*, 1st edn, London: Baillière, Tindall & Cox, 2nd edn, 1958.

Sears, W.G. (1953), *Medicine for Nurses*, 1st edn, London: Edward Arnold, 13 edns 1953–1979 (11th edn with Winwood, R.S.).

Smith, E.M. (1929), *Notes on Practical Nursing*, London: Faber & Gwyer.

Stewart, I. and Cuff, H.E. (1899), 1st edn, *Practical Nursing*, Edinburgh and London: William Blackwood & Sons; 2nd edn, 1903; new edn, 1904; 3rd edn, 1910; 4th edn revised Cuff, H.E. and Gordon Pugh, W.T., 1913.

Toohey, M. (1953), *Medicine for Nurses*, 1st edn, Edinburgh: E. & S. Livingstone, 14 edns 1953–1986.

Vivian, M. (1920), *Lectures to Nurses in Training*, London: Scientific Press.

Voysey, M.H.A. (1905), *Nursing: Hints to Probationers on Practical Work*, London: Scientific Press, new and revised edn, 1911.

Watson, J.K. (1899), *A Handbook for Nurses*, 1st edn, London: Faber & Gwyer Ltd. (The Scientific Press), 12 edns 1899–1946.

Watson, J.K. (1926), *A Handbook for Senior Nurses and Midwives*, 1st edn, London: Humphrey Milford, Oxford University Press, 2nd edn, 1931.

Williams, R. and A. Fisher (1877), *Hints for Hospital Nurses*, Edinburgh: MacLachlan & Stewart; London: Simpkin, Marshall & Co.; Dublin: Fannin & Co.

Wood, C.J. (undated, c. 1887), *A Handbook of Nursing for the Home and the Hospital*, 8th edn, London: Cassell & Co.

Government and professional reports

Bonham Carter, H. (1888), *Is a General Register of Nurses Desirable?*, London.

Bonham Carter, H. (ed.) (1892) *Memorandum on the Registration of Nurses and the Royal British Nurses' Association*, London.

British Hospitals Association (1948), *Memorandum of Comment on the Report of the Working Party on the Recruitment and Training of Nurses Submitted to the Minister of Health*, Wettenhall J.P. , Secretary, London: British Hospitals Association, February.

Cohen, J. (1948), *Working Party on the Recruitment and Training of Nurses, Minority Report*, London: HMSO.

English National Board for Nursing, Midwifery and Health Visiting (1983), *The End of the Beginning*, London: ENB.

'In the Privy Council' (undated, c. 1892), *Re The Petition for a Charter for the Incorporation of the Royal British Nurses' Association: Case in Opposition to the Petition and Appendix*, London: Cookson, Wainewright & Pennington.

King Edward's Hospital Fund for London (1947), *Comments on the Report of the Working Party on the Recruitment and Training of Nurses Submitted to the Minister of Health*, London: King Edward's Hospital Fund, November.

King's Fund Hospital Centre (1968), *A Study of Student Nurses' Progress*, King's Fund: London, November.

The Lancet Commission on Nursing: Final Report (1932), London: The Lancet Ltd.

Ministry of Health Board of Education (1939), *Interdepartmental Committee on Nursing Services: Interim Report*, the Rt. Hon. The Earl of Athlone, Chairman, London: HMSO.

Ministry of Health, Department of Health for Scotland, Ministry of Labour and National Service (1947), *Report of the Working Party on the Recruitment and Training of Nurses*, Sir Robert Wood, Chairman, London: HMSO.

Ministry of Health, Department of Health for Scotland (1954), *Report of the Committee Set Up to Consider the Function, Status and Training of Nurse Tutors*, Janet K. Aitken, Chairman, London: HMSO.

Minister of Health, National Health Service (1968), *Findings and Recommendations following Enquiries into Allegations Concerning the Care of Elderly Patients in Certain Hospitals*, London: HMSO, July.

Ministry of Health, Central Health Services Council (1961), *The Pattern of the In-patient's Day*, HMSO: London.

Ministry of Health Scottish Home and Health Department (1966), *Report of the Committee on Senior Nursing Staff*, Brian Salmon, Chairman, London: HMSO.

Nuffield Provincial Hospitals Trust (1948), *Observations Submitted to the Ministry of Health on the Ministry's Working Party on the Recruitment and Training of Nurses*, Oxford: Oxford University Press.

Nuffield Provincial Hospitals Trust (1953), *The Work of Nurses in Hospital Wards: Report of a Job-analysis*, Goddard, H.A., Director, London: Nuffield Lodge, Regent's Park.

Report of the Committee on Nursing (1972), Professor Asa Briggs, Chairman, Cmnd.5115, London: HMSO.

Royal College of Nursing, *Nursing Reconstruction Committee Report and Supplements*, Lord Horder, Chairman, London, Royal College of Nursing; Section I, The Assistant Nurse (1942), Section II, Education and Training (1943), Section III, Recruitment (1943), Section IV, The Social and Economic Conditions of the Nurse (1949).

Royal College of Nursing (1948), *Memorandum on the Report of the Working Party on the Recruitment and Training of Nurses*, London: Royal College of Nursing.

Royal College of Nursing (1953), *Comment on the Nuffield Provincial Hospitals Trust Job Analysis of the Work of Nurses in Hospital Wards*, London: Royal College of Nursing, November.

Royal College of Nursing (1956), *Observations and Objectives: A Statement on Nursing Policy*, London: Royal College of Nursing.

Royal College of Nursing and National Council of Nurses of the United Kingdom (1964), *A Reform of Nursing Education: First Report of a Special Committee on Nurse Education*, Sir Harry Platt, Chairman, London: Royal College of Nursing and National Council of Nurses of the United Kingdom.

Royal College of Nursing and National Council of Nurses of the United Kingdom (1971), *Rcn Evidence to the Committee on Nursing*, London: Royal College of Nursing and National Council of Nurses of the United Kingdom.

Royal College of Nursing and National Council of Nurses of the United Kingdom (1973), *Rcn Comment on the Report of the Committee on Nursing*, London: Royal College of Nursing and National Council of Nurses of the United Kingdom, February.

Royal Commission on the National Health Service (1979), Sir Alec Merrison, Chairman, Cmnd. 7615, London: HMSO.

The Ten Group (1948), *Working Party Report on the Recruitment and Training of Nurses: Comments Submitted to the Minister of Health by the Ten Group*, Croyden, Surrey: Grubb, February.

United Kingdom Central Council for Nursing, Midwifery and Health Visiting (1986), *Project 2000: A New Preparation for Practice*, London: UKCC.

Chapters and articles

' "Existing" Nurses: A Settlement at Last' (1923), *Nursing Times*, pp. 665–666, July 14.

'... and Criticism' (1967), letter, *Nursing Mirror*, p. 252, December 8.

'A Fit and Proper Person' (1963), editorial, *Nursing Times*, p. 1623, December 27.
'A New Beginning' (1970), editorial, *Nursing Times*, p. 385, March 26.
'A Question of Faith', letters (1964), *Nursing Mirror*, p. 584, September 25.
'A Question of Faith', letters (1964), *Nursing Mirror*, p. 46, October 9.
'A Reform of Nursing Education' (1964), *Nursing Mirror*, pp. 130, 147, November 6.
'A Reform of Nursing Education' (1964), *Nursing Times*, pp. 813–814, June 19
'A Reform of Nursing Education' (1964), *Nursing Times*, pp. 873–877, July 3.
'A Shocking Situation' (1961), editorial, *Nursing Mirror*, p. 1399, July 28.
'Allocation of Ward Duties' (1953), editorial, *Nursing Times*, p. 225, March 7.
'An Outward Look' (1963), *Nursing Times*, p. 689, May 31.
'Anthropology of Man' (1965), letters, *Nursing Mirror*: p. 269, June 11; p. 310, June 25.
'Arrival of the Wounded in the Bosphorus' (1854), *The Times*, p. 8, October 9; 'From our Own Correspondent' (1854), *The Times*, p. 7, October 12; editorial (1854), *The Times*, p. 6, October 12; 'From our Own Correspondent' (1854), *The Times*, p. 8, October 13; 'Hospital Assistants in the East' (1854), letter, *The Times*, p. 7, October 14.
'Bedside Nursing' (1965), letters, *Nursing Mirror*, p. 533, August 27; p. 151, October 15.
'Bendall on Briggs' (1972), *Nursing Times*, p. 1403, November 9.
'Briggs on Nursing' (1970), *Nursing Times*, pp. 1566–1567, December 3.
'British Hospitals Association on Working Party's Report' (1948), *Nursing Mirror*, p. 418, March 13.
'By Briggs out of Nightingale' (1972), editorial, *Nursing Times*, p. 1401, November 9.
'Change of Direction?' (1953), editorial, *Nursing Times*, p. 253, March 14.
'Christianity and Nursing Today' (1965), *Nursing Mirror*, p. 346, January 8.
'College Conference on the Job Analysis' (1953), editorial, *Nursing Times*, pp. 1233–1234, December 5.
'Conference Discusses Supply and Demand' (1965), *Nursing Mirror*, pp. 387–389, July 16.
'Conference on Nursing Education', *British Journal of Nursing* (1921), pp. 266–272, May 7; 'The General Nursing Council of England and Wales' (1921), *Nursing Mirror and Midwives' Journal*, pp. 90–92, May 7; 'Making the Future Nurse: Great Conference on the Syllabus of Training and Affiliation Schemes' (1921), *Nursing Times*, pp. 498–512, May 7.
'Defence Mechanisms in Nursing' (1960), review, R.M.N., *Nursing Times*, pp. 1078–1079, September 2.
'Discussing the Working Party Report: A Talk by Miss E. Cockayne, Matron, Royal Free Hospital' (1947), *Nursing Times*, pp. 910–911, December 27.
'Edinburgh University – the First Research Fellowship in Nursing' (1953), *Nursing Times*, p. 311, March 28.
'Editorial' (1963), *Nursing Mirror*, p. 311, January 11.
'Editorial' (1963), *Nursing Mirror*, p. 45, April 19.
'Editorial' (1963), *Nursing Mirror*, p. 87, May 3.
'Editorial' (1963), *Nursing Mirror*, p. 313, July 12.
'Editorial' (1964), *Nursing Mirror*, p. 251, June 19.
'Editorial' (1964), *Nursing Mirror*, p. 299, July 3.
'Editorial' (1965), *Nursing Mirror*, p. 1, October 1.
'Editorial' (1965), *Nursing Mirror*, p. 275, November 19.
'Editorial' (1965), *Nursing Mirror*, p. 323, December 3.
'Editorial' (1965), *Nursing Mirror*, p. 217, December 9.
'Editorial' (1965), *Nursing Mirror*, p. 375, January 22.
'Editorial' (1965), *Nursing Mirror*, p. 471, February 19.

'Editorial' (1965), *Nursing Mirror*, p. 365, July 16.
'Editorial' (1965), *Nursing Mirror*, p. 475, August 13.
'Editorial' (1966), *Nursing Mirror*, p. 57, April 22.
'Editorial' (1967), *Nursing Mirror*, p. 155, November 17.
'Editorial' (1967), *Nursing Mirror*, p. 83, October 27.
'Educating for Nursing – Aims and Objectives' (1966), *Nursing Mirror*, pp. 528, 549–550, February 4.
'Ethics and Public Health Nursing' (1954), *Nursing Times*: pp. 264–267, March 11; pp. 294–295, March 18.
'Evolution and Christianity' (1965), letters, *Nursing Mirror*: p. 593, March 19; p. 594, March 19.
'Extracts of the Report will be Published in this and Subsequent Issues of this Journal: Introduction' (1953), *Nursing Times*, pp. 177–178, February 21.
'Facts about Nursing' (1953), leading article, *Lancet*, pp. 379–380, February 21.
'Facts for 1948' (1948), editorial, *Nursing Mirror*, pp. 271–272, January 17.
'For Immediate Action' (1964), editorial, *Nursing Times*, p. 849, July 7.
'For Whom the Train Stopped' (1962), editorial, *Nursing Mirror*, p. 481, September 21.
'Function, Status and Training of Nurse Tutors' (1955), *Nursing Times*, pp. 145–149, February 11.
'G.N.C. (England and Wales), Report on W.P. R.' (1948), *Nursing Mirror*, p. 201, June 26.
'General Nursing Council for England and Wales' (1965), *Nursing Times*, pp. 1353–1354, October 1.
'Giving a Lead' (1963), editorial, *Nursing Times*, p. 665, May 31.
'Gone are the Days' (1948), letter, M.C.S., *Nursing Mirror*, p. 46, October 16.
'Helen Downton' (1994), *Daily Telegraph*, p. 29, November 23.
'Hospital Job Analysis' (1953), editorial, *Nursing Times*, p. 173, February 21.
'House of Lords Debate on Nursing, Job Analysis Theme' (1953), *Nursing Mirror*, pp. 503–504, 522, May 22.
'I Use the Word Nursing for the Want of a Better' (1970), editorial, *Nursing Times*, 66, 40, p. 1249, October 1.
'In Reply to Agnostic Nurse' (1967), letters, *Nursing Mirror*, pp. 200–201, November 24,
'Job Analysis' (1948), editorial, *Nursing Mirror*, pp. 97–98, May 15.
'Job Analysis on Nursing: "The Work of Nurses in Hospital Wards"' (1953), *Nursing Mirror*, pp. 456–458, February 20;
'Job Analysis Report' (1953), *Nursing Mirror*, pp. 163–162 (concluded opposite page), April 17;
'Job Analysis Report' (1953), *Nursing Mirror*, pp. 502, 522, May 22;
'Job Analysis Study Conference' (1953), editorial, *Nursing Times*, p. 455, May 9;
'Ministry of Health Allegations about Care of Elderly Patients in Seven Hospitals' (1968), *Nursing Times*, p. 943, July 12.
'Miss Lonsdale and the Nursing at Guy's Hospital' (1880), editorial, *British Medical Journal*, pp. 706–707, May 8.
'Miss Loveridge of Bart's: A Profile' (1967), *Nursing Times*, p. 1032, August 4.
'Miss Virginia Henderson in London' (1963), *Nursing Mirror*, p. 243–244, June 14.
'Morale in the Ward' (1964), editorial, *Nursing Times*, p. 421, April 3.
'More Ado about Working Party's Report' (1948), *Nursing Mirror*, pp. 390–391. February 28;
'New Comments for Consideration' (1948), editorial, *Nursing Times*, pp. 1–2, January 3.
'News from Westminster: Next Move to Improve Nurses' Status' (1964), *Nursing Mirror*, p. 207, November 27.

'News of the Week. 1,000 March on Whitehall' (1968), *Nursing Times*, p. 1126, August 23.
'No Sense of Vocation Today?' (1961), editorial, *Nursing Mirror*, pp. 99,120, November 10.
'No to Platt' (1965), *Nursing Times*, p. 1330, October 1.
'Notable memorandum on W.P. Report' (1948), *Nursing Mirror*, pp. 25–26, April 10.
'Nurse and Patient by E.Pearce, Third Edition', T.A.K. (1969), *Nursing Mirror*, pp. 44–45, September 26.
'Nurse and Patient by Evelyn Pearce, Second Edition.', K.L.B. (1963), *Nursing Mirror*, p. vii, November 8.
'Nurse and Patient: A Study in Human Relationships. Evelyn C. Pearce' (1953), *Lancet*, p. 380, August 22.
'Nurses and Doctors: Edinburgh Infirmary Nursing, by One of the Staff' (1880), *Edinburgh Medical Journal*, 25, 11, pp. 1051–1052, May.
'Nurses and Doctors: Systems of Nursing, by a Nurse' (1880), *Edinburgh Medical Journal*, 25, 11, pp. 1048–1050, May.
'Nurses Comment on W.P. Report' (1948), editorial, *Nursing Mirror*, pp. 17–18, April 10.
'Nurses Discuss the Platt Report' (1964), *Nursing Mirror*, p. 313, July 3.
'Nursing – Neurosis or Vocation?' (1960), letter, Animus, *Nursing Times*, p. 1513, December 2.
'Nursing at Guy's Hospital' (1879), editorial, *British Medical Journal*, pp. 1027–1028, December 27.
'Nursing at Guy's Hospital' (1880), editorial, *British Medical Journal*, p. 374, March 6.
'Nursing Difficulties' (1880), editorial, *British Medical Journal*, pp. 289–290, February 21.
'Nursing Problems in the Provinces' (1953), leading article, *Lancet*, p. 1292, June 27.
'Pairs of Hands' (1965), editorial, *Nursing Times*, p. 11, May 7.
'Pattern of Nursing Education: Report of W.H.O. Working Conference' (1954), *Nursing Mirror*, pp. 426,434, May 15.
'Pattern of the In-patient's Day' (1961), *Nursing Times*, p. 392, March 31; 'Ward Time-table: Revised Pattern (1961), *Nursing Times*, p. 398–399, March 31; The Pattern of the In-patient's Day (1961), *Nursing Times*, p. 440–442, April 7.
'Platt and the Student Nurse' (1964), *Nursing Times*, p. 1550, November 20.
'Pointers for 1962' (1961), editorial, *Nursing Mirror*, pp. 233, 250, December 29.
'Preparation for Platt' (1964), editorial, *Nursing Times*, 1964, p. 1487, November 13.
'Professional Roots' (1961), editorial, *Nursing Times*, p. 1557, December 1.
'Raise the Roof!' (1968), editorial, *Nursing Times*, p. 753, June 7.
'Realism and Idealism' (1948), letter, Two S.R.N.s, *Nursing Mirror*, p. 79, October 30.
'Recruitment – a Social Problem' (1952), editorial, *Nursing Times*, pp. 601–602, June 21.
'Regional Action on Platt Report' (1964), *Nursing Mirror*, pp. 169–170, November 13.
'Religion for Nurses' (1967), letter, *Nursing Mirror*, pp. 174–175. November 17.
'Religion for Nurses' (1967), letter, *Nursing Mirror*, p. 199, November 24.
'Research into Basic Nursing' (1961), editorial, *Nursing Times*, p. 327, March 17.
'Selection and Training of Nurses', A Nurse (1960), *Nursing Times*, 1960, p. 857, July 8.
'Selection of Letters from Readers on our Controversial Series of "Platitudes" (1960), *Nursing Mirror*, p. 65, October 7; p. 352, October 28.
'Staff Nurses Conference' (1958), *Nursing Times*, pp. 500–502, May 2.
'Student Nurse Assessment' (1969), *Nursing Times*, pp. 119–120, July 24.
'Student Nurses' Association Discusses Platt' (1964), *Nursing Mirror*, p. 174, November 20.
'Student Nurses Speak Out' (1965), *Nursing Times*, p. 1328, September 24.
'Study Conference – "The first step"' (1953), editorial, *Nursing Times*, pp. 479–480, May 16.
'Talking Point', Cyclops (1960), *Nursing Times*, p. 810, July 1.

'Talking Point', Wrangler (1960), *Nursing Times*, p. 600, May 13.
'Teaching and Learning' (1960), editorial, *Nursing Times*, p. 771, June 24.
'The Basic Things of Nursing 1: A Relationship between two People' (1953), *Nursing Mirror*, p. 1598, September 18; 'The Basic Things of Nursing 2: Profession or Vocation?' (1953), *Nursing* Mirror, p. 1662, September 25; 'The Basic Things of Nursing 3: Service and Satisfaction' (1953), *Nursing Mirror*, p. 28, October 2.
'The Bedpan Round' (1963), editorial, *Nursing Times*, p. 281, March 8.
'The Changing Scene' (1955), *Nursing Times*, pp. 1225–1228, October 28.
'The College Council Meets' (1954), *Nursing Times*, pp. 1044–1045, September 25.
'The College Prayer' (1954), *Nursing Times*, p. 750, July 10.
'The Decline in Nursing' (1946), *British Journal of Nursing*, editorial, G.M.H., 94, 2140, pp. 121–122, November.
'The General Nursing Council for England and Wales' (1921), *The British Journal of Nursing*, pp. 187–189, April 2.
'The General Nursing Council for England and Wales' (1923), *Nursing Times*, pp. 271–276, March 24.
'The GNC and Platt' (1965), Iconclast, letter, *Nursing Times*, pp. 1416–1417, October 15.
'The Hospital Nursing Service' (1932), editorial, *British Medical Journal*, pp. 344–346, February 20.
'The Image' (1972), editorial, *Nursing Times*, p. 1535, December 7.
'The Job Analysis Report' (1953), *Nursing Times*, pp. 1238–1240, December 5.
'The Job Analysis Report' (1953), *Nursing Times*, pp. 1273–1275, December 12.
'The Job Analysis Study Conference' (1953), *Nursing Times*, pp. 482–484, May 16.
'The Job Analysis Study Conference' (1953), *Nursing Times*, p. 506–508, May 23.
'The Labour Conference' (1903), *British Journal of Nursing*, 75, 1927, pp. 42–44, February.
'The Labour Conference' (1903), *British Journal of Nursing*, 75, 1903, 1927, pp. 42–44, February.
'The Lancet Commission on Nursing' (1933), editorial, *Lancet*, pp. 369–370, February 18.
'The Means at our Disposal' (1954), *Nursing Times*, pp. 1230–1231, November 5.
'The Nursing at Guy's Hospital' (1880), editorial, *British Medical Journal*, pp. 525–526, April 3.
'The Nursing at Guy's Hospital' (1880), editorial, *British Medical Journal*, p. 563, April 10.
'The Nursing Question at Guy's Hospital' (1879), editorial, *British Medical Journal*, p. 871, November 29.
'The Nursing Question at Guy's Hospital' (1879), editorial, *British Medical Journal*, p. 918, December 6.
'The Nursing Staff at Guy's Hospital' (1879), editorial, *The British Medical Journal*, p. 898, December 6.
'The Nursing Team' (1956), Annotations, *Lancet*, p. 1090, November 24.
'The Philosophy of Briggs' (1972), editorial, *Nursing Times*, p. 1305, October 19.
'The Platt Committee Report' (1964), editorial, *Nursing Times*, pp. 783–784, June 19.
'The Platt Report – A Vital Document' (1964), *Nursing Mirror*: pp. 271–273, June 19; pp. 287–289, June 26; pp. 307–309, July 3.
'The Proper Task of a Hospital Nurse' (1953), editorial, *Nursing Mirror*, pp. 480, 496, February 27.
'The Proper Task of the Nursing Profession' (1953), editorial, *Nursing Mirror*, p. 512, March 13.
'The Royal College of Nursing Memorandum on the Report of the Working Party on the Recruitment and Training of Nurses' (1948), *Nursing Times*, pp. 260–262, April 10.

'The Student Life: The Philosophy of Sir William Osler edited by Richard E. Verney, M.B., F.R.C.P. E., D.R.' (1958), *Nursing Times* p. 152, February 9.

'The Student Nurse and the Bedpan Round' (1963), *Nursing Times*, p. 311, March 8.

'The Summer of our Discontent' (1968), editorial, *Nursing Times*, p. 1125, August 23.

'The Vigil and the Vow' (1960), editorial, *Nursing Mirror,* p. 1141, December 30.

'The Work of Nurses in Hospital Wards' (1953), *Nursing Times*, pp. 750–755, July 25.

'The Work of Nurses in Hospital Wards: Abstract of a Job Analysis Undertaken by the Nuffield Provincial Hospital Trust, continued' (1953), *Nursing Times*, pp. 259–264, March 14;

'The Work of Nurses in Hospital Wards: Abstract of the Report of a Job Analysis Undertaken by the Nuffield Provincial Hospital Trust' (1953), *Nursing Times*, pp. 203–206, 211, February 28.

'The Work of Nurses in Hospital Wards: Abstract of the Report of a Job Analysis Undertaken by the Nuffield Provincial Hospital Trust, concluded' (1953), *Nursing Times*, pp. 233–237, March 7;

'The Work of Nurses in Hospital Wards: Report of a Job Analysis Undertaken by the Nuffield Provincial Hospital Trust (1953), *Nursing* Times, pp. 176–177, February 21.

'To the Rt Hon. Kenneth Robinson MP Minister of Health' (1968), *Nursing Times*, p. 512, April 12.

'Trade Unions and the Nursing Profession' (1926), editorial, *Nursing Times*, 1129, pp. 1165–1166, December 18.

'Training Nurses' (1955), editorial, *The Times*, p. 7, August 22.

'University Co-operation' (1954), editorial, *Nursing Times*, pp. 1085–1086, October 8.

'Vale Atque Ave' (1962), editorial, *Nursing Mirror*, p. 267, December 28.

'Vespers', 'Religion for Nurses' (1967), letter, *Nursing Mirror*, p. 174, November 17.

'View of an Agnostic Nurse' (1967), *Nursing Mirror*, p. 149, November 10.

'Vocation *or* Profession' (1961), letter, W.C., *Nursing Times*, p. 157, February 3.

'Ward Teaching' (1954), *Nursing Times*, pp. 1283–1285, November 19.

'What is Wrong with Apprenticeship?' (1960), *Nursing Mirror and Midwives Journal*, 110, 2881, p. 2185, September 16.

'Who will Nurse the Patients of Tomorrow?' (1961), *Nursing Times*, 1961, pp. 946–947, July 21.

'Why Briggs? asks Lady Summerskill' (1970), *Nursing Times*, p. 354, March 19.

'Wolfson School of Nursing' (1961), *Nursing Times*, p. 392, March 31.

'Working Conference at St Andrew's University for Trained Nurses in any Field Organized by the Scottish Board of the Royal College of Nursing' (1954), *Nursing Times*, pp. 421–422, 430–431, April 17.

'You Hear it Said, Platitude 1, Nurses are different!' (1960), *Nursing Mirror*, p. 1915, August 26; 'Platitude 2. Nurses are Practical People' (1960), *Nursing Mirror*, p. 2005, September 2; 'Platitude 3. Nurses Have to be Tough!' (1960), *Nursing Mirror*, p. 2105, September 9; 'Platitude 4. Nurses Find it Hard to Express Themselves!' (1960), *Nursing Mirror*, p. 2197, September 16; 'Platitude 5. Nurses are Not What They Used to Be' (1960), *Nursing Mirror*, p. 2287, September 23; 'Platitude 6. Nurses Need Discipline' (1960), *Nursing Mirror*, p. 2370, September 30; 'Platitude 7. Nurses are not Professionally Minded' (1960), *Nursing Mirror*, p. 64, October 7.

Abel-Smith, B. (1961), 'Crisis in Nursing – 5: The Sociologist's View', *Nursing Times*, pp. 1262–1263, September 29.

Abel-Smith, B. (1964), 'The Platt Report: Some Implications', *Nursing Times*, pp. 925–926, July 17.

Abell, G. (1961), 'The Ministry of the Christian Nurse', *Nursing Mirror*, p. 156, April 14; p. 254, April 21; p. 338, April 28; p. 432, May 5; p. 542, May 12; p. 554, May 19.

Akester, J. (1954),'The Education of the Nurse', *Nursing Times*, pp. 918–200, August 19.

Akester, J.M. (1957), 'Future of Nursing', letter, *Lancet*, p. 96, January 12.

Allen, H.O. (1972),'A General Textbook of Nursing', *Nursing Times*, p. 639, May 25.

Altschul A. (1966), 'Value of Research' (1966), letter, *Nursing Mirror*, p. 234, June 10.

Anderson, T. (1953), 'The Training of Nurses', letter, *Lancet*, pp. 1047–1048, May 23.

Anderson, T. (1957),'The Future of Nursing', letter, *Lancet*, p. 45, January 5.

Anonymous (1961), 'Crisis in Nursing – 7: A Nurse's View', *Nursing Times*, pp. 1324–1325, October 13.

Anonymous (1961), 'Crisis in Nursing – 8: A Nurse's View 2. Long-term Policy', *Nursing Times*, pp. 1358–1359, October 20.

Ashe, E.J. (1960), 'Nursing – Neurosis or Vocation?', letter, *Nursing Times*, p. 1576, December 16.

Baly, M.E. (1965),'The Reform of Nursing Education', *Nursing Times*, pp. 867–868, June 25; pp. 955–956, July 9; pp. 977–978, July 16.

Barton, D.R. (1965), 'Open Forum: Views on the Platt Report: 2. The Attack', *Nursing Mirror*, pp. 477–478, February 19.

Bedford Fenwick, E. (1893),'Nursing at the World's Fair', *Nursing Record*, pp. 52–59, January 26;

Bedford Fenwick, E. (1896),'American Nurses', editorial, *Nursing Record and Hospital World*, pp. 205–206, March 14.

Bedford Fenwick, E. (1896),'Women', *Nursing Record and Hospital World*, p. 423, May 23.

Bedford Fenwick, E. (1900),'A Selfish Age', editorial, *Nursing Record and Hospital World*, p. 145, August 25.

Bedford Fenwick, E. (1924),'Nurses Keep your Souls Alive!', editorial, *British Journal of Nursing*, p. 1, January.

Bedford Fenwick, E. (1933),'The Sacred Vocation of Nursing', editorial, *British Journal of Nursing*, p. 149, June.

Bedford Fenwick, E. (1937),'The Life of the Spirit in Hospitals', editorial, *British Journal of Nursing*, p. 29, February.

Bedford Fenwick, E. (1899), 'Religious Liberty', editorial, *Nursing Record and Hospital World*, pp. 345–346, October 28.

Bedford Fenwick, E. (1931), 'Patients First: is Nursing a Profession or a Trade?', editorial, *British Journal of Nursing*, p. 57, March.

Bell, F. (1953), 'Nursing is a vocation', letter, *Nursing Mirror*, 1953, p. 244, October 23.

Bell, F.W. (1966), 'Life and Living it', *Nursing Mirror*, pp. 309–310, July 1.

Bell. F.W. 'All the World's a Stage' (1966), *Nursing Mirror*, p. 561, September 9; 'No Standing on the Top Deck', p. 586, September 16; 'It all Adds up to Something', p. 602, September 23; 'This Side of Innocence', p. 622, September 30; 'All the World's a Stage and all the Men and Women Merely ...', p. 16, October 7.

Belsey, C. (1967), 'How can I nurse ...', *Nursing Times*, p. 573, April 28.

Bendall, E.R.D. (1969),'The Next Fifty Years', *Nursing Times*, p. 152, January 30.

Bendall, E.R.D. (1977), 'The Future of British Nurse Education', *Journal of Advanced Nursing*, 2, pp. 171–181.

Bendall, E.R.D. (1983),'Commitment to What?', in *A Time for Commitment*, Baroness Cox of Queensbury, Chairman, pp. 35–42, London: ENB, November 15.

Bennett, B.A. (1960),'A Sociologist Looks at Nursing (in England and Wales since 1800),', *Nursing Mirror*, pp. 2289–2290, September 23.

Benton, A. (1966), 'Drug Addiction in a 19-year-old Youth', *Nursing Mirror*, p. 562, February 11.

Bishop of Lichfield (1962), 'The Festival of Love and Worship. Series of three articles on the meaning of Christmas', *Nursing Mirror*, p. 244, December 14; p. 264, December 21; p. 280, December 28.

Bishop, D. (1972), 'Why Do You Wish to be a Nurse?', *Nursing Mirror*, p. 44, August 25.

Bocock, E.J. (1954), 'The Education of Nurses', *Nursing Times*, 1954, p. 601, June 5.

Bodgener, J.H. (1960), 'Some Familiar Hymns', *Nursing Mirror*, p. 426, April 29; p. 605, May 13; p. 691, May 20; p. 774, May 27; p. 869, June 3.

Bonham Carter, H. (1880), 'Nursing Organisation in Hospitals', correspondence, *The British Medical Journal*, p. 225, February 7.

Booth, H. (1963), 'A Chaplain's Diary', *Nursing Times*, p. 658, May 24.

Bowman, M.P. (1983), 'Nursing by Lamplight', *Health Services*, pp. 10–11.

Boyle, E.S. (1961), 'Vocation or Profession', letter, *Nursing Times*, 1961, p. 221, February 17.

Braxton Hicks, J. (1880), 'On Nursing Systems', correspondence, *British Medical Journal*, pp. 11–12, January 3.

Breay, M. (1897), 'Duty', *The Nursing Record and Hospital World*, pp. 335–336, April 24.

Briggs, A. (1979), 'The Essence of Briggs', *Nursing Times*, p. 345, March 1.

Briggs, A. (1983), 'The Commitment of the Briggs Committee', in *A Time for Commitment*, Baroness Cox of Queensbury, Chairman, pp. 2–11, London: English National Board for Nursing, Midwifery and Health Visiting, November 15.

Brooke, H. (1958),'In Search of Ideas', *Nursing Times*, pp. 680–681, June 13.

Brown, J.P. (1965), 'Faith and Nursing', *Nursing Times*, p. 1428, October 15.

Buckley, D.A. (1963), 'A Question of Vocation', letter, *Nursing Mirror*, p. 102, May 3.

Burkinshaw, S.M. (1954),'Trends in Nursing Education', *Nursing Times*, pp. 204–205, February 20.

Buxton, O.V. (1960), 'A Day Off in the Life of a Matron', *Nursing Mirror*, p. 641, November 18.

Campbell, M.L. (1961), 'Home Thoughts from Abroad', letter, *Nursing Times*, p. 156, February 3.

Carr, A. (1964),'It is not Professional', *Nursing Mirror*, p. 258, June 19.

Carter Hall, S.C. (1861), 'Something of What Florence Nightingale has Done and is Doing', *St James's Magazine*, vol. 1, pp. 29–40, April–July.

Carter, G.B. (1953),'Windsor, Ontario, Experimental School: A Review of Dr. Lord's Evaluation', *Nursing Times*, pp. 316–318, March 28.

Carter, G.B. (1953), 'Collegiate Education for Nursing: A Review of Dr. Margaret Bridgeman's Book', *Nursing Times*, pp. 812–813, August 15.

Carter, G.B. (1954), 'Experimental Training for Nurses', *Nursing Times*, pp. 6–8, January 2.

Castle, B. (1988), 'No Kitchen Cabinet', in Maitland, S. (ed.), *Very Heaven*, pp. 47–58, London: Virago Press.

Chillman, J.H. (1955), 'Training Nurses', letter, *The Times*, p. 9, August 25.

Clarke, M. (1963), 'Nurse and Patient, Human Relations in Nursing, Second Edition. Evelyn Pearce', *Nursing Times*, pp. 1422–1423, November 8.

Cole, A. (1993), 'Castles in the Air', *Nursing Times*, pp. 16–17, July 21.

Collins, S.M. (1964),'Exchange of Nurse Teachers', *Nursing Times*, pp. 370–372, March 6.

Corbishley, T. (1964), 'Christian Humanism', *Nursing Mirror*, p. 237, June 12.

Crawford, T. (1975), 'Foreword', in Powell, M., *Patients are People*, pp. 9–11, Reading: Educational Explorers.

Creelman, L. (1965), 'There is no Change without Challenge, *Nursing Mirror*, pp. 127–130, May 7; pp. 160–162, May 14.

Dainty, E. (1960), 'Back to School at Thirty-Seven', *Nursing Mirror*, pp. 59,64, October 7; pp. 167–168, October 14.

Daniels, S. (1972), 'What *are* Nursing Duties?', *Nursing Times*, p. 121, January 27.

Dann, T.L. (1972), 'The Briggs Debate', letter, *Nursing Times*, p. 1422, November 9.

Dannatt, A. (1888), 'What Constitutes an Efficient Nurse', *Nursing Record*, pp. 87–90, May 24;

Darnell, L. (1955), 'The Education of the Nurse: Further Considerations', *Nursing Times*, pp. 1056–1058, September 23.

Davie, M. (1964),'Mental Illness', *Nursing Mirror*, p. 464, August 21.

Davies, C. (1976),'Experience of Dependency and Control in Work: The Case of Nurses', *Journal of Advanced Nursing*, 1, pp. 273–282.

Davies, C. (1977),'Continuities in the Development of Hospital Nursing in Britain', *Journal of Advanced Nursing*, 2, pp. 479–493.

Davies, C. (1980),'Past and Present in Nursing Education', *Nursing Times*, pp. 1703–1707, September 25.

Davis, A. (1960), 'Moral Re-armament', letter, *Nursing Times*, p. 479, April 15.

de la Cuesta, C. (1983), 'The Nursing Process: From Development to Implementation', *Journal of Advanced Nursing*, 8, pp. 365–371.

Dibb, M. 'Research Waste' (1966), letter, *Nursing Mirror*, p. 163, May 20.

Dock, L.L. (1895),'Nurses Directories', *Nursing Record and Hospital World*, pp. 255–256, April 20.

Dock, L.L. (1896),'A National Association for Nurses and its Legal Organisation', *Nursing Record and Hospital World*, p. 208–209, March 14; Letter from Miss Lavinia L. Dock, R.N., in Bedford Fenwick, E. (1943), 'A Demand for Justice for the State Registered Nurse', editorial, *British Journal of Nursing*, p. 61, June.

Dolan, V. (1967), 'How can I Nurse without Knowing my Lord?', *Nursing Times*, p. 398, March 24

Downton, H. (1959), 'Divine Healing: The Nurse and Spiritual Healing', *Nursing Times*, p. 851, September 11.

Duncan, I.G. (1961), 'Home Thoughts from Abroad', letter, *Nursing Times*, p. 252, February 24.

Earle, N. (1962), 'The Resurrection Appearances of Jesus', *Nursing Mirror*, p. x, April 27; p. 88, May 4; p. xvi, May 11; p. 136, May 18; p. xvi, May 25.

Edwards, M.M. (1961), 'Becoming a Nurse', *Nursing Times*, p. 1198, September 15.

Ellicott, B. (1965), 'The G.N.C. and Platt', letter, *Nursing Mirror*, p. 219, October 29.

Elton, Lord (1939), 'Florence Nightingale', *Nursing Times*, pp. 1442–1443, December 2.

Enoch, M.D. (1967), 'Afterword, Ready for the Scrapheap' in Robb, B., *Sans Everything*, pp. 36–140, London: Thomas Nelson & Sons.

Farnworth, M. (1952), 'The Social Prestige of Nursing', *Nursing Times*, pp. 604–605, June 21; pp. 628–631, June 28; pp. 688–690, July 12.

Fawkes, B.N. (1954),'A Year at Teachers College, Columbia University, New York 1: Introduction', *Nursing Times*, pp. 1017–1019, September 18; 'A Year at Teachers College, Columbia University, New York 2: Public Health in Basic Training', *Nursing Times*, pp. 1075–1076, October 1; 'A Year at Teachers College, Columbia University, New York 3: Personnel and Counselling Problems', *Nursing Times*, pp. 1140–1141, October 15.

Fawkes, B.N. (1972), 'Needs of Education and Training in Nursing', *Nursing Times*, pp. 69–71, May 4.

Fisher, R. (1969),'Raising the Roof', letter, *Nursing Times*, pp. 1559–1560, December 4.
Fletcher, R. (1958),'A Changed Society and its Effects on Nursing', *Nursing Times*, pp. 530–532, May 9.
Fluker, J. (1966), 'Venereal Disease and the Young Woman', *Nursing Mirror*, pp. 633–636, March 4; pp. 663–666, March 11.
Foster, J. (1960), 'Christian Witness in the Early Centuries', *Nursing Mirror*, p. 1230, January 8; p. 1316, January 15; p. 1406, January 22; p. 1496, January 29; p. 1590, February 15.
Fothergill, A. (1966), 'Why Education for Nurses?', *Nursing Mirror*, p. 695, March 18.
Fox, E.M. (1912), 'Nursing Ethics', *Nursing Times*, pp. 475–478, May 4.
Fretwell, J.E. (1980), 'Hospital Ward Routine – Friend or Foe?', *Journal of Advanced Nursing*, 5, pp. 625–636.
Friend, P. (1966), 'Nursing in a Technological Age', *Nursing Mirror*, p. 145, November 11.
Gainsborough, H. (1961), 'Crisis in Nursing – 4: The Physician's View', *Nursing Times*, pp. 1228–1229, September 22.
General Nursing Council for England and Wales (1965), 'Memorandum on the Platt Report', *Nursing Times*, pp. 1347–1349, October 1.
General Nursing Council for England and Wales (1965), 'The G.N.C. Comments on the Platt Report', *Nursing Mirror*, pp. 17–19, October 1.
Goodland, N. (1967), 'Is Nursing a "Vocation"?', *Nursing Mirror*, pp. 372–373, January 20.
Gordon, J.E. (1963), 'The Nurse's Contribution to the Community', *Nursing Mirror*, pp. 92–94, May 3; pp. 113–115, May 10; pp. 139–141, May 17; pp. 161–162, May 24.
Gull, W.W. (1880), 'On the Nursing Crisis at Guy's Hospital I', *Nineteenth Century*, vii, 39, pp. 884–891, May.
Habershon, S.O. (1880), 'On the Nursing Crisis at Guy's Hospital II', *Nineteenth Century*, vii, 39, pp. 892–901, May.
Hancock, C. (1998), 'The Lady of the Lamp', *Guardian*, p. 22, November 20.
Hanham, H.J. (1965), 'Politics in Nursing', *Nursing Mirror*, pp. 553–555, September 3.
Harrison-Thomas, M. (1967), 'Vocation', letter, *Nursing Mirror*, p. 467, February 17.
Hart, F. (1961), 'Crisis in Nursing – 1: The Administrator's View', *Nursing Times*, pp. 1119–1120, September 1.
Harvey, S. (1958), 'Vocation', letter, *Nursing Times*, p. 816, July 11.
Haward, L.R.C. (1960), 'Selection of Nurses: A New Approach', *Nursing Times*, pp. 776–778, June 24.
Hayward, J.C. (1982), 'Nursing Research', in Allan, P. and M. Jolley (eds), *Nursing, Midwifery and Health Visiting Since 1900*, pp. 196–214, London: Faber & Faber.
Haywood, S.C. Jefford, R.E. MacGregor, R.B.K. Stevenson, K. Wooding Jones, G.D.E. (1961), 'The Patient's View of the Hospital: An Experimental Survey,' *Hospital*, 57, pp. 644–650, October.
Headberry, J.E. (1966), 'Florence Nightingale and Modern Nursing', *Nursing Mirror*, 1966, p. xiii, September 2.
Hector, W. (1972), 'The Role and Preparation of the Teacher', *Nursing Times*, pp. 1460–1461, November 16.
Henriques, A.G. (1880), 'On the Nursing Crisis at Guy's Hospital III', *Nineteenth Century*, vii, 39, pp. 902–904, May.
Hill, S.G. (1964), 'A Reform of Nursing Education', *Nursing Times*, pp. 858–859, July 3.
Hodsoll, E.H. (1950),'The Assistant Nurse', *Nursing Times*, p. 733–734, July 15.
Holder, S. (1972), 'Masterly Report? Managerial Waffle?', *Nursing Times*, pp. 1374–5, November 2.
Holder, S. (1994), 'Leader with a Common Touch', *Nursing Standard*, 8, 19, p. 46, February 2.

Holt, R. (1969), 'Raising the Roof', letter, *Nursing Times*, p. 1559, December 4.
Home, J.E. (1955),'Ideals and Education', letter, *Nursing Times*, p. 1259, November 4.
Hovenier, B. (1967), 'Un-Christian Attitude', letters, *Nursing Mirror*, p. 252, December 8.
Hulme, M. (1967), 'Dictatorial Leader', letter, *Nursing Mirror*, p. 225, December 1.
Illing, M. (1972), 'Briggs Debate', letter, *Nursing Times*, p. 1388, November 2.
James, P.D. (1975), 'A Breath of Fresh Air', *Times Literary Supplement*, p. 517, May 9.
Johnson, S.M. (1964),'Fallen Angels', *Nursing Mirror*, p. xvi, August 7.
Jones, A. (1966), 'Careerist or Vocationalist', *Nursing Mirror*, p. 576, September 16.
Kirkpatrick, W.J. (1965), 'A Proper Nurse', letter, *Nursing Times*, p. 1114,
Kitchin, K.F. (1943), 'Nursing the Individual', *Nursing Times*, pp. 772–773, October 16.
Kremsdorf, D. (1953), 'An American Nurse Looks at British Nursing', *Nursing Mirror*, p. 145, May 15.
Lamb, M. (1969),'The Image of British Nursing', *Nursing Times*, pp. 1523–1524, November 27.
Lance, G. (1953), 'Staff Shortage has not Affected the Modern Training of the Nurse', Point of View, *Nursing Mirror*, p. 1216, August 7.
Lawrence, J.A.G. (1961), 'Vocation or Profession?', letter, *Nursing Times*, p. 97, January 20.
Laws, E.M. (1964), 'What are Nurses for?' *Nursing Mirror*, 1964, pp. 178–180, November 20.
Letters (1963), *Nursing Times*, p. 687, May 31, pp. 715–716, June 7, p. 756, June 14, pp. 786–787, June 21, p. 816, June 28, p. 849, July 5.
Letters (1968), *Nursing Times*, p. 1150, August 23; p. 1180, August 30; p. 1211, September 6; p. 1250, September 13, pp. 1279–1280, September 20.
Lloyd, H.M. (1962), 'The Service of the Five Candles', *Nursing Mirror*, 1962, p. 480, March 16; p. xvi, March 23; p. x, March 30; p. 13, April 6; p. 35, April 13; p. 54, April 20.
Lockyer, E. (1963), 'Taking a Vocation Too Far', letter, *Nursing Mirror*, p. 59, April 19.
Lonsdale, M. (1880), 'Doctors and Nurses III', *Nineteenth Century*, 7, 40, pp. 1105–1108, June.
Lonsdale, M. (1880), 'The Present Crisis at Guy's Hospital' *Nineteenth Century*, 7, 38, pp. 677–684, April.
Macbeth, R. (1957), 'Future of Nursing', letter, *Lancet*, p. 96, January 12.
MacDougall, A. (1958), 'Vocation', letter, *Nursing Times*, p. 870, July 25.
MacGuire, J.M. (1961), 'From Student to Nurse', *Nursing Times*, pp. 1297–1298, October 6.
Mackenzie, N. (1953),'Needs and Resources in the Nursing Profession I: The Means to the End', *Nursing Times*, pp. 1236–1237, December 5; 'Needs and Resources in the Nursing Profession II: The Pattern of Ward Life', *Nursing Times*, pp. 1267–1268, December 12; 'Needs and Resources in the Nursing Profession III: The Pattern of the Classroom, *Nursing Times*, pp. 1288–1290, December 19.
Mackie, J. (1961), 'Home Thoughts from Abroad', letter, *Nursing Times*, pp. 315–316, March 10.
Macleod, G. (1964), 'Confession is Good for the Soul', *Nursing Mirror*, p. 376, January 24; 'Intercession', p. 417, February 7; 'Interior Prayer', p. 500, February 28; 'What Happens when you Shut your Eyes?', p. 3569, January 17.
MacManus, E.E.P. (1947),'The Working Party Report – a Critical Survey', *Nursing Times*, pp. 834, 839, November 29.
Malkin, S.A.S. (1961), 'Crisis in Nursing – 2: The Surgeon's View', *Nursing Times*, pp. 1150–1151, September 8.
Marriott, C.H. (1880), 'Guy's Hospital', correspondence, *British Medical Journal*, 1879, p. 1045, December 27.

Marriott, C.H. (1880), 'Nursing Systems', correspondence, *British Medical Journal*, 1880, p. 73, January 10.

Martin, J.L. (1965), 'West Indian Pupil Nurses and their Problems in Training', *Nursing Times*, pp. 1079–1082, August 6.

Martin, J.M. (1965), 'The GNC and Platt', letter, *Nursing Times*, p. 1417, October 15.

May, M.F. (1908),'The Relation of the Nurse to Doctor and Patient', in *The Science and Art of Nursing: A Guide to the Various Branches of Nursing, Theoretical and Practical*, vol. 1, p. 109–115, London, Paris, New York, Toronto and Melbourne: Cassell & Co.

McFarlane, J.K. (1983),'The Commitment of the First English National Board for Nursing, Midwifery and Health Visiting', in *A Time for Commitment*, Baroness Cox of Queensbury, Chairman, pp. 13–19, 45, London: ENB, November 15.

McMillan, A. (1965), 'The GNC and Platt', letter, *Nursing Times*, p. 1417, October 15.

Meir, E.M. (1958),'Nurses with Degrees', *Nursing Times*, p. 629, May 30.

Menzies, I.E.P. (1960), 'A Case Study in the Functioning of Social Systems as a Defence Against Anxiety: A Report on a Study of the Nursing Service of a General Hospital, *Human Relations*, 13, pp. 95–121.

Menzies, I.E.P. (1961),'Nurses under Stress', *Nursing Times*, 1, pp. 141–142, February 3; *Nursing Times*, 2, pp. 173–174, February 10; *Nursing Times*, 3, pp. 206–208, February 17.

Messenger Bradley, S. (1880), 'Miss Lonsdale on the Present Crisis at Guy's Hospital', correspondence, *British Medical Journal*, 1880, pp. 605–606, April 17.

Messer, E. (1962), 'Nursing is a Job', letter, *Nursing Mirror*, p. 34, April 13.

Mole, E.A. (1962), 'A Vocation and Profession', letter, *Nursing Mirror*, p. 89, May 4.

Mollett, M. (1888),'Discipline', *The Nursing Record*, 1,9, pp. 99–101, May 31.

Montacute, C. (1969), 'The Next Fifty Years', *Nursing Times*, pp. 153–154, January 30.

Moxon, W. (1888), 'Miss Lonsdale on Guy's Hospital' *Contemporary Review*, xxxvii, pp. 872–892.

Mullen, C. (1968), 'Protest March', letter, *Nursing Times*, p. 1211, September 6.

Murray, R. (1956), 'Looking Ahead – The Education of the Student Nurse', *Nursing Times*, 1956, pp. 362–366, May 4.

Neale, J.E. (1880), 'On Nursing Systems', correspondence, *British Medical Journal*, p. 90, January 17.

Nicusane (Northern Ireland, Canada, United States of America, Nurse–Teacher Exchange), 1960–1962 (1963), *Report of the Advisory Committee on a Pilot Scheme for the Exchange of Nurse Teachers*, Belfast: Northern Ireland Hospitals Authority, Royal Victoria Hospital; Boston: Massachusetts General Hospital; Toronto: Toronto Western Hospital.

Nightingale, F. (1882), 'Nurses, Training of; Nursing the Sick' in Quain, R. (ed.), *A Dictionary of Medicine*, 1st edn, pp. 1038–1049 (part 2); London: Longmans, Green & Co.

Nightingale, F. (1892), 'The Reform of Sick Nursing and the Late Mrs Wardroper', *British Medical Journal*, p. 1448, December 31.

Nightingale, F. (1893), 'Sick Nursing and Health Nursing' in Hampton, I.A. (ed.), *Nursing of the Sick*, pp. 24–37, New York: McGraw-Hill Book Company, inc.

Nightingale, F. (1894), 'Nurses, Training of; Nursing the Sick' in Quain, R. (ed.), *A Dictionary of Medicine*, 2nd edn, pp. 231–244, London: Longmans, Green & Co.

Nightingale, F. (1902), 'Nursing the sick' in Murray, M. (ed.), *Quain's Dictionary of Medicine*, 3rd edn, 1097–1103, London: Longmans, Green, and Co.

Norton, D. (1965), 'Research for Progress', *Nursing Mirror*, 1965, pp. 390–393, January 22.

Parry-Jones, W.Ll. (1971), 'Human Relations Training in the General Hospital', *International Journal of Nursing Studies*, 8, pp. 153–162.

Patey, E. (1963), 'Has Science made Religion out of Date?', *Nursing Mirror*, p. 476, March 1; 'Can We Prove the Existence of God?', p. 514, March 15; 'The Search for Truth, pp. 385–386, August 2.

Patey, E. (1967), 'All in it Together', *Nursing Mirror*, p. 573, March 24; 'A Time for Revaluation', p. 282, December 22.

Paul, F.T. (1880), 'Nursing Institutions', correspondence, *British Medical Journal*, pp. 125–126, January 24.

Paulley, J.W. (1971), 'Is it Too Late to Scrap Salmon – A Charter for Incompetents?', *Nursing Times*, pp. 212–213, February 18.

Paulley, J.W. (1973), 'Masterly Report? Managerial Waffle?', *Nursing Times*, pp. 1374–5, November 2.

Peake, M.W. (1965), 'A Proper Nurse?', letter, *Nursing Times*, p. 1087, August 6.

Pearce, M.M. (1967), 'Un-Christian Attitude', letters, *Nursing Mirror*, p. 252, December 8.

Pearce, M.M. (1969),'The Next Fifty Years', *Nursing Times*, p. 153, January 30.

Penny, E. (1880), 'The Nursing at Guy's Hospital', correspondence, *British Medical Journal*, correspondence, p. 230, February 7.

Perowne, S. (1960), 'Paul – An Apostle of Jesus Christ', *Nursing Mirror*, p. 2194, September 16; p. 2292, September 23; p. 2372, September 30; p. 56, October 7; p. 180, October 14; p. 269, October 21.

Pitter, R. (1960), 'In the Service of God', *Nursing Mirror*, p. 2070, March 11; p. 2162, March 18; p. 2250, March 25; p. 55, April 1; p. 166, April 8.

Pooley, E. (1953), 'Wanted – Nurse with a Vocation', letter, *Nursing Mirror*, 1953, p. 38, October 2.

Potter, A. (1968),'Protest March', letter, *Nursing Times*, p. 1150, August 23.

Potter, A. (1968), 'Protest March', letter, *Nursing Times*, p. 1250, September 13.

Powell, M. (1967), 'The Challenge of Nursing Education', *Nursing Mirror*, pp. 551–554, March 17; pp. 581–584, March 24.

Powell, M. (1968), 'Nursing Education', letter, *Nursing Times*, p. 574, April 26.

Powell, M.B. (1963), 'Nursing Training and Standards of Care', *Nursing Times*, pp. 1081–1082, August 30.

Powell, M.B. (1969), 'Nursing – its Contribution to Society', *Nursing Times*, Part 1, 1969, pp. 113–116, July 17; Part 2, pp. 117–118, July 24.

Price, J.B. (1965), 'The GNC and Platt', letter, *Nursing Times*, p. 1416, October 15.

Raphael, W. (1965), 'Patient Care', *Nursing Times*: pp. 1606–1608, November 26; pp. 1654–1656, December 3; pp. 1686–1687, December 10; pp. 1725–1727, December 17; pp. 1759–1761, December 24.

Raven, K.A. (1961), 'The Future of the Nursing Profession', *Nursing Mirror*, 1961, pp. 739–740, May 26; pp. 843–845, June 2.

Rayner, C. (1963), 'Chastity and Charity', letter, *Nursing Times*, pp. 715–716, June 7.

Reindorp, G. (1961), 'Hold Fast That Which Thou Hast', *Nursing Mirror*, 1961, pp. 137–138, November 17.

Reindorp, G. (1963), 'How do you Read your Bible?', *Nursing Mirror*, 1963, p. 538, March 22; 'Tiresome Types', p. 560, March 29; 'No Work Today', p. 32, April 12; 'The Waters of Comfort', p. 75, April 26; 'Remember Lot's Wife' p. 134, May 17.

Repton, D. (1964),'Spiritual Help', *Nursing Mirror*, p. 538, September 11.

Rhodes, P. (1965), 'Society, Culture and Reproduction,' *Nursing Mirror*, pp. iv–vi,xvi, May 28; pp. vii–ix, June 4; pp. i–iii, June 11.

Ritchie Russell, W. (1956), 'The Future of Nursing', letter, *Lancet*, p. 1261, December 15.

Roberts, E.M. (1965),'Open Forum: Views on the Platt Report: 1. The Defence', *Nursing Mirror*, 1965, p. 477, February 19.

Robertson, C.M. (1966), 'Education for Nurses', letter, *Nursing Mirror*, p. 43, April 8.

Robinson, J. (1961), 'The Gift of the Spirit', *Nursing Mirror*, p. 1544, September 8; p. 1566, September 15; p. 1580, September 22; p. 1594, September 29; p. 15, October 6; p. 6, October 20.

Robinson, K. (1961), 'Crisis in Nursing – 3: The Politician's View', *Nursing Times*, pp. 1195–1196, September 15.

Rose, D.J. (1957), 'Future of Nursing', letter, *Lancet*, 1957, p. 97, January 12.

Russell, C.A. (1953),'The Nurse Must Choose Whether She Wants to be Nurse or Administrator', Point of View, *Nursing Mirror*, p. iv, August 21.

Sangar, R. (1967), 'Nurses and Religion', letter, *Nursing Mirror*, pp. 150–151, November 10.

Scales, M. (1948),'A Ward Sister's View', correspondence, *Nursing Times*, p. 804, October 30.

Schuster, G. (1962), 'Service of Dedication to Workers in Oxford', *Nursing Mirror*, p. 184, November 23; p. 203, November 30.

Scott Wright, M. (1965), 'Politics in Nursing', *Nursing Mirror*, pp. 163–170, October 15.

Scott, B.B. (1964), 'The Platt Report', *Nursing Times*, pp. 1017–1018, August 7.

Seale, J. (1961), 'Crisis in Nursing – 6: The Medical Economists's View', *Nursing Times*, pp. 1286–1288, October 6.

Seymer, L.R. (1948), 'Florence Nightingale's Writings on Nursing' *Nursing Mirror*, pp. 81–82, May 8

Seymer, L.R. (1954), 'The Function of the Training School is not only to Teach the Mind but to form the Character' *Nursing Times*, pp. 871–872, August 14.

Sharkey, S.J. (1880), 'Doctors and Nurses II', *The Nineteenth Century*, 7, 40, pp. 1097–1104, June.

Sharpe, G. (1953), 'New Trends in Curricula for Schools of Nursing 1: In Canada', *Nursing Times*, pp. 814–815, August 15.

Shout, M.G. (1948), 'Teaching Practical Nursing', *Nursing Times*, pp. 761,764, October 16.

Simson, M. (1953), 'Is Nursing a Vocation?', *Nursing Times*, pp. 899–900, September 5.

Singh, A. (1970), 'The Student Nurse on Experimental Courses – I: Attitudes Towards Nursing as a Career', *International Journal of Nursing Studies*, 7, pp. 201–224.

Singh, A. (1971),'The Student Nurse on Experimental Courses – II: Personality Patterns', *International Journal of Nursing Studies*, 8, pp. 189–205.

Singh, A. (1971), 'The Student Nurse on Experimental Courses – III: Basic Values', *International Journal of Nursing Studies*, 8, pp. 207–218.

Singh, A. MacGuire, J. (1971),'Occupational Values and Stereotypes in a Group of Trained Nurses', *Nursing Times*, pp. 165–168, October 21.

Smith, D. (1967), 'How Can I Nurse ...', letter, *Nursing Times*, p. 496, April 14.

Smith, J.P. (1965), 'Promiscuity, Morality and all That', *Nursing Mirror*, p. iv, January 1.

Smith, J.P. (1972), 'The Briggs Debate', letter, *Nursing Times*, p. 1422, November 9.

Smith, S.M. (1969),'Raising the Roof', letter, *Nursing Times*, p. 1499, November 20.

Spalding, I. (1955), 'Professional Ideals,' *Nursing Times*, pp. 1198–1200, October 21.

Stalford, D.D. (1958),'Vocation' letter, *Nursing Times*, 1958, p. 932, August 8.

Stephens, W.E.D. (1964), 'An Educationist Looks at Platt', *Nursing Times*, pp. 1373–1374, October 16.

Stevens Fisher, E.D. (1954),'American letter – 13: A Series of Personal Views and Comments on Life in America', *Nursing Times*, p. 286, March 18.

Stevens, A. (1963), 'So You're Going to be a Nurse', *Nursing Mirror*, pp. 280–281, June 28.

Stewart, D. (1961), 'The Parables of Jesus', *Nursing Mirror*, p. 1823, February 17; p. 1906, February 24; p. 2004, March 3; p. 2118, March 10; p. 2216, March 17; p. 2308, March 24.

Stocks, M. (1960), 'The Unread Best-seller', *Nursing Mirror*, p. 1488, July 22; p. 1568, July 29; p. 1654, August 5; p. 1752, August 12; p. 1832, August 19; p. 1918, August 26.

Stocks, M. (1961), 'Favourite Tales from the Old Testament', *Nursing Mirror*, 1961, p. 1036, June 16; p. 1144, June 23; p. 1232, June 30; p. 1324, July 7; p. 1378, July 14; p. 1396, July 21.

Stocks, M. (1962), 'Living World of the Bible', *Nursing Mirror*, p. 394, August 17; p. 415, August 24; p. 436, August 31; p. 456, September 7; p. 480, September 15.

Sturges, O. (1880), 'Doctors and Nurses I', *Nineteenth Century* vii, 40, pp. 1089–1096, June.

Sykes, M. (1961), 'Profession or Vocation?', letter, *Nursing Times*, p. 314, March 10.

The Probationer's Page (1912), 'Nursing Ethics I', *Nursing Times*, p. 769, July 27; 'Nursing Ethics II', *Nursing Times*, p. 862, August 24; 'Nursing Ethics III', *Nursing* Times, p. 929, September 14.

Thornton, I.W. (1967), 'No Christian Names', letter, *Nursing Mirror*, p. 175, November 17.

Unmack, A. (1963),'Chastity and Charity', *Nursing Times*, p. 651–652, May 24.

Watkin, B. (1956),'The Future of Nursing', letter, *Lancet*, p. 1354, December 29.

Wauchope, G.M. Ottley, C.M. (1957), 'Future of Nursing', letter, *The Lancet*, p. 96–97, January 12.

White R. (1963), 'Chastity and Charity', letter, *Nursing Times*, pp. 786–787, June 21.

White, R. (1968), 'Protest March', letter, *Nursing Times*, p. 1180, August 30.

Whittaker, D. (1948), 'Patients First', letter, *Nursing Mirror*, p. 238, July 10.

Whyte, B.B. (1960), 'Home Thoughts from Abroad', *Nursing Times*, pp. 1351–1352, December 9.

Whyte, B.B. (1961),'Worm's Eye View', *Nursing Times*, pp. 332–333, March 17.

Wilfred Vilning, C. (1956),'The Future of Nursing', letter, *Lancet*, 1956, pp. 1353–1354, December 29.

Wilkey, H. (1968), 'Two Types of Letters', letter, *Nursing Times*, p. 1249, September 13.

Wilson, M. (1960), 'Religion, Life and Healing', *Nursing Mirror*, p. 1156, December 30; 1961, p. 1251, January 6; p. 1348, January 13; p. 1444, January 20; p. 1538, January 27; p. 1632, February 3.

Wilson, M. (1962), 'The Purpose and Practice of Prayer', *Nursing Mirror*, p. 13, October 5; p. 38, October 12; p. 63, October 19; p. 88, October 26; p. 110, November 2; p. 136, November 9.

Wolfenden, J. (1958), 'Moral Values in a Changing Society', *Nursing Times*, pp. 794–797, July 11.

Wood, T. (1968), 'Protest March', letter, *Nursing Times*, p. 1211, September 6.

Wyatt, J.F. (1978), 'Sociological Perspectives on Socialization into a Profession: A Study of Student Nurses and their Definition of Learning', *British Journal of Educational Studies*, 3, pp. 263–276, October 3.

Parliamentary proceedings

Report of the Select Committee of the House of Lords on Metropolitan Hospitals with Minutes of Evidence, Appendix and Index (1890), vol. xvi, London, HMSO, Irish University Press Series of British Parliamentary Papers (eds) , Ford, P. and G. Ford, vol. 12, Shannon, Ireland: Irish University Press.

Second Report of the Select Committee of the House of Lords on Metropolitan Hospitals with Minutes of Evidence, Appendix and Index (1891), vol. xvi, London, HMSO, Irish University Press Series of British Parliamentary Papers (eds) , Ford, P. and G. Ford, vol. 13, Shannon, Ireland: Irish University Press,

Report from the Select Committee on Registration of Nurses together with the Proceedings of the Committee, Minutes of Evidence and Appendix (1904), House of Commons, London: HMSO.

Report from the Select Committee on Registration of Nurses together with the Proceedings of the Committee, Minutes of Evidence and Appendix (1905), House of Commons, London: HMSO.

Report from the Select Committee on the General Nursing Council together with the Proceedings of the Committee and Minutes of Evidence (1925), House of Commons, London: HMSO.

House of Lords Parliamentary Debates (Hansard) (1948), *Shortage of Nurses*, London, HMSO, 1948.

House of Lords Parliamentary Debates (Hansard) (1953), *Hospital Nursing Services*, London, HMSO.

House of Lords Parliamentary Debates (Hansard) (1978), *Queen's Speech*, London: HMSO.

House of Commons Parliamentary Debates (Hansard) (1978), *Nurses, Midwives and Health Visitors Bill*, London: HMSO.

House of Commons Parliamentary Debates (Hansard) (1979), *Nurses, Midwives and Health Visitors Bill*, London: HMSO.

General Nursing Council syllabuses

General Nursing Council for England and Wales (1923), *Syllabus of Lectures and Demonstrations for Education and Training in General Nursing*, London: General Nursing Council for England and Wales.

General Nursing Council for England and Wales (1923), *Syllabus of Subjects for Examination for the Certificate of General Nursing*, London: General Nursing Council for England and Wales; revised 1925, 1933, 1939, 1952, 1955.

General Nursing Council for England and Wales (1952), *Syllabus of Subjects for Examination for the Certificate of General Nursing*, London: General Nursing Council for England and Wales, revised 1958.

General Nursing Council for England and Wales (1952), *Syllabus of Subjects for Examination for the Certificate of General Nursing for Male nurses*, London: General Nursing Council for England and Wales, revised 1958.

General Nursing Council for England and Wales (undated) *Record of Practical Instruction and Experience for the Certificate of General Nursing*, London: General Nursing Council for England and Wales.

General Nursing Council for England and Wales (undated), *Guide to the Syllabus of Examination for the General Register*, London: General Nursing Council for England and Wales.

General Nursing Council for England and Wales (1962), *Guide to the Syllabus of Subjects for Examination for the Certificate of General Nursing*, London: General Nursing Council.

General Nursing Council for England and Wales (1962), *Syllabus of Subjects for Examination for the Certificate of General Nursing*, London: General Nursing Council.

General Nursing Council for England and Wales (1969), *Syllabus of Subjects for Examination and Record of Practical Instruction and Experience for the Certificate of General Nursing*, London: General Nursing Council, reprinted 1973, 1974, 1976.

General Nursing Council for England and Wales (1977), *Training Syllabus Register of Nurses: General Nursing*, London: General Nursing Council, Amended.

General Nursing Council for England and Wales (1977), *Educational Policy: Syllabus and Practical Experiences Required for Admission to the General Part of the Register, Revising Council's Circular 69/4/3, 77/19/B*, London: General Nursing Council.

Bodleian Library, Oxford, Royal College of Nursing, London

Books

Nursing Textbooks

Journals

Nursing Times
Nursing Mirror
Nursing Record and Hospital World
British Nursing Journal
British Medical Journal
Lancet

London, Public Record Office: official papers

MH 55/2070, Responses from Nursing Organisations, 1948, to Ministry of Health, Department of Health for Scotland, Ministry of Labour and National Service (1947), *Report of the Working Party on the Recruitment and Training of Nurses*, Sir Robert Wood, Chairman, London: HMSO.

MH 55/2063, Response from Government, 1948, to Ministry of Health, Department of Health for Scotland, Ministry of Labour and National Service (1947), *Report of the Working Party on the Recruitment and Training of Nurses*, Sir Robert Wood, Chairman, London: HMSO.

MH 55/2070, The General Nursing Council for England and Wales (1948) *Memorandum of the General Nursing Council for England and Wales on the Report of the Working Party on the Recruitment and Training of Nurses*, London: GNC, January.

MH 55/2063, Letter from N.D. Walker to J. McCree Esq. (1948), Ministry of Health, Whitehall, London, S.W.1., 9 April.

MH 55/2063, Letter from J. McCree to N.D. Walker (1948), Department of Health for Scotland, St Andrew's House, Edinburgh 1., 12 April.

MH 55/2063, Minister of Health (1948), 'Summary of Comments by Interested Organisations to the Minister of State for Scotland'.

Oxford University, Bodleian Library

Acland Papers MS Acland d.70

Letter from Sir Henry Acland to Mr Wakley, MS Ackland d. 70, 23 July, 1889.

Burdett Papers MS Eng. 5930–5938

Letter from Florence Nightingale to Sir Henry Acland, MS Acland d.70, 27 February, 1872.

Letter from Florence Nightingale to Sir Henry Acland, MS Acland d.70, 28 April, 1893.

Burdett Papers, Correspondence related to nursing.

Letters from Florence Nightingale to Sir Henry Acland, MS Acland d.70, 7 July, 1889; 24 July, 1889.

Letter from Sir Arthur Stanley to Sir Henry Burdett, 28 February, 1917, *Burdett Papers*, College of Nursing Ltd. correspondence 1916–1919, Folio 11; Letter from Sir Henry Burdett to Sir Cooper Perry, 6 February, 1919, *Burdett Papers*, College of Nursing, correspondence 1916–1919, Folio 85; Letter from Sir Henry Burdett to Sir Arthur Stanley, 6 February 1919, *Burdett Papers*, College of Nursing Ltd., correspondence 1916–1919, Folio 87; Sir Henry Burdett, 'Points Arising out of Miss Cox-Davies' Letter dated 20th February 1919 to Sir Cooper Perry, and the Joint Report of Miss Cox-Davies and Miss Finch' *Burdett Papers*, College of Nursing, correspondence 1916–1919, Folio 102.

Letter from Sir Henry Burdett to Sir Cooper Perry 13 April, 1916, *Burdett Papers*, College of Nursing Ltd., correspondence 1916–1919, Folio 6.

University College, London

Nightingale, Florence. *Letters and addresses to the Probationer Nurses in the 'Nightingale Fund' School at St Thomas's Hospital and Nurses who were formerly trained there* (1873–1897), Original letters and prints for private circulation.

Letters to author

Letter from Lord Briggs to Ann Bradshaw, 3 November 1994.

Letter from Lindsay L. Brook, Research Director, SCPR, to Ann Bradshaw, 19 September 1995.

Secondary sources

Books

Abel-Smith, B. (1960), *A History of the Nursing Profession*, London: Heinemann.

Baly, M.E. (1973), *Nursing and Social Change*, London: William Heinemann Medical Books.

Baly, M.E. (1980), *Nursing and Social Change*, 2nd edn, London: William Heinemann Medical Books.

Baly, M.E. (1986), *Florence Nightingale and the Nursing Legacy*, London: Croom Helm.

Bendall, E.R.D. and E. Raybould (1969), *A History of the General Nursing Council for England and Wales 1919–1969*, London: H.K. Lewis & Co.

Bradshaw, A. (1994), *Lighting the Lamp*, London: Scutari Press.

Cook, E.T. (1913), *The Life of Florence Nightingale*, volumes 1 and 2, London: Macmillan & Co.

Coventry, S. (1990), *Images of a Nightingale*, Rustington, W. Sussex: Beauclerk Publishing.

Davies, C. (ed.) (1980), *Rewriting Nursing History*, London: Croom Helm.

Dingwall, R., A.M. Raffertyand C. Webster (1988), *An Introduction to the Social History of Nursing*, Routledge: London.

Dossey, B.H. (1999), *Florence Nightingale: Mystic, Visionary, Healer*, Springhouse, Penn.: Springhouse Corporation.

Emmet, D.M. (1958), *Function, Purpose and Powers*, London: Macmillan & Co., Ltd.

Emmet, D.M. (1966), *Rules Roles and Relations*, London: Macmillan and Co.

Freidson, E. (1970), *Profession of Medicine*, New York: Harper & Row.

Ham, C. (1992), *Health Policy in Britain*, Houndmills, Basingstoke: Macmillan.

Heasman, K. (1962), *Evangelicals in Action*, London: Geoffrey Bles.

Hector, W. (1973), *The Life of Mrs Bedford Fenwick and the Rise of Professional Nursing*, London: Royal College of Nursing.

Maggs, C.J. (1983), *The Origins of General Nursing*, London: Croom Helm.

Moore, J. (1988), *A Zeal for Responsibility*, Athens: University of Georgia Press.

Quinn, E.V. and J.M. Prest (1987), *Dear Miss Nightingale*, Oxford: Clarendon Press.

Rafferty, A.M. (1996), *The Politics of Nursing Knowledge*, London: Routledge.

Rivett G. (1998), *From Cradle to Grave: 50 years of the NHS*, London: King's Fund.

Seymer, L.R. (1953), *Dame Alicia Lloyd Still 1869–1944*, London, The Nightingale Fellowship, St Thomas's Hospital, for private circulation only.

Seymer, L.R. (1960), *Florence Nightingale's Nurses*, London: Pitman Medical.

Skretkowicz V. (ed.) (1992), *Nightingale, F. Notes on Nursing*, 1861, London: Scutari Press.

Smith, F.B. (1982), *Florence Nightingale: Reputation and Power*, London: Croom Helm.

Smith, J.P. (1989),*Virginia Henderson: The First Ninety Years*, London: Scutari Press.

Titmuss, R.M. (1963), *Essays on 'The Welfare State'*, London: George Allen & Unwin.

Wake, R. (1998), *The Nightingale Training School 1860–1996*, London: Haggerston Press.

Watkin, B. (1978), *The National Health Service: the First Phase*, London: George Allen & Unwin.

Weber, M. (1976), *The Protestant Ethic and the Spirit of Capitalism*, Giddens, A. (intro), 2nd edn, London: George Allen & Unwin.

White, R. (1985), *The Effects of the National Health Service on the Nursing Profession, 1948–1961*, London: King Edward's Hospital Fund for London.

Woodham-Smith, C. (1955), *Florence Nightingale*, Harmondsworth: Penguin.

Articles and chapters

Baker, M. (1996),'Starched Collars and Starch Baths', *Nursing Times*, pp. 50–51, January 17.

Davis, F. (1975), 'Professional Socialization as Subjective Experience: The Process of Doctrinal Conversion among Student Nurses', in Cox, C. and A. Mead (eds), *A Sociology of Medical Practice*, p. 116–131, London: Collier-Macmillan.

Emmet, D.M. (1967),'Professional Ethics' in Macquarrie J. and J.F Childress (eds), *A New Dictionary of Christian Ethics*, pp. 502–504, London: SCM Press.

Grell, O.P. (1997), 'The Protestant Imperative of Christian care and Neighbourly Love', in Grell, O.P. and A. Cunningham (eds), *Health Care and Poor Relief in Protestant Europe 1500–1700*, pp. 43–65, London: Routledge.

Jarvis, P. (1996), 'Commentary on A Case Study of a Patient-Centred Nurse', in Fulford, K.W.M., S. Ersser and T. Hope (eds), *Essential Practice in Patient-Centred Care*, pp. 193–197, Oxford: Blackwell Science.

Nightingale, F. letter to Julia Ann Elizabeth Roundell, 4 August, 1896, in Vicinus, M. and B. Nergaard (1989) (eds) , *Ever Yours, Florence Nightingale*, pp. 433–435, London: Virago Press.

Saunders, C. (1986), 'The Modern Hospice', in *In Quest of the Spiritual Component of Care for the Terminally Ill: Proceedings of a Colloquium*, Wald, F.S. (ed.), pp. 41–48, Yale University School of Nursing, May 3–4.

Saunders, C. (1998), 'What Made the Nightingales so Special?', *Nursing Times*, p. 14, May 20.

Seymer, L.R., M. Houghton and M.L. Wenger (1971), 'Nursing', *Encyclopaedia Britiannica*, vol. 16, pp. 791–795, Chicago: William Benton.

Summers, A. (1991), 'The Costs and Benefits of Caring: Nursing Charities, c. 1830–c. 1860', in Barry, J. and C. Jones (eds) , *Medicine and Charity before the Welfare State*, pp. 133–148, Routledge: London.

Taylor, A.J.P. (1965), *English History 1914–1945*, Oxford: Oxford University Press.

Taylor, A.J.P. (1967), 'Seventy Years On', in Barker, L.M. (ed.), *Pears Cyclopaedia 1967–68*, pp. vii–x, London: Pelham Books.

White, R. (1985),'Political Regulators in British Nursing', in White, R. (ed.), *Political Issues in Nursing*, vol. 1, pp. 19–43, Chichester: John Wiley.

White, R. (1986), 'From Matron to Manager: The Political Construct of Reality', in White, R. (ed.), *Political Issues in Nursing*, vol. 2, pp. 45–68, Chichester: John Wiley.

Wolstenholme, G.E.W. (1971), 'Florence Nightingale: New Lamps for Old' in Shaw, R.M., R.A. Bowen and G.E. Paget (eds), *All Heal*, pp. 201–215, London: William Heinemann Medical Books, for the Royal Society of Medicine.

Unpublished thesis

Prince, J. (1982), 'Florence Nightingale's Reforms of Nursing 1860–1887', London School of Economics, PhD thesis.

Index

Printed in Great Britain
by Amazon

18529672R00160